Handbook for Prescribing Medications

W9-DDF-724

Handbook for Prescribing Medications During Pregnancy

Second Edition

Richard L. Berkowitz, M.D., M.P.H.

Professor and Chairman, Department of Obstetrics-Gynecology and Reproductive Science, Mount Sinai School of Medicine of the City University of New York; Chief of Obstetrics and Gynecology and Director of Maternal-Fetal Medicine, Mount Sinai Medical Center, New York, New York

Donald R. Coustan, M.D.

Professor of Obstetrics and Gynecology, Brown University Program in Medicine; Director of Maternal-Fetal Medicine, Women and Infants Hospital of Rhode Island, Providence, Rhode Island

Tara K. Mochizuki, Pharm.D., J.D.

Attorney-at-law, Bronson, Bronson, and McKinnon, San Francisco; formerly Assistant Clinical Professor of Pharmacy, University of California, San Francisco, School of Pharmacy, San Francisco, and Pediatric Pharmacist, University of California Medical Center, San Diego, California

Little, Brown and Company
Boston/Toronto

Library of Congress Catalog Card No. 86-81745

ISBN 0-316-09199-5

Printed in the United States of America

FG

Second Printing

Contents

Contributors to the Second Edition

Gaetano Bello, M.D.

Gertrud S. Berkowitz, Ph.D.

Richard L. Berkowitz, M.D., M.P.H.

Donald R. Coustan, M.D.

Jane E. Gordon, Ph.D.

Lauren Lynch, M.D.

Tara K. Mochizuki, Pharm.D., J.D.

Isabelle Wilkins, M.D.

Contributors to the First Edition

Richard L. Berkowitz, M.D.

Elizabeth A. Capriotti, R.Ph.

John R. Cote, Pharm.D.

Donald R. Coustan, M.D.

Ronald A. Cwik, M.D.

Alan H. DeCherney, M.D.

Greggory R. DeVore, M.D.

Allan D. DiCamillo, R.Ph.

Arnold J. Friedman, M.D.

Joel A. Giuditta, R.Ph.

Peter A. Grannum, M.D.

Robert J. Harrison, R.Ph.

Thomas K. Hazlet, Pharm.D.

Joyce M. Heineman, R.Ph.

Brian D. Hotchkiss, R.Ph.

David J. Iamkis, R.Ph.

Daniel J. Kazienko, R.Ph.

Phyllis C. Leppert, M.D.

Mark C. Malzer, M.D.

Mary Jane Minkin, M.D.

Tara K. Mochizuki, Pharm.D.

William O'Brien, M.D.

Phillip H. Radell, M.D.

Peter L. Ricupero, R.Ph.

Roberto J. Romero, M.D.

Paul J. Roszko, R.Ph.

Bonnie R. Saks, M.D.

C. Robert Sturwold, R.Ph.

Khalil Tabsh, M.D.

C. Edward Todd, R.Ph.

Ellen M. Todesca, R.Ph.

Cecily R. Victor, R.Ph.

Preface to the Second Edition

Our stated purpose for creating the first edition of *Handbook for Prescribing Medications During Pregnancy* was to provide clinicians with an up-to-date desktop reference on the use of drugs in pregnancy. The popular and critical success of that effort suggests that readers have found this handbook to be useful, and as a result, we have been encouraged to prepare a second edition. In order to remain relevant, this book must continue to incorporate the most currently available data. This, of course, means that periodic updating of the material is mandatory in order to add new information and maintain the validity of the recommendations being made.

The format used in the first edition has been preserved in the main body of the text. All of the original 140 entries have been reviewed, updated, and in many cases, substantially rewritten. Furthermore, 54 new drugs have been added. The appendix containing 17 vitamins and minerals has also been thoroughly updated. A new appendix containing 12 antineoplastic agents has been added. These drugs are discussed as a separate group because they all have the potential of being harmful to the developing fetus but sometimes must be administered for overriding maternal considerations. In that difficult setting, it is clearly beneficial to know which agent maximizes benefit to the mother while minimizing risk to her fetus. Finally, an appendix containing data on the effects of 30 industrial chemicals on obstetric patients has been added, as well as an appendix on immunization.

The authors have been responsible for the updating of all the material that appeared in the first edition and have written the new drug entries. Dr. Berkowitz was greatly assisted in this task by Dr. Gaetano Bello, Dr. Isabelle Wilkins, and Dr. Lauren Lynch, all of the Mount Sinai Medical Center. Dr. Coustan and Dr. Mochizuki worked alone. The extremely complex appendix on industrial chemicals was written by Dr. Gertrud S. Berkowitz and Dr. Jane E. Gordon.

The reader is encouraged to read the Preface to the First Edition because it describes the layout of each entry, the types of recommendations made, and the organization of the indexes. All of this remains relevant for the second edition. The only portion of the original preface that no longer applies is the last paragraph. All of the authors were at the Yale University School of Medicine when the first edition was published. Dr. Berkowitz and Dr. Coustan have since moved to New York City and Providence, Rhode Island, respectively, where they still function as practicing perinatologists. Dr. Mochizuki has moved to San Francisco and has obtained a law degree. She currently works at the interface of our legal system and the pharmaceutical industry. As in the first edition, however, each entry in this book has been reviewed by all three authors.

We sincerely hope that the second edition of *Handbook for Prescribing Medications During Pregnancy* proves to be of practical benefit to our readers and their patients. It must be noted, however, that the caveats in the Preface to the First Edition still apply. Our recommendations are based on currently available information, and they may require revision as more is learned. Furthermore, some published data may have escaped our attention despite our best efforts to be comprehensive. Many readers have contacted us with suggestions, questions, and comments regarding the first edition. We request that this continue and stress that if anyone is aware of relevant data that have been overlooked, he or she should not hesitate to contact us so that appropriate additions can be made in future editions.

Finally, the authors thank the contributors mentioned above as well as the outstanding staff at Little, Brown and Company for helping to make this book possible. It truly could not have been done without them.

R.L.B.
D.R.C.
T.K.M.

Preface to the First Edition

This book was inspired by the frequent phone calls received by each of the editors regarding the administering of drugs to pregnant women. Its purpose is to provide clinicians with an up-to-date desktop reference on the use of drugs during pregnancy. The publication of new data in multiple journals makes it very difficult to stay abreast of current work in this dynamic field. Furthermore, no major reference work has been devoted specifically to this subject. Since the pharmacological actions of drugs administered during pregnancy may have effects that reach far beyond the therapeutic intent for which they were prescribed, few areas of information have more practical importance.

Because of the bewildering variety of pharmacological preparations currently available in the United States, we have made no attempt to be comprehensive. Instead we have tried to select widely available and frequently prescribed preparations as well as those specifically indicated for uncommon conditions that can affect obstetrical patients. We have also included discussions of some drugs that are not indicated during pregnancy because they might be inadvertently taken before conception has been confirmed.

This book is not intended to rival standard pharmacological textbooks in terms of detailed descriptions of mechanisms of action, metabolic degradation pathways, stoichiometric parameters, and the like. It is a synopsis of the most current relevant information about the effects of individual drugs on the pregnant woman. In addition, we have attempted to present data concerning both the mutagenic and teratogenic potential of each agent on the developing fetus. Each entry begins with the indications for use of that particular drug and the author's specific recommendations. If the drug is absolutely contraindicated during pregnancy, or relatively contraindicated because other therapeutic agents are preferable, this is stated and explained. Drugs that do not fall into these categories are divided into those that are (1) safe for use during pregnancy, (2) indicated only for specific conditions, or (3) the subject of ongoing controversy. In any of these cases a further discussion ensues. A section on special considerations during pregnancy discusses effects that are specifically related to the pregnancy. These include sequelae to both mother and fetus as well as the impact on breastfeeding infants. Appropriate dosages are then presented, followed by a listing of potential general adverse effects. The drug's pharmacological properties are next described in terms of major mechanisms of action, and its absorption and biotransformation are summarized. Finally, each entry concludes with a few relevant recommended readings.

The problems of studying the effects on the fetus of drugs administered to the mother are formidable. In many cases this information is simply not known. Many pharmacological agents have been released by the FDA without specific approval for use during pregnancy. The *Physicians' Desk Reference* frequently offers the familiar caveat: "The safety of _____ in human pregnancy has not been established. The use of the drug in pregnancy requires that the expected therapeutic benefit be weighed against possible hazard to mother and infant." This is not terribly helpful. Obviously, pharmacological agents should not be given during the first trimester, when embryogenesis is occurring, unless absolutely necessary. Another important principle, however, is that medically indicated drug therapy should not be withheld from pregnant women. We have offered specific recommendations about the advisability of utilizing particular drugs with the understanding that they never should be administered frivolously during pregnancy. Our suggestions are based on currently available information, and they may need revision as more is learned. Furthermore, despite our efforts to be thorough, it is certainly possible that some published reports may have escaped our attention. We plan to continue to maintain an active surveillance of the literature and hope to update the material with subsequent editions. If a reader is aware of any data that have been overlooked, he or she should not hesitate to contact the editors so that appropriate additions can be made in the future.

Our approach has been to consider each drug individually. We have not tried to write a manual of therapeutics. Consequently, this book is not particularly intended for the reader who is attempting to formulate a treatment plan for a specific complex problem, such as asthma or hypertension. If, however, the reader is interested in knowing whether a particular drug, such as ephedrine, should be prescribed for the pregnant asthmatic, this can quickly be determined. If a drug is not recommended because another one is considered preferable, the preferred alternative is cited.

The entries are arranged alphabetically by generic name. Some of the more common brand names are also presented with each drug. A general index includes both generic and trade names, while a classification index subdivides the drugs into functional groups by generic name only. Groups of related drugs, such as the penicillins, are sometimes presented in a single entry. The individual constituents of these families, however, are listed separately in the general index and are also considered independently within the entry when this is warranted. Over-the-counter (OTC) preparations are listed according to their major generic ingredients. Tobacco, alcohol (ethyl), and marijuana are separate entries. Vitamin and mineral requirements during pregnancy are discussed in the Appendix.

The individual entries were prepared by house staff and faculty members in the Department of Obstetrics and Gynecology of the Yale University School of Medicine and staff members of the Department of Pharmacy Services of the Yale—New Haven Medical Center. (The author's initials can be found in parentheses following each entry.) All entries were reviewed by the three editors, two of whom are practicing perinatologists, while the third is a clinical pharmacist. Some recommendations concerning drug preference, dosage schedules, and routes of administration reflect approaches that are utilized on the obstetric service of the Yale—New Haven Medical Center, in preference to other acceptable alternatives. Whenever this is the case, it has been so stated in the text.

R.L.B.
D.R.C.
T.K.M.

Handbook for Prescribing
Medications During Pregnancy

Notice

The indications and dosages of all drugs in this book have been recommended in the medical literature and conform to the practices of the general medical community. The medications described do not necessarily have specific approval by the Food and Drug Administration for use in the diseases and dosages for which they are recommended. The package insert for each drug should be consulted for use and dosage as approved by the FDA. Because standards for usage change, it is advisable to keep abreast of revised recommendations, particularly those concerning new drugs.

Acetaminophen (Datril®, Nebs®, Tempra®, Tylenol®)

Indications and Recommendations

Acetaminophen is safe to use during pregnancy in therapeutic dosages. Maternal overusage may cause significant sequelae, including hepatic necrosis. Although this compound does cross the placenta, available evidence suggests that congenital malformations are not associated with maternal use. The use of large dosages by a pregnant woman, however, has been anecdotally reported to result in fetal renal changes similar to those seen in adults. Because of concern about the fetal effects of aspirin, acetaminophen is the analgesic and antipyretic of choice during pregnancy.

Special Considerations in Pregnancy

There are no unique maternal problems when acetaminophen is taken in recommended dosages during pregnancy. Although it crosses the placenta, no adverse effects on the fetus have been reported. No formal clinical or epidemiologic studies of adverse effects in pregnancy have been conducted. Fetal hemolytic anemia and methemoglobinemia are theoretic possibilities but are unlikely since a single 2-g dose converts less than 3% of the total circulating hemoglobin to methemoglobin, a level of methemoglobin of little clinical significance. Renal abnormalities were noted in a newborn whose mother ingested 1.3 g acetaminophen daily throughout the pregnancy.

Dosage

The usual dose of acetaminophen is 325–650 mg every 4 hours, with a maximum dosage of 2.6 g/day. The drug is available in tablets and suppositories (120, 325, and 650 mg) and in elixir and syrup (120 mg/5 ml).

Adverse Effects

A variety of central nervous system (CNS) symptoms have been attributed to acetaminophen, including relaxation and drowsiness as well as stimulation and euphoria. Patients occasionally complain of lightheadedness, dizziness, and a sense of unreality and detachment. An erythematous or urticarial skin rash associated with a drug fever can occur. Idiosyncratic responses include neutropenia, leukopenia, pancytopenia, and thrombocytopenia. Methemoglobinemia and hemolytic anemia may occur as acute toxic reactions, but they are usually seen in association with chronic overdosage. Hepatic necrosis may occur with overdosage. Nephrotoxicity secondary to papillary necrosis and chronic interstitial nephritis have been described in chronic abusers. Excessive ingestion can also cause hypoglycemic coma and myocardial damage.

Mechanism of Action

Both the antipyretic and analgesic actions of acetaminophen seem to be due to a direct hypothalamic effect. The effect of endogenous

1

pyrogens on CNS heat regulatory centers is inhibited, which results in peripheral vasodilatation with subsequent loss of body heat. The analgesic actions are less well understood.

Absorption and Biotransformation

Acetaminophen is rapidly absorbed from the gastrointestinal tract and reaches peak plasma concentrations in 0.5–1.0 hour. It becomes evenly distributed among all body fluids. The plasma half-life is 1–3 hours, but may exceed 12 hours in an overdose. Approximately 3% is excreted unchanged in the urine while 80% is metabolized in the liver to inactive conjugates and to a hepatotoxic intermediate metabolite. The intermediate is detoxified by glutathione, and all metabolites are excreted by the kidneys.

Recommended Reading

Collins, E. Maternal and fetal effects of acetaminophen and salicylates in pregnancy. *Obstet. Gynecol.* 58:57S, 1981.

Gilman, A. G., Goodman, L. S., and Gilman, A. *The Pharmacological Basis of Therapeutics* (6th ed.). New York: Macmillan, 1980. Pp. 701–705.

Nelson, M. M., and Forfar, J. O. Associations between drugs administered during pregnancy and congenital abnormalities of the fetus. *Br. Med. J.* 1:523, 1971.

Niederhoff, H., and Zahradnik, H. Analgesics during pregnancy. *Am. J. Med.* 75:117, 1983.

Schenkel, B., and Vorherr, H. Non-prescription drugs during pregnancy: Potential teratogenic and toxic effects upon embryo and fetus. *J. Reprod. Med.* 12:27, 1974.

Acetazolamide (Diamox®)

Indications and Recommendations

The use of acetazolamide during pregnancy should be limited to adjunctive therapy for increased intraocular pressure and the treatment of increased intracranial pressure caused by pseudotumor cerebri. It may also be used in the prophylactic management of petit mal epilepsy in women whose seizures increase at the time of menstruation. Although animal data implicate the drug as a teratogen, no human data support this. Periodic monitoring of electrolyte balance is recommended when this drug is given during pregnancy.

Special Considerations in Pregnancy

Acetazolamide has been shown to cause forelimb malformations in some offspring of pregnant rats receiving doses of 200 mg/kg. This is greater than 10 times the usual adult human dosage. Ectrodactyly has also been seen in the offspring of golden hamsters and mice exposed to this drug in utero. Furthermore, prenatal exposure of the mouse to high doses of acetazolamide has caused posteriad extension of portions of one or both frontal bones. As of yet, retrospective data have not shown any significant incidence of malformations in infants whose mothers have received therapeutic doses of acetazolamide during pregnancy. There is, however, an isolated report of sacrococcygeal teratoma in a 27-week-old stillborn whose mother was treated with acetazolamide up to the nineteenth week of gestation. It is not known whether acetazolamide enters human breast milk.

Dosage

The recommended adult dose of acetazolamide for adjunctive treatment of open-angle glaucoma is 250 mg taken orally qd–qid or a 500-mg sustained-release capsule taken bid. For rapid lowering of intraocular pressure, 500 mg may be given parenterally. As an adjunct in the prophylactic management of epilepsy, the suggested dose is 8–30 mg/kg/day in divided doses in addition to other anticonvulsants.

Adverse Effects

Serious side effects are rare. Most adverse reactions are dose dependent and usually respond to a decrease in the amount being administered or to withdrawal of the drug. Patients may experience drowsiness, temporary myopia, skin rashes, anorexia, and nausea. The most common side effects are changes in fluid and electrolyte balance, especially metabolic acidosis and hypokalemia. More serious, but rarer, adverse reactions include hypersensitivity reactions, bone marrow depression, and renal toxicity.

Mechanism of Action

Acetazolamide acts by a noncompetitive inhibition of carbonic anhydrase to reduce the formation of hydrogen ion and bicarbonate ion from carbon dioxide and water. This inhibition results in decreased production of aqueous humor, increased renal excretion of bicarbonate ion with alkalinization of the urine, and increased excretion of sodium and potassium with resultant diuresis. Plasma bicarbonate is decreased and plasma chloride increased.

The anticonvulsant activity of acetazolamide is thought to be due to the induced metabolic acidosis. Another postulated mechanism is a direct action on the brain by increased carbon dioxide tension, which has been shown to retard neuronal conduction. In addition, cerebrospinal fluid formation may be decreased.

Absorption and Biotransformation

Acetazolamide is readily absorbed from the gastrointestinal tract with peak plasma concentrations occurring within 2 hours. Onset of action after an oral dose is approximately 1 hour later, while its duration is 8–12 hours. A time-release preparation is available, the duration of which is 18–24 hours. When given intravenously, onset of action occurs within 2 minutes, peak effect occurs at 15 minutes, and duration is 4–5 hours. Its major route of elimination is via the kidney, where it undergoes active tubular secretion.

Recommended Reading

Beck, S. L. Another special effect of prenatal acetazolamide exposure in the mouse. *Teratology* 27:51, 1983.

Beck, S. L. Assessment of adult skeletons to detect prenatal exposure to acetazolamide in mice. *Teratology* 28:45, 1983.

Gilman, A. G., Goodman, L. S., and Gilman, A. *The Pharmacological Basis of Therapeutics* (6th ed.). New York: Macmillan, 1980. Pp. 896–899.

Heinonen, O. P., Slone, D., and Shapiro, S. *Birth Defects and Drugs in Pregnancy.* Littleton, Mass.: Publishing Sciences Group, 1977. Pp. 372, 441, 495.

Layton, W., and Hallesy, D. W. Deformity of forelimb in rats: Association with high doses of acetazolamide. *Science* 149:306, 1965.

Long, J. W. *The Essential Guide to Prescription Drugs.* New York: Harper & Row, 1977. Pp. 265–267.

Worsham, F., Jr., Beckman, E. N., and Mitchell, E. H. Sacrococcygeal teratoma in a neonate. Association with maternal use of acetazolamide. *J.A.M.A.* 240:251, 1978.

Albumin (Albuminar®, Albuspan®, Albutein®)

Indications and Recommendations

The use of albumin during pregnancy should be limited to the treatment of acute oliguria secondary to hypovolemia. It can also be used as a temporary plasma expander during hypovolemic states secondary to hemorrhage if blood is not immediately available. Central venous pressure should be carefully monitored when albumin is administered during pregnancy.

Special Considerations in Pregnancy

Albumin does not cross the placenta. Pregnancy is generally accompanied by an increase in maternal intravascular volume; in severe pregnancy-induced hypertension, however, hypovolemia often occurs. In this situation, albumin may occasionally be used to increase oncotic pressure and improve renal perfusion. If albumin is given, central pressures should be monitored in order to document hypovolemia and to prevent the development of heart failure due to secondary intravascular overload.

Dosage

Albumin is supplied in 25% solution, with 50 ml containing 12.5 g albumin and 100 ml containing 25 g. The onset of action is immediate since it is given intravenously.

Adverse Effects

Albumin is inert. The major side effect is intravascular overload, especially in the patient with compromised cardiovascular status; congestive heart failure may occur in this setting.

Mechanism of Action

Normal human serum albumin is a sterile preparation from the fractionated blood of healthy donors. It is generally free of the hepatitis virus.

The intravenous administration of albumin raises the oncotic pressure of the intravascular space. Extracellular fluid is thus drawn into the intravascular compartment. Hypotension is improved, and renal perfusion is increased, with a resultant increase in urinary output.

Recommended Reading

Berkowitz, R. L. (ed.). The Management of Hypertensive Crises During Pregnancy. In *Critical Care of the Obstetric Patient.* New York: Churchill Livingstone, 1983. P. 299.

Gifford, R. W., Jr. A guide to the practical use of diuretics. *J.A.M.A.* 235:1890, 1976.

Gilman, A. G., Goodman, L. S., and Gilman, A. *The Pharmacological Basis of Therapeutics* (6th ed.). New York: Macmillan, 1980. Pp. 859–862.

Alcohol, Ethyl (Ethanol)

Indications and Recommendations

Ethyl alcohol has been administered to pregnant women for the treatment of premature labor, but its use for this indication has been largely supplanted by newer tocolytic agents (ritodrine, terbutaline, $MgSO_4$). Ethanol is also taken socially, and its chronic use in large doses (>2.2 g absolute alcohol [AA] per kilogram of body weight per day) has been associated with a constellation of fetal anomalies, the fetal alcohol syndrome (FAS). Although chronic ingestion of greater than 2.2 g/kg AA per day throughout pregnancy is absolutely contraindicated, not enough data are available to determine whether an occasional social drink (<1 ounce AA per day) is harmful to the fetus. No recommendation can therefore be made in regard to social drinking during pregnancy. Although ethanol may be effective in the treatment of premature labor, beta-mimetic agents or $MgSO_4$ is preferred in this situation.

Special Considerations in Pregnancy

Chronic ethanol ingestion has been associated with FAS. According to criteria developed by the Fetal Alcohol Study Group of the Research Society on Alcoholism in 1980, FAS is diagnosed when there are abnormalities in each of the following three categories: (1) prenatal or postnatal growth retardation; (2) central nervous system (neurologic abnormality, developmental delay, or intellectual impairment); and (3) characteristic facial dysmorphology with at least two of the following three signs: (a) microcephaly, (b) microophthalmia or short palpebral fissures, and (c) poorly developed philtrum, thin upper lip, or flattening of the maxillary area.

It is not clear whether alcohol itself or its metabolite acetaldehyde is acting as the toxin to produce abnormalities. Both substances cross the placenta, and in animal studies, both affect somites, deforming the brain and spinal cord and producing severe growth retardation. The quantity and regularity of alcohol consumption around the time of conception and during various stages of pregnancy may have different effects. It is likely that heavy regular drinking during the first trimester has the greatest effect on fetal maldevelopment, whereas excessive alcohol consumption later in pregnancy may have greater impact on fetal nutrition and size. In a single series of 43 pregnant "problem drinkers" followed in a special clinic in Finland, three neonates had talipes, a significantly higher number when compared with the overall incidence in Finland (0.12%).

Studies have shown that chronic alcohol ingestion of greater than 2.2 g/kg/day AA increases the frequency of abnormalities associated with FAS. For the average pregnant woman, this quantity is approximately equivalent to 4.5 ounces of pure alcohol, 9 ounces of 100-proof liquor, nine 4-ounce portions of 12% table wine, or nine 12-ounce containers of beer per day. Estimates of the incidence of FAS among offspring of alcoholic mothers range from a high of 40% (in a series of case reports) to as low as 2.5–10.0% in the few prospective series available. In addition to those children with full-blown FAS, there are evidently a large number who have "fetal alcohol effects" but who do not satisfy all of the criteria for the syndrome. It is impossible at present to estimate the incidence of these problems, since many of the manifestations (most notably growth retardation) are not specific to alcohol.

Although a few studies have reported an increased miscarriage rate among moderate but frequent drinkers, there are no convincing data implicating an occasional drink (<1 ounce AA per day) with any adverse outcome of pregnancy. In a large prospective study of 31,604 pregnancies, the consumption of at least one to two drinks daily was associated with a substantially increased risk of producing a growth-retarded infant, and the reduction in mean birth weight was dose related. In this study, the consumption of less than one drink daily had no demonstrable effect on birth weight. Thus, although it would be very difficult to establish the daily alcohol consumption below which there is *no* risk, the existing data do not warrant advising pregnant women that they must drink no alcohol at all or, more particularly, instilling a sense of guilt over past alcohol use.

In a blinded study, the infants of eight mothers who drank a mean of 21 ounces AA per week were compared with the infants of 29 mothers who never drank and of 15 mothers who drank but stopped in the second trimester. Neurobehavioral examinations on the third day of life showed significantly more tremors, hypertonia, restlessness, excessive mouthing movements, inconsolable crying, and reflex abnormalities among the infants of mothers who drank throughout pregnancy compared to those in the two control groups. None of these infants had FAS. The authors conclude that there may be neonatal withdrawal from alcohol among non-FAS infants of those who drink "moderately" throughout pregnancy.

Ethanol has been used in the treatment of premature labor in the third trimester, although beta-mimetic agents or $MgSO_4$ is preferred in this situation. There is some evidence implicating alcohol treatment within 12 hours of delivery in lower 1-minute Apgar scores and an increased incidence of respiratory distress syndrome, and possibly in developmental problems. Because of the potential fetal risk from chronic maternal alcohol ingestion and the lack of evidence that chronic oral tocolysis, administered once premature labor has been stopped, is critical in forestalling preterm delivery, chronic oral alcohol therapy for successfully treated preterm labor is not recommended.

Adverse Effects

Side effects of alcohol consumption include nausea and vomiting (with the potential for aspiration pneumonia), hypoglycemia, central nervous system depression, and mild hypotension. These effects are seen whether the alcohol is taken orally or intravenously (as in the treatment of premature labor). The complications of excessive consumption include increased blood lactate, hyperlipemia, and fatty liver. The continued use of large amounts of alcohol can lead to alcoholic hepatitis and cirrhosis. There are, however, individual differences in response to alcohol; in particular, not all heavy drinkers develop hepatitis and cirrhosis.

Mechanism of Action

Ethanol inhibits release of the neurohypophyseal hormones oxytocin and vasopressin from the posterior pituitary gland. Intravenous or oral administration in early premature labor (with intact membranes) will postpone labor in two-thirds of cases. This is somewhat better than results in women in control groups who were given intravenous glucose. It is assumed that the effect of alcohol on labor is due to inhibition of oxytocin release.

The central nervous system is most markedly affected with the social ingestion of alcohol. Ethanol is a primary and continuous depressant of the central nervous system. The apparent stimulation gained from social drinking results from the unrestrained activity of parts of the brain when inhibitory control mechanisms for those parts are depressed. It is this "stimulation" that gives ethanol-containing products their high potential for abuse. Other physiologic effects include vasodilatation, stimulation of gastric secretions, and diuresis due to inhibition of the antidiuretic hormone.

Absorption and Biotransformation

Ethyl alcohol is absorbed from the stomach, small intestine, and colon. Absorption from the small intestine is rapid and complete. In the liver, ethanol is metabolized to acetaldehyde at a rate of 10 ml/hour. Acetaldehyde is then normally oxidized to acetyl coenzyme A, which is in turn metabolized in the citric acid cycle.

Recommended Reading

American College of Obstetricians and Gynecologists (A.C.O.G.). *Alcohol and Your Unborn Baby* (patient information booklet). Washington, D.C.: A.C.O.G., 1982.

Hanson, J. W., Jones, K. L., and Smith, D. W. Fetal alcohol syndrome. *J.A.M.A.* 235:1458, 1976.

Harlap, S., and Shiono, P. H. Alcohol, smoking and incidence of spontaneous abortions in the first and second trimester. *Lancet* 2:173, 1980.

Kline, J., et al. Drinking during pregnancy and spontaneous abortion. *Lancet* 2:176, 1980.

Mills, J. L., et al. Maternal alcohol consumption and birth weight: How much drinking during pregnancy is safe? *J.A.M.A.* 252:1875, 1984.

Ouellette, E., et al. Adverse effects on offspring of maternal alcohol abuse during pregnancy. *N. Engl. J. Med.* 297:528, 1977.

Rosett, H. L., et al. Patterns of alcohol consumption and fetal development. *Obstet. Gynecol.* 61:539, 1983.

Rosett, H. L., and Weiner, L. *Alcohol and the Fetus.* New York: Oxford University, 1984.

Sisenwein, F. E., et al. Effects of maternal ethanol administration during pregnancy on the growth and development of children at four to seven years of age. *Am. J. Obstet. Gynecol.* 147:52, 1983.

Sokol, R. J., et al. The Cleveland NIAAA prospective alcohol-in-pregnancy study: The first year. *Neurobehav. Toxicol. Teratol.* 3:203, 1981.

Zervoudakis, I. A., et al. Infants of mothers treated with ethanol for premature labor. *Am. J. Obstet. Gynecol.* 137:713, 1980.

Allopurinol (Zyloprim®)

Indications and Recommendations

The use of allopurinol is relatively contraindicated during pregnancy because other therapeutic agents are preferable (for example, probenecid). It is used for the treatment of both the primary hyperuricemia of gout and hyperuricemia secondary to hematologic disorders and antineoplastic therapy.

Allopurinol and its metabolite, alloxanthine, inhibit xanthine oxidase, the enzyme that catalyzes the conversion of hypoxanthine to xanthine and xanthine to uric acid. Thus, serum and urine levels of uric acid are decreased while levels of the more soluble oxypurine precursors are increased. The decrease in serum urate levels occurs during the first 1–3 weeks of therapy.

Attacks of gout may occur more frequently during the initial months of therapy. Hypersensitivity reactions, predominantly erythematous, pruritic, or maculopapular cutaneous eruptions, may occur. Occasionally these lesions may be exfoliative, urticarial, or purpuric. Fever, malaise, and muscle aches may also become manifest. Transient leukopenia, leukocytosis, and eosinophilia are rare reactions but may require cessation of therapy. Headache, drowsiness, nausea and vomiting, diarrhea, and gastric irritation occur occasionally.

Allopurinol is not teratogenic in mice. Due to its structural similarity to purines, there is a theoretical possibility that this drug or one of its metabolites may be incorporated into nucleic acids. It has been shown, however, that neither allopurinol nor alloxanthine is incorporated into DNA during any stage of replication and that neither produces any mutagenic effect. Allopurinol's effects on the human fetus are unknown.

Gout is uncommon in women and is rarely seen before menopause. Elevated serum uric acid is common in toxemia but rarely requires therapy. Probenecid has been safely used and is indicated for treatment of hyperuricemia in pregnancy.

Recommended Reading

Gilman, A. G., Goodman, L. S., and Gilman, A. *The Pharmacological Basis of Therapeutics* (6th ed.). New York: Macmillan, 1980. Pp. 720–722.

Stevenson, A. C., Silcock, S. R., and Scott, J. T. Absence of chromosome damage in human lymphocytes exposed to allopurinol and oxipurinol. *Ann. Rheum. Dis.* 35:143, 1976.

Alphaprodine (Nisentil®)

Indications and Recommendations

Alphaprodine may be used as an analgesic in patients in the active phase of labor at term. A synthetic narcotic indicated for the relief of moderate to severe pain, its onset of action is faster than that of morphine or meperidine when given subcutaneously, but its duration of analgesia is shorter. In most cases there is no significant advantage to using alphaprodine rather than morphine or meperidine. The safe use of alphaprodine in pregnancy, other than during labor, has not been established.

It is recommended that if this drug is used during labor, the lowest effective dose should be administered. Infants born to mothers who have received alphaprodine as antepartum analgesia should be observed for respiratory depression. Should this occur, it can be reversed by naloxone.

The degree of neonatal respiratory depression produced by any narcotic administered during labor depends on the gestational age and condition of the infant. The magnitude of this effect is inversely proportional to gestational age and may be potentiated by birth asphyxia. Alphaprodine, therefore, should be used with extreme caution, if at all, during a labor that will produce a premature infant.

Special Considerations in Pregnancy

Most clinical reports indicate that alphaprodine does not interfere with the active phase of labor. *Any* narcotic administered during the latent phase, however, may result in uterine inertia. When meperidine was compared to alphaprodine in one study, no significant difference in duration of labor was noted.

All narcotics cross the placental barrier, and neonatal respiratory depression has been seen with the use of alphaprodine during labor. This may be due to vasoconstriction of placental vessels, as well as to a direct depressant effect on the infant's respiratory center. Bonica states that the degree of neonatal depression caused by all narcotics during their peak action is about the same when the drug is given to the mother in equianalgesic doses. The peak effect of most narcotics following subcutaneous or intramuscular administration is seen in 2–3 hours. Therefore, infants born less than 1 hour or more than 4 hours after a single dose of narcotic is administered to the mother usually show little or no effects. Since alphaprodine exerts its analgesic effect more rapidly than morphine or meperidine, it probably has a depressant effect on the fetus earlier. Even though its duration of action in the mother is shorter than these other drugs, however, it is possible that the fetal depressant effects may be of a duration similar to the others. If neonatal respiratory depression occurs in an alphaprodine-exposed newborn, naloxone should be immediately administered to the baby.

Petrie and associates reported that administration of alphaprodine, 20 mg given intravenously over 2 minutes, was followed by a statistically significant decrease in fetal heart rate variability in 10 in 14 (71%) patients studied. Both short-term and long-term variability were affected; these indices demonstrated a return toward normal values at 25 and 30 minutes, respectively.

After giving 40–60 mg alphaprodine intramuscularly to women in labor at 36 weeks' gestation or later, Gray and colleagues noted that sinusoidal fetal heart rate patterns developed in 17 in 40 (42.5%) patients. This pattern appeared approximately 20 minutes after administration of the drug and persisted for about 60 minutes. In this study, 15 in 17 babies with sinusoidal heart rates during labor had 1- and 5-minute Apgar scores of 7 or greater. The other two had low 1-minute Apgar scores that were directly associated with complications at delivery. The authors conclude that sinusoidal patterns developing during labor following the administration of alphaprodine are not associated with increased perinatal morbidity or mortality.

Dosage

Clinical trials in patients with postoperative pain have suggested the following approximate equivalent analgesic potencies.

Alphaprodine	Morphine sulfate	Meperidine
30 mg	6 mg	50 mg
40 mg	8 mg	75 mg
50 mg	10 mg	100 mg

The optimum dose range of alphaprodine for women in labor is 40–50 mg SQ, 30–40 mg IM, or 15–20 mg IV. The onset of action is rapid, but the duration is shorter than that of other narcotics. Adequate analgesia usually only lasts 2–3 hours after subcutaneous administration and 1.5–2.0 hours after intramuscular or intravenous administration. Despite this, however, it is recommended that alphaprodine *not* be given more frequently than every 4 hours because of the potential for fetal depression in excess of observed analgesic effects in the mother. Bonica notes that the advantages of more rapid absorption and, therefore, more prompt analgesia over other narcotics when alphaprodine is given subcutaneously are lessened with intramuscular administration and eliminated when the drug is given intravenously.

Adverse Effects

In equianalgesic dosages, the side effects of alphaprodine for the mother are very similar to those seen when morphine is used but are of shorter duration. It may cause respiratory depression, orthostatic hypotension, and urinary retention. Gastric emptying can be delayed, and constipation may result from a decrease in secretions and propulsive movements of the small and large bowel. Biliary tract smooth muscle tone is increased and spasm may result with large dosages. Alphaprodine may cause less vomiting than some of the other narcotics.

Mechanism of Action

Alphaprodine, like the other narcotics, exerts its analgesic effect on the central nervous system. It produces analgesia, drowsiness, changes in mood, and mental clouding.

Absorption and Biotransformation

Alphaprodine is relatively ineffective orally but may be administered by subcutaneous, intramuscular, or intravenous routes. It is primarily metabolized in the liver. Like meperidine, alphaprodine probably undergoes hydrolysis and conjugation and is mainly excreted in the urine as the free drug or its glucuronide conjugate.

Recommended Reading

Bonica, J. J. *Principles and Practice of Obstetric Analgesia and Anesthesia.* Philadelphia: Davis, 1967. Vol. 1, pp. 238–250.

Gillam, J. S., Hunter, G. W., Darner, C. B., and Thompson, G. R. Meperidine hydrochloride and alphaprodine hydrochloride as obstetric analgesic agents. *Am. J. Obstet. Gynecol.* 75:1105, 1958.

Gray, J. H., et al. Sinusoidal fetal heart rate pattern associated with alphaprodine administration. *Obstet. Gynecol.* 52:678, 1978.

Miller, F. C., Mueller, E., and McCart, D. Maternal and fetal response to alphaprodine during labor. A preliminary study. *J. Reprod. Med.* 27:439, 1982.

Petrie, R. H., et al. The effect of drugs on fetal heart rate variability. *Am. J. Obstet. Gynecol.* 130:294, 1978.

Amantadine (Symmetrel®)

Indications and Recommendations

The use of amantadine is relatively contraindicated in pregnancy because other therapeutic agents are preferable. It is an antiviral agent used in the prevention and symptomatic treatment of influenza A respiratory tract illness in patients who, because of underlying disease (e.g., cardiovascular, pulmonary, metabolic, neuromuscular), are at high risk for complications and dangerous sequelae of viral infections. In addition, it is occasionally used in the treatment of Parkinson's disease and drug-induced extrapyramidal reactions.

Its antiviral activity, specific to influenza A virus, is not fully understood. In parkinsonism, it is thought to release dopamine from dopaminergic terminals, and it is less effective than levodopa.

No large-scale studies of amantadine use in pregnancy have been performed. In an isolated case report, however, its use in the first trimester was associated with the development of a complex cardiovascular lesion in the infant. It was hypothesized that agents that inhibit lymphocyte stimulation, such as amantadine and thalidomide, share teratogenic potential.

Because it is unlikely that women of childbearing age will suffer either from Parkinson's disease or a chronic disease that creates a high risk for influenza A, amantadine use during pregnancy will rarely be necessary. Should the indication arise, other safer agents such as anticholinergics for treatment of drug-induced extrapyramidal symptoms and symptomatic treatment for influenza A respiratory infections are recommended.

Recommended Reading

Coulson, A. A. Amantadine and teratogenesis (letter). *Lancet* 2:1044, 1975.
Monto, A. S. Prevention and drug treatment of influenza. *Am. Fam. Phys.* 28:165, 1983.
Nora, J. J., Nora, A. H., and Way, G. L. Cardiovascular maldevelopment associated with maternal exposure to amantadine (letter). *Lancet* 2:607, 1975.

Aminocaproic Acid (Amicar®)

Indications and Recommendations

The use of epsilon aminocaproic acid (EACA) is contraindicated during pregnancy. It inhibits fibrinolysis and has been used in the treatment of excessive bleeding secondary to systemic and urinary hyperfibrinolysis. It has also been used in the treatment of acute exacerbations of hereditary angioneurotic edema.

Epsilon aminocaproic acid is a competitive inhibitor of plasminogen activators and to a lesser degree directly inhibits the action of plasmin. Any interference with plasmin activity results in a diminished capacity to hydrolyze fibrin, fibrinogen, and other clotting components. The thrombogenic capability of EACA is responsible for its most serious side effects, which include pulmonary emboli, intrapleural clot formation, and renal failure secondary to glomerular capillary thrombosis.

Patients with hereditary angioneurotic edema have a deficiency of C1 inhibitor, a substance that interferes with the activation of the first component of complement. Without this inhibitor, several components of the complement system combine to form a peptide that, when cleaved by plasmin, increases the permeability of postcapillary venules and produces angioedema. It is by thus reducing plasminogenolysis that EACA produces beneficial effects in these patients. It should be noted that two cases of painful muscle necrosis have been reported in patients with hereditary angioneurotic edema whose conditions were treated with EACA.

Epsilon aminocaproic acid has been reported to be teratogenic in animals; no congenital anomalies in humans have yet been reported.

It should not be used during pregnancy unless a coagulopathy develops that can be proved to be caused by primary fibrinolysis. Hereditary angioneurotic edema tends to be a mild disease during pregnancy, and investigators at the National Institutes of Health have recommended that EACA not be used to treat this condition in obstetric patients.

Recommended Reading

Gilman, A. G., Goodman, L. S., and Gilman, A. *The Pharmacological Basis of Therapeutics* (6th ed.). New York: Macmillan, 1980. P. 1362.
Nilsson, I. M., Andersson, L., and Bjorkman, S. E. Epsilon-aminocaproic

acid (E-ACA) as a therapeutic agent based on 5 years clinical experience. *Acta Med. Scand.* 180(Suppl. 448):1, 1966.

Aminoglycosides: Amikacin (Amikin®), Gentamicin (Garamycin®), Kanamycin (Kantrex®), Streptomycin, Tobramycin (Nebcin®)

Indications and Recommendations

The aminoglycosides should be given during pregnancy only when serious gram-negative infections are suspected. Streptomycin has been used to treat enterococcal and *Streptococcus viridans* endocarditis, tuberculosis, plague, tularemia, and brucellosis. Kanamycin is used to treat serious, aerobic gram-negative infections in which *Pseudomonas aeruginosa* is not suspected as an etiologic agent. Gentamicin, tobramycin, amikacin, and netilmicin are used to treat aerobic gram-negative infections, including those caused by *P. aeruginosa*.

Gentamicin is preferable to tobramycin, amikacin, or netilmicin because it has been more extensively studied. Tobramycin may be valuable in treating *Pseudomonas* infections in patients with cystic fibrosis.

Special Considerations in Pregnancy

There are no unusual effects on the mother during pregnancy, but serum aminoglycoside levels are usually lower in pregnant than in nonpregnant patients receiving equivalent doses. Thus, it is important to monitor levels frequently to prevent subtherapeutic dosing.

All of these drugs cross the placenta but have lower concentrations in fetal blood when tested at full term than in simultaneously obtained maternal samples.

Streptomycin and kanamycin have been noted to be associated with congenital deafness in the offspring of mothers who take these drugs during pregnancy. They should therefore not be administered during the first trimester or in dosages exceeding a total of 20 g during the last half of pregnancy. Ototoxicity has been reported with doses as low as 1 g streptomycin biweekly for 8 weeks during the first trimester. Studies of effects of aminoglycoside administration during labor have not demonstrated toxicity to the fetus.

Dosage

Drug	Route	Dose (mg/kg/day)*	Interval
Neomycin	IM	15	q6h
Streptomycin	IM	15–25	q12h
Kanamycin	IM/IV	15	q8–12h
Gentamicin	IM/IV	3–5	q8h
Tobramycin	IM/IV	3–5	q8h
Amikacin	IM/IV	15	q8–12h
Netilmicin	IM/IV	3.0–6.5	q12h

*Dosage must be adjusted in the face of renal impairment.

Adverse Effects

STREPTOMYCIN

Permanent vestibular eighth nerve damage may occur, as already noted. Paresthesias, rash, fever, pruritus, renal damage, and anaphylaxis are occasionally noted. Rarely, blood dyscrasias, optic neuritis, myocarditis, and hepatic necrosis may develop. Neuromuscular blockade and apnea have been reported with parenteral administration of the drug.

Nephrotoxicity may be increased when the drug is given with cephaloridine, cephalothin, or polymyxins. Ototoxicity may be increased by interaction with ethacrynic acid and neuromuscular blockade with curariform drugs.

KANAMYCIN

Occasionally, auditory eighth nerve damage will occur. This may remain undetected until after therapy has been stopped and can be irreversible. Renal damage, rash, and peripheral neuritis also have been noted. Parenteral or intraperitoneal administration may produce neuromuscular blockade or apnea.

Effects of drug interactions include increased nephrotoxicity with cephalosporins and polymyxins, ototoxicity with ethacrynic acid, and neuromuscular blockade with curariform drugs.

GENTAMICIN

Occasionally, vestibular eighth nerve damage, rash, and renal impairment may occur. Rarely, auditory damage has been noted. Neuromuscular blockade and apnea may develop.

Effects of drug interactions include increased nephrotoxicity with cephalosporins and polymyxins, ototoxicity with ethacrynic acid, and neuromuscular blockade with curariform drugs.

Tobramycin and amikacin produce essentially the same side effects of gentamicin. They are newer drugs, however, and additional adverse sequelae may become evident in the future.

Mechanism of Action

The aminoglycoside antibiotics penetrate the cell wall and cytoplasmic membrane of susceptible microorganisms and act on the bacterial ribosomes. They bind to the ribosomes and cause a misreading of the microorganism's genetic code, which leads to the production of abnormal proteins and ultimately cell death.

Absorption and Biotransformation

These antibiotics are polycations, and their polarity is believed to be responsible for the pharmacokinetic properties common to the entire group. These include poor absorption after oral administration, poor penetration into the cerebrospinal fluid, and rapid excretion by the normal kidney. The aminoglycosides do not bind well to plasma proteins. Because their clearance is related to the glomerular filtration rate, dosage must be readjusted in the face of abnormal renal function.

Recommended Reading

Handbook of Antimicrobial Therapy. The Medical Letter on Drugs and Therapeutics (revised ed.). New Rochelle, N.Y.: The Medical Letter, 1978.

Jones, H. C. Intrauterine ototoxicity: A case report and review of literature. *J. Natl. Med. Assoc.* 65:201, 1973.

Landers, D. V., Green, J. R., and Sweet, R. L. Antibiotic use during pregnancy and the postpartum period. *Clin. Obstet. Gynecol.* 26:391, 1983.

Robinson, G. C., and Cambon, K. G. Hearing loss in infants of tuberculous mothers treated with streptomycin during pregnancy. *N. Engl. J. Med.* 271:949, 1964.

Weinstein, A. J., Gibbs, R. S., and Gallagher, M. Placental transfer of clindamycin and gentamicin in term pregnancy. *Am. J. Obstet. Gynecol.* 124:688, 1976.

Yoshioka, H., Monma, T., and Matsuda, S. Placental transfer of gentamicin. *J. Pediatr.* 80:121, 1972.

Zaske, D. E., et al. Rapid gentamicin elimination in obstetric patients. *Obstet. Gynecol.* 56:559, 1980.

Aminosalicylate Sodium (PAS)

Indications and Recommendations

Aminosalicylate sodium (PAS) may be used during pregnancy for the treatment of tuberculosis that is not amenable to treatment with more effective antitubercular agents.

Special Considerations in Pregnancy

Although not commonly used, PAS has been prescribed for the treatment of tuberculosis in pregnant women. Retrospective reports do not suggest that it is teratogenic, but large-scale prospective studies are lacking.

Should PAS be prescribed during pregnancy, it is important to note that it may interfere with absorption of oral folic acid and vitamin B_{12}. Parenteral supplementation of these compounds may therefore be necessary.

Aminosalicylate sodium attains levels of approximately 70 mg/liter in maternal serum. Simultaneously measured breast milk levels are 1.1 mg/liter, and therefore the drug could be considered safe. Nevertheless, infants exposed to PAS through breast milk should be monitored for symptoms of toxicity.

Dosage

The usual adult dose is 14–16 g/day PO divided bid or tid. As PAS may inhibit the absorption of rifampin, the doses of each should be separated by 8–12 hours.

Adverse Effects

The most common side effects are nausea, vomiting, diarrhea, and abdominal pain. Less common is hypersensitivity reaction, which may include fever, rashes, leukopenia, agranulocytosis, thrombocytopenia, and infectious mononucleosis–like symptoms. In addition, goiter, both with and without myxedema, has been reported.

Mechanism of Action

The mechanism of PAS as an antitubercular agent is unknown. It is bacteriostatic to *Mycobacterium tuberculosis* and inhibits the onset of bacterial resistance to isoniazid and streptomycin.

Absorption and Biotransformation

Aminosalicylate sodium is readily absorbed from the gastrointestinal tract and widely distributed to all parts of the body. It is concentrated in pleural and caseous tissue. Its half-life is approximately 1 hour. It undergoes metabolism in the liver, and 80% is excreted in the urine as either metabolite or free acid. Excretion is diminished in the presence of renal dysfunction.

Recommended Reading

de March, A. P. Tuberculosis and pregnancy. Five to ten year review of 215 patients in their fertile age. *Chest* 68:800, 1975.

Good, J. T., et al. Tuberculosis in association with pregnancy. *Am. J. Obstet. Gynecol.* 140:492, 1981.

Holdiness, M. R. Antituberculosis drugs and breast feeding (letter). *Arch. Intern. Med.* 144:1888, 1984.

Lowe, C. R. Congenital defects among children born to women under supervision or treatment for pulmonary tuberculosis. *Br. J. Prev. Soc. Med.* 18:14, 1964.

Wilson, E. A., Thelin, T. J., and Dilts, P. V., Jr. Tuberculosis complicated by pregnancy. *Am. J. Obstet. Gynecol.* 115:526, 1973.

Ammonium Chloride
(P-V-Tussin®, Quelidrine®)

Indications and Recommendations

Ammonium chloride should only be used during pregnancy as an acidifying agent in the treatment of significant maternal metabolic alkalosis and in initiating a forced acid diuresis in specific instances of drug intoxication (e.g., quinine or amphetamines). The ammonium ion is thought to exert an expectorant action and is contained in some cough syrups, but it should not be administered to obstetric patients for this purpose.

Data regarding the effects of ammonium chloride salts in pregnancy are limited. When experimentally administered orally for up to 24 days in pregnant women, a metabolic acidosis was produced that resulted in reduced fetal oxygen saturations and pH along with increased fetal PCO_2 values. The acute intravenous administration of ammonium chloride to pregnant women has been shown to cause fetal and subsequent neonatal hypoxemia despite relatively unchanged maternal concentrations of oxygen. The degree of the fetal and neonatal responses appears to be proportional to the severity of the maternal acidosis. Therefore, in view of the limited experience with this compound during pregnancy and the alterations in fetal acid-base status that it may cause, its use should be limited to life-threatening situations in which safer alternatives are not available.

Recommended Reading

Blechner, J. N., et al. Oxygenation of the human fetus and newborn infant during maternal metabolic acidosis. *Am. J. Obstet. Gynecol.* 108:47, 1970.

Gilman, A. G., Goodman, L. S., and Gilman, A. *The Pharmacological Basis of Therapeutics* (6th ed.). New York: Macmillan, 1980. Pp. 869–870.

Goodlin, R. C., and Kaiser, I. H. The effect of ammonium chloride induced maternal acidosis on the human fetus at term: I. pH, hemoglobin, blood gases. *Am. J. Med. Sci.* 233:662, 1957.

Amobarbital (Amytal®)

Indications and Recommendations

Amobarbital is contraindicated for use during pregnancy since other therapeutic agents are preferable. It is most frequently used as a short-acting sedative-hypnotic in a similar fashion to phenobarbital. Based on data from the Collaborative Perinatal Project, use of amobarbital in the first trimester of pregnancy might be associated with an increased incidence of cardiovascular malformations, polydactyly in black offspring, genitourinary problems other than hypospadias, inguinal hernia, and clubfoot.

Amobarbital freely crosses the placenta with levels in cord serum being similar to those in the mother. Either single or multiple dosing of mothers near term, however, results in neontal half-lives that are up to 2.5-fold those in the maternal serum. This phenomenon is due to the fact that fetal-neonatal liver hydroxylation is not induced by the drug, and its elimination is prolonged in the neonate.

Recommended Reading

Draffan, G. H., et al. Maternal and neonatal elimination of amobarbital after treatment of the mother with barbiturates during late pregnancy. *Clin. Pharmacol. Ther.* 19:271, 1976.

Gilman, A. G., Goodman, L. S., and Gilman, A. *The Pharmacological Basis of Therapeutics* (6th ed.). New York: Macmillan, 1980. Pp. 350, 1670.

Heinonen, O. P., Slone, D., and Shapiro, S. *Birth Defects and Drugs in Pregnancy.* Littleton, Mass.: Publishing Sciences Group, 1977. Pp. 336, 344, 438.

Kraver, B., et al. Elimination kinetics of amobarbital in mothers and newborn infants. *Clin. Pharmacol. Ther.* 14:442, 1973.

Amphetamines: Amphetamine Sulfate (Benzedrine®), Dextroamphetamine Sulfate (Dexedrine®)

Indications and Recommendations

Amphetamines should not be used during pregnancy. These central sympathomimetic agents have been used as appetite suppressants, antifatigue agents, and in the treatment of narcolepsy. Although the data are conflicting, there are studies that show an increased incidence of cardiac defects and cleft palate after fetal exposure to amphetamine. At present, weight reduction and fatigue prevention are not valid indications for amphetamine therapy. Thus, narcolepsy is the only clinical situation in which these drugs might be considered in the pregnant woman, and methylphenidate is probably a better choice for this rare condition (see *Methylphenidate Hydrochloride*).

Recommended Reading

Gilman, A. G., Goodman, L. S., and Gilman, A. *The Pharmacological Basis of Therapeutics* (6th ed.). New York: Macmillan, 1980. Pp. 159–163.

Goodner, D. M. Teratology for the obstetrician. *Clin. Obstet. Gynecol.* 18:245, 1975.

Milkovich, L., and van den Berg, B. J. Effects of antenatal exposure to anorectic drugs. *Am. J. Obstet. Gynecol.* 129:637, 1977.

Amphotericin B (Fungizone®)

Indications and Recommendations

The use of amphotericin B during pregnancy should be limited to the treatment of life-threatening fungal infections such as cryptococcosis, blastomycosis, coccidioidomycosis, histoplasmosis, mucormycosis, aspergillosis, and disseminated candidiasis. The safety of this drug during pregnancy has not been established. Patients receiving amphotericin B should be hospitalized and their renal function monitored at least once a week. While theoretic risks to the fetus are of some concern, the effective treatment of these serious maternal infections is of overwhelming importance.

Special Considerations in Pregnancy

Generally, the side effects of amphotericin B are no worse in the pregnant than in the nonpregnant woman. In pregnant patients, however, preexisting anemia may be exacerbated by the anemia caused by amphotericin B and may necessitate transfusion.

Amphotericin B crosses the placenta and reaches cord levels of approximately one-third maternal levels. A study of teratogenic effects in mammals showed no developmental toxicity attributable to this drug. The literature contains several individual case reports of mothers who received amphotericin B during all stages of pregnancy. While some births were normal, others were complicated by such conditions as spontaneous abortion, prematurity, and small size for gestational age. There does not seem to be a correlation between the trimester of treatment and outcome of the pregnancy.

Dosage

The recommended starting dose is 0.25 mg/kg/day, which is then gradually increased to 1 mg/kg/day as tolerance to the common side effects (chills and fever) develops. The maximum dose, given in severe infections, is 1.5 mg/kg/day. The usual duration of therapy is from 6 weeks to 4 months but may be shorter if adverse effects require discontinuation. The drug is administered intravenously in a concentration of 0.1 mg/ml over 4–6 hours. Because of the long plasma half-life, alternate-day dosing is feasible.

Adverse Effects

Chills, fever (up to 40°C), vomiting, anorexia, and headache are commonly observed in patients during the infusion period. With repeated infusions, thrombophlebitis, anemia, and nephrotoxicity frequently occur. The severity of renal impairment is dose related, generally not reaching clinical significance unless the cumulative dose is 4 g. Mild manifestations are reversible with cessation of therapy. Hypersensitivity reactions have included anaphylaxis, thrombocytopenia, flushing, generalized pain, and convulsions.

Absorption and Biotransformation

Amphotericin B is poorly absorbed from the gastrointestinal tract and is, therefore, given intravenously for the treatment of systemic infections. The plasma half-life is 24 hours. A small fraction of the dose appears in the urine and is detectable for as long as 7–8 weeks after therapy is discontinued. No abnormal accumulation is seen in patients with renal failure. The drug appears to be stored in the body, very slowly released, metabolized, and then slowly excreted by the kidneys. No specific metabolites have been identified.

Recommended Reading

Attkin, G. W., and Symonds, E. M. Cryptococcal meningitis in pregnancy treated with amphotericin B: A case report. *J. Obstet. Gynaecol. Br. Commonw.* 69:677, 1962.

Bindschadler, D. D., and Bennett, J. E. A pharmacologic guide to the clinical use of amphotericin B. *J. Infect. Dis.* 120:427, 1969.

Curole, D. N. Cryptococcal meningitis in pregnancy. *J. Reprod. Med.* 26:317, 1981.

Feldman, R. Cryptococcosis of the central nervous system treated with amphotericin B during pregnancy. *South. Med. J.* 52:1415, 1959.

Gilman, A. G., Goodman, L. S., and Gilman, A. *The Pharmacological Basis of Therapeutics* (6th ed.). New York: Macmillan, 1980. Pp. 1233–1236.

Ismail, M. A., and Lerner, S. A. Disseminated blastomycosis in a pregnant woman. Review of amphotericin B usage in pregnancy. *Am. Rev. Respir. Dis.* 126:350, 1982.

Philpot, C. R. Cryptococcal meningitis in pregnancy. *Med. J. Aust.* 2:1005, 1972.

Ruo, P. A case of torulosis of the CNS during pregnancy. *Med. J. Aust.* 1:558, 1962.

Stafford, C. R., et al. Cryptococcal meningitis in pregnancy. *Obstet. Gynecol.* 62:355, 1983.

Anal Analgesics (Anugesic®, Anusol® Suppository or Ointment, Anusol-HC®)

Indications and Recommendations

Anusol® suppositories and ointment are safe to use during pregnancy. These preparations are used for the symptomatic relief of pain or discomfort related to external or internal hemorrhoids, proctitis, cryptitis, fissures, and incomplete fistulas and for relief of local pain following anorectal surgery. The use of Anusol-HC® and Anugesic® is controversial and if used at all should be restricted to very specific situations.

Special Considerations in Pregnancy

Anusol-HC® contains 10 mg hydrocortisone acetate and is often used for severe acute discomfort. Because topical steroids are absorbed systemically, this drug should be used during pregnancy with the same precautions as other steroid preparations.

Dosage

One Anusol® suppository may be inserted rectally in the morning, another at bedtime, and one after each bowel movement. Anusol® ointment can be applied externally or inserted rectally with a plastic applicator. The ointment should be applied every 3–4 hours.

Mechanism of Action and Adverse Effects

Anusol® contains bismuth subgallate, bismuth resorcin, benzyl benzoate, Peruvian balsam, and zinc oxide. This combination provides a soothing, lubricating action on the mucous membranes, which relieves discomfort secondary to the passage of stool. No side effects have been noted.

Anugesic® contains pramoxine hydrochloride, which may cause a skin sensitivity reaction. This preparation therefore should be used with caution.

Recommended Reading

Gerbie, A. B., and Sciarra, J. J. *Gynecology and Obstetrics.* Hagerstown, Md.: Harper & Row, 1978. Vol. 2, chap. 12:8.

Physicians' Desk Reference (33rd ed.). Oradell, N.J.: Medical Economics, 1979. Pp. 1809–1810.

Antacids (over-the-counter): Aluminum Hydroxide, Calcium Carbonate, Magnesium Compounds, Sodium Bicarbonate

Many over-the-counter (OTC) preparations include a combination of gastric antacids. The different components of these preparations are described separately.

One retrospective study suggested an association between the administration of aluminum hydroxide, calcium carbonate, and magnesium compound antacids during the first 56 days of gestation and the occurrence of major and minor congenital anomalies. It should be noted, however, that this was a heterogeneous group of anomalies. It was found that 5.9% of 458 mothers giving birth to anomalous babies took antacids during the first trimester, while 2.6% of 911 mothers of normal babies took these drugs. No causality can be inferred, and no substantiating data have followed.

ALUMINUM HYDROXIDE

Indications and Recommendations

Aluminum hydroxide is safe to use during pregnancy in the last two trimesters. It is used to neutralize gastric acid and to treat phosphate nephrolithiasis.

Dosage

Aluminum hydroxide comes in tablets containing 300–600 mg. A 600-mg dose will neutralize 2–10 mEq acid in 30 minutes.

Adverse Effects

Side effects of aluminum hydroxide include constipation; transient hypophosphatemia and hypophosphaturia; phosphate depletion syndrome with chronic use; increased calcium absorption, possibly leading to hypercalcemia and hypercalciuria; and hypomagnesemia. Aluminum hydroxide will decrease the absorption of tetracycline, chlorpromazine, acetylsalicylic acid, anticholinergic agents, pentobarbital, and sulfadiazine. The absorption of both penicillin and pseudoephedrine is increased, and there is a slight decrease in the absorption of amino acids, ascorbic acid, vitamin A, and glucose.

Mechanism of Action

Aluminum hydroxide reacts with hydrochloric acid in the stomach to form aluminum chloride. Nonabsorbed aluminum hydroxide is converted to insoluble aluminum phosphate in the gastrointestinal tract, making this a useful substance in the treatment of phosphate nephrolithiasis.

Absorption and Biotransformation

Between 17 and 31% of an oral dose of aluminum hydroxide may be recovered in the urine.

CALCIUM CARBONATE

Indications and Recommendations

Calcium carbonate is safe to use during pregnancy in the last two trimesters as long as chronic high doses are avoided. It is used to neutralize acid in the stomach.

Special Considerations in Pregnancy

Fetal hypomagnesemia, increased deep tendon reflexes, and increased muscle tone have been reported.

Dosage

The average dose of calcium carbonate is 1,000 mg; this dose will neutralize 13 mEq acid in 30 minutes.

Adverse Effects

Side effects include constipation, nausea, and belching. In predisposed persons, hypercalciuria with nephrolithiasis and azotemia may occur. Patients taking calcium carbonate for the treatment of ulcer disease may note "rebound" aggravation of their ulcer symptoms. In the milk-alkali syndrome, caused by the excessive intake of milk or soluble alkali, there is mild alkalosis, hypercalcemia, band keratopathy, distaste for food, nausea, vomiting, headache, and weakness. The condition is generally reversible after the calcium carbonate is discontinued.

Mechanism of Action

Calcium carbonate reacts with hydrochloric acid in the stomach to form calcium chloride, carbon dioxide, and water.

Absorption and Biotransformation

Calcium carbonate is absorbed at a rate of 10–15% by healthy individuals and 10–35% by persons with peptic ulcer disease. A transitory hypercalcemia is noted after an oral dose of calcium carbonate, but this effect is less marked if it is taken chronically by a person with normal renal function.

MAGNESIUM COMPOUNDS

Indications and Recommendations

Magnesium trisilicate, magnesium carbonate, and magnesium hydroxide are safe to use during pregnancy in the last two trimesters as long as chronic high doses are avoided. They are used to neutralize acid in the stomach.

Special Considerations in Pregnancy

Neonatal hypermagnesemia with drowsiness, decreased muscle tone, respiratory distress, and cardiovascular impairment has been reported in newborns exposed in utero to chronic high maternal magnesium levels. Silicaceous nephrolithiasis has also been reported in newborns whose mothers were chronic magnesium trisilicate takers.

Dosage

Magnesium trisilicate is taken in 500-mg tablets. The usual dose is two tablets, chewed thoroughly. This dose should neutralize 13–17 mEq acid in 30 minutes. Magnesium hydroxide can be taken as a 310-mg tablet (neutralizes 10.7 mEq acid) or as an 8% aqueous suspension (milk of magnesia); the usual dose is 5 ml, neutralizing 13.5 mEq acid. When given in 15–30-ml doses, it is used as a cathartic.

Adverse Effects

In patients with renal insufficiency, the magnesium compounds may cause hypermagnesemia, with its associated muscle weakness and hypotonia, sedation, confusion, and in some cases, cardiovascular effects such as complete heart block. These compounds also may augment the absorption of warfarin compounds but decrease the absorption of barbiturates, quinidine, and digoxin. Chronic ingestion of magnesium trisilicate has been reported to result in formation of silicaceous stones in the urinary tract. Magnesium hydroxide acts as a cathartic when ingested in high doses.

Mechanism of Action

Magnesium trisilicate reacts with hydrochloric acid to form silicon dioxide and magnesium. The former substance, a gelatinous compound, may provide an adherent coating to an ulcer crater. Magnesium hydroxide (milk of magnesia 8%) reacts with hydrochloric acid to form magnesium chloride. Magnesium carbonate reacts with hydrochloric acid to form carbon dioxide and magnesium chloride.

Absorption and Biotransformation

Approximately 5% of the magnesium in magnesium trisilicate is absorbed. In both magnesium hydroxide and magnesium carbonate, 5–10% of the magnesium is absorbed.

SODIUM BICARBONATE

Indications and Recommendations

The use of sodium bicarbonate is relatively contraindicated during pregnancy because other therapeutic agents are preferable. It is used to neutralize stomach acid but is absorbed systemically (unlike most of the other antacid agents). The systemic absorption leads to a short duration of action, with a resultant rebound increase in symptoms. Chronic use also leads to systemic alkalosis. The sodium load that is absorbed can also cause edema and weight gain. For these reasons, it is recommended that other, less systemically active agents be used if antacid therapy is considered necessary.

An exception to this relative contraindication is the use of sodium citrate as a preoperative antacid for patients undergoing cesarean section. Sodium citrate, available in combination with citric acid, is metabolized to sodium bicarbonate and thus acts as a buffer. Because other antacids contain particulate matter, which may cause bronchopneumonia if aspirated, many anesthesiologists prefer to give a clear antacid, sodium citrate. Since this preparation is only used acutely, the problems listed in the previous paragraph are unlikely in this clinical situation.

Recommended Reading

Gibbs, C. P., and Banner, T. C. Effectiveness of Bicitra® as a preoperative antacid. *Anesthesiology* 61:97, 1984.

Gilman, A. G., Goodman, L. S., and Gilman, A. *The Pharmacological Basis of Therapeutics* (6th ed.). New York: Macmillan, 1980. Pp. 988–1001.

McElnay, J. C., et al. The interaction of digoxin with antacid constituents. *Br. Med. J.* 1:1554, 1978.

Nelson, M. M., and Forfar, J. O. Associations between drugs administered during pregnancy and congenital abnormalities of the fetus. *Br. Med. J.* 1:523, 1971.

Schenkel, B., and Vorherr, H. Non-prescription drugs during pregnancy: Potential teratogenic and toxic effects upon embryo and fetus. *J. Reprod. Med.* 12:27, 1974.

Anticholinesterases: Ambenonium (Mytelase®), Edrophonium (Tensilon®), Neostigmine (Prostigmin®), Physostigmine (Eserine), Pyridostigmine (Mestinon®)

Indications and Recommendations

Reports of the use of ambenonium and edrophonium in obstetric patients are limited, and while these drugs are probably safe, they are relatively contraindicated because the other agents in this group have been used more extensively. Neostigmine or pyridostigmine is safe to use for the treatment of myasthenia gravis. It is preferable to avoid physostigmine for this indication because it has a greater theoretic propensity to cross the placenta.

These agents are reversible anticholinesterase compounds. By inhibiting acetylcholinesterase, they result in the accumulation of acetylcholine at cholinergic receptor sites and are therefore capable of causing effects that resemble excessive cholinergic stimulation throughout the central and peripheral nervous systems. These drugs are used therapeutically in the treatment of glaucoma, myasthenia gravis, atony of intestinal and bladder smooth muscle, and to terminate the effects of competitive neuromuscular-blocking drugs.

Special Considerations in Pregnancy

Although the reversible cholinesterase inhibitors have been shown to cause vertebral malformations and leg muscle hypoplasia in quail and chick embryos, there is no evidence for their teratogenicity in humans to date. Furthermore, despite theoretic concerns that these agents might promote premature labor, there is no evidence that this occurs, even when the drugs are given parenterally.

No congenital defects were noted in one report of 22 first-trimester exposures to neostigmine. In another study, 27 gravidas were given small doses of neostigmine for 3 days before the fourteenth week of pregnancy. One patient miscarried, and the other 26 delivered at or near term without reported complications or anomalies.

Unlike neostigmine and pyridostigmine, which are quaternary compounds, physostigmine is a tertiary ammonium compound that easily crosses both the blood-brain and placental barriers. In one study, this drug was given intravenously to laboring patients to reverse scopolamine delirium. All of the 15 women in this series became cooperative and oriented within 3–5 minutes, and all of their infants had 5-minute Apgar scores of 8 or greater.

Cholinesterase inhibitors may affect the neonates of myasthenic mothers treated with these agents throughout pregnancy. From 15–20% of newborns born to myasthenic women develop transient muscular weakness, and some authors have postulated that the anticholinesterases may contribute to this short-lived phenomenon.

Contrary to an earlier report, as well as what would be predicted from physicochemical laws of membrane transport, pyridostigmine has been shown to enter breast milk. Postpartum milk concentrations have been found to approximate those found in maternal plasma. By the sixtieth postpartum day, milk concentrations were noted to be 40% of those in maternal plasma. The amount of drug ingested by this route is negligible, but these data demonstrate that presumably ionized quaternary ammonium compounds do enter breast milk, and therefore may also traverse the placenta.

Dosage

In the treatment of myasthenia gravis, the optimal single dose of an anticholinesterase is determined by observing the patient's response to graduated doses. After establishing baseline values of vital capacity and muscular strength, an oral dose of 7.5 mg neostigmine or 30 mg pyridostigmine is given. Improvements in muscular strength are noted at frequent intervals until there is a return to the basal state. One hour later, the drug is again given, with the dose increased by 50% over the initial amount, and the observational process is repeated. This sequence is continued with increasing increments of one-half the initial dose until an optimal effect is achieved. The ideal single oral dose may range from the initial doses cited to more than 10 times these amounts.

An alternate approach is to give successive low-dose intravenous injections of neostigmine (0.125 mg) or pyridostigmine (0.5 mg) at intervals of several minutes while monitoring muscle strength in the same fashion as described previously. If the parenteral approach is used, the patient should be premedicated with 0.4–0.6 mg atropine to prevent muscarinic side effects. When the maximally effective total intravenous dosage has been established, the optimal single oral dose is approximately 30 times that amount.

Neostigmine is available in 15-mg oral tablets, usually taken every 2–4 hours. Pyridostigmine is available for oral use in 60-mg tablets taken every 3–6 hours or in a 180-mg sustained-release tablet for use at beatime. Ambenonium is marketed in 10-mg tablets and is taken every 3–6 hours.

Physostigmine salicylate is available in various strengths as an ophthalmic solution either alone or in combination with pilocarpine nitrate.

Adverse Effects

Anticholinesterase compounds cause multiple side effects at both nicotinic and muscarinic sites. At autonomic effectors, miosis, spasm of accommodation, reduction of intraocular pressure, decreased heart rate, dilatation of blood vessels, increased gastrointestinal motility and secretion, and stimulation of secretory glands can occur. Skeletal muscle shows increased strength of contraction and occasionally fibrillation. Central nervous system effects include confusion and ataxia. Overdosage may lead to death from respiratory failure. It is sometimes difficult to know whether a patient's weakness is due to her mysasthenia or to overdosage with an anticholinesterase. In this situation, a neurologist should be urgently consulted and asked to evaluate the patient. Edrophonium may be used to differentiate between these two conditions, but extreme caution must be exercised since this drug can cause a respiratory arrest if the weakness is cholinergic in origin.

Mechanism of Action

All of these agents reversibly inhibit acetylcholinesterase. Physostigmine is a naturally occurring tertiary amine and neostigmine is a synthetic quaternary compound. Both have a carbamyl ester linkage and are hydrolyzed by acetylcholinesterase, but much more slowly than is acetylcholine. The duration of acetylcholinesterase inhibition by the carbamylating agents is 3–4 hours. Pyridostigmine is a close congener of neostigmine. Edrophonium is an analog of neostigmine that lacks the carbamyl group. It has a brief duration of action because of the reversibility of its binding to acetylcholinesterase and rapid elimination by the kidneys after systemic administration. Because of its short action, edrophonium is often used in the "Tensilon® test" to diagnose or verify optimization of dosage in the treatment of myasthenia gravis. Ambenonium is a potent bis-quaternary compound that is also used in the treatment of myasthenia gravis.

Absorption and Biotransformation

Physostigmine is readily absorbed from the intestines, subcutaneous tissues, and mucous membranes. The conjunctival instillation of this drug may cause systemic effects if measures are not taken to prevent absorption from the nasal mucosa. Physostigmine is largely destroyed by hydrolytic cleavage at the ester linkage by cholinesterases, and renal excretion plays only a minor role in its disposal. A 1-mg dose injected subcutaneously is largely destroyed within 2 hours.

Neostigmine and the related quaternary ammonium compounds are absorbed poorly after oral administration, which is why much larger doses are necessary than when they are administered parenterally. Neostigmine is destroyed by plasma esterases and the quaternary alcohol and parent compound are excreted in the urine. Pyridostigmine and its quaternary alcohol are also excreted by the kidneys.

Recommended Reading

Blackhall, M. I., et al. Drug-induced neonatal myasthenia. *J. Obstet. Gynaecol. Br. Commonw.* 76:157, 1969.

Buckley, G. A., et al. Drug-induced neonatal myasthenia. *Br. J. Pharmacol.* 34:203P, 1968.

Gilman, A. G., Goodman, L. S., and Gilman, A. *The Pharmacological Basis of Therapeutics* (6th ed.). New York: Macmillan, 1980. Pp. 100–119.

Landauer, W. Cholinomimetic teratogens: Studies with chicken embryos. *Teratology* 12:125, 1975.

McNall, P. G., and Jafarnia, M. R. Management of myasthenia gravis in the obstetrical patient. *Am. J. Obstet. Gynecol.* 92:518, 1965.

Meiniel, R. Neuromuscular blocking agents and axial teratogenesis in the avian embryo. Can axial morphogenetic disorders be explained by pharmacological action upon muscle tissue? *Teratology* 23:259, 1981.

Smiller, B. G., et al. Physostigmine reversal of scopolamine delirium in obstetric patients. *Am. J. Obstet. Gynecol.* 116:326, 1973.

Wise, G. A., and McQuillen, M. R. Transient myasthenia of the newborn. Clinical and electromyographic studies. *Trans. Am. Neurol. Assoc.* 94:100, 1969.

Antihistamines (over-the-counter): Brompheniramine, Chlorpheniramine, Cyclizine, Doxylamine, Meclizine, Phenindamine, Pheniramine, Pyrilamine

Indications and Recommendations

Antihistamines in pregnancy should be limited to their use in the treatment of allergic symptoms, the prophylaxis of motion sickness, and as sedatives. The antihistamine compounds available in over-the-counter (OTC) preparations, with the exception of brompheniramine, have not been implicated as having deleterious effects in the pregnant woman or fetus. As with any drug, however, antihistamines should be used only when absolutely necessary during pregnancy. Chlorpheniramine does not appear to have teratogenic effects at recommended dosages; however, no prospective studies are available. These drugs are not recommended for use by lactating women.

Special Considerations in Pregnancy

A large-scale study of drugs that could possibly have a teratogenic effect if taken during pregnancy included the following antihistamines available in OTC preparations: chlorpheniramine,

pheniramine, and brompheniramine. Of these, only with brompheniramine was there a statistically significant increased risk of teratogenicity. Animal studies have implicated meclizine and cyclizine as teratogenic agents. Large-scale studies in humans, however, have not shown an increased incidence of death or malformations in children of women who used any of these drugs during pregnancy. When, as is usual, they are found in combination products, the potential effects of all ingredients must be considered.

Due to its anticholinergic properties, chlorpheniramine may inhibit lactation. In addition, small amounts may be secreted into breast milk. This drug and all antihistamines, therefore, should be avoided by the lactating mother.

Dosage

The dosage amount of any of these antihistamines varies with the particular preparation in which it is found. They are often found combined with other ingredients.

Adverse Effects

Side effects of antihistamines are most commonly anticholinergic in nature and include dryness of the mouth, difficulty in voiding, and, rarely, impotence. Dizziness, lassitude, incoordination, fatigue, blurred vision, and nervousness also occur. Digestive tract effects include anorexia, nausea, vomiting, constipation, and diarrhea, all of which may be avoided by taking the drug with meals. Leukopenia and agranulocytosis are rarely seen. Toxic doses result in hallucinations, ataxia, athetosis, and convulsions. Death may result from cardiorespiratory collapse.

Mechanism of Action

Antihistamines act by competitive antagonism to prevent histamine from exerting its vasodilatory and bronchoconstrictive effects. They are effective in suppressing the symptoms of seasonal rhinitis but are less effective in the treatment of perennial rhinitis. They may also be effective in the treatment of certain allergic dermatoses. Antihistamines also have central effects that account for their sedative properties and their efficacy in the prevention of motion sickness.

Absorption and Biotransformation

The pharmacokinetics of these drugs are not well known. They are well absorbed from the gastrointestinal tract. As a group, they seem to be metabolized in the liver with little if any being excreted unchanged in the urine.

Recommended Reading

Gilman, A. G., Goodman, L. S., and Gilman, A. *The Pharmacological Basis of Therapeutics* (6th ed.). New York: Macmillan, 1980. Pp. 622–629.

Greenberger, P., and Patterson, R. Safety of therapy for allergic symptoms during pregnancy. *Ann. Intern. Med.* 89:234, 1978.

Heinonen, O. P., Slone, D., and Shapiro, S. *Birth Defects and Drugs in Pregnancy.* Littleton, Mass.: Publishing Sciences Group, 1977. Pp. 322–334.

Aspartame (Equal®, Nutrasweet®)

Indications and Recommendations

Aspartame, a nonnutritive artificial sweetener that is a combination of aspartic acid and phenylalanine, is safe to use during pregnancy. The FDA has approved the use of aspartame by the general population, including pregnant and lactating women. This compound should be avoided by individuals with phenylketonuria who are pregnant, as should all phenylalanine-containing foods.

Special Considerations in Pregnancy

There is no evidence for teratogenicity of this drug in animals.

High maternal serum levels of phenylalanine have been associated with mental retardation and microcephaly in infants of mothers with phenylketonuria who did not restrict their diets during pregnancy. Since aspartame contains phenylalanine, there has been concern that the ingestion of large amounts of this food additive by pregnant women may be deleterious to the fetus. In hearings before marketing approval for aspartame, the FDA arbitrarily considered the toxic threshold for phenylalanine to be 100 μmol/dl in adults and 50 μmol/dl (because fetal phenylalanine levels are approximately twice maternal levels) in pregnant women. Clinical testing showed that the average 60-kg adult would have to consume 600 aspartame tablets (or 24 liters of aspartame-sweetened beverage) at a single sitting to reach this level. Additionally, it should be noted that phenylalanine is a normal dietary component. If one ingests aspartame at the projected 99th percentile of consumption, the overall daily phenylalanine intake would only increase by 6%.

Another concern was the finding that aspartame may decompose if stored at high temperatures or for long time periods, with the production of methanol and diketopiperazine (DKP). Methanol is a common decomposition product of dietary constituents. In fact, a liter of fruit juice would yield almost 3 times the methanol of a liter of aspartame-sweetened beverage, even if all of the aspartame decomposed. No measurable increases in blood levels of methanol occurred until single administered doses substantially exceeded the 99th percentile of expected aspartame use. Diketopiperazine is an uncommon constituent of foods, so that numerous animal studies were carried out with this compound. There was no evidence of teratogenicity, mutagenicity, or reproductive effects for DKP in laboratory animals, even at dosages far exceeding those that would be produced by complete decomposition of aspartame consumed at the 99th percentile of expected intake.

In studies of lactating laboratory animals, barely detectable increases in phenylalanine and aspartate levels were found in the milk of mothers fed very large amounts of aspartame.

Dosage

Aspartame is available in tablet form, with one tablet containing 19 mg aspartame, the sweetening equivalent of 1 teaspoon sugar. A granulated form is also available. Many carbonated beverages are made with aspartame as the sweetener; these drinks contain approximately 700 mg/liter. A multitude of other foods are now available with aspartame as the sweetening agent. The projected 99th percentile of aspartame intake in the general population is 34 mg/kg/day, or approximately 1,700 mg for a 50-kg individual. This amount is equal to 2.5 liters of aspartame-sweetened beverage, or approximately 89 packets or tablets of aspartame.

Adverse Effects

No adverse effects of aspartame have been documented to date. However, the Centers for Disease Control (CDC) has investigated 231 consumer complaints, which included headaches, dizziness, mood alterations, gastrointestinal symptoms, and allergic and dermatologic manifestations. The conclusions are as follows:

> This investigation of consumer complaints of symptoms experienced after consumption of aspartame-containing products identified no specific constellation of symptoms clearly related to aspartame consumption. The overrepresentation of women reporting symptoms could not be explained with available data. Despite great variety overall, the majority of frequently reported symptoms were mild and are symptoms that are common in the general populace. While some reports are undoubtedly due to the coincidence of symptoms and aspartame consumption, and others may be due to the suggestibility of some persons, still others may be attributable to some as yet undefined sensitivity of some individuals to aspartame in commonly consumed amounts. The only way these possibilities can be thoroughly evaluated would be through focused clinical studies.

> In summary, currently available information, based on data with limitations as described in the report, indicates a wide variety of complaints that are generally of a mild nature. Although it may be that certain individuals have an unusual sensitivity to the product, these data do not provide evidence for the existence of serious, widespread, adverse health consequences attendant to the use of aspartame.

Mechanism of Action

Aspartame, the methyl ester of aspartyl-phenylalanine, has a sweetening potential approximately 200 times that of sucrose.

Absorption and Biotransformation

Studies in monkeys have shown that aspartame is digested in the same way as natural constituents of the diet. The methyl group is hydrolyzed by intestinal esterases to methanol, which is oxidized to CO_2. The resultant dipeptide is split at the mucosal surface of the intestine by dipeptidases and the free amino acids are absorbed. The aspartic acid moiety is mainly transformed to CO_2 via the tricarboxylic acid cycle, while phenylalanine is incorporated into body protein unchanged or as the major metabolite, tyrosine.

Recommended Reading

Centers for Disease Control. Evaluation of consumer complaints related to aspartame use. *M.M.W.R.* 33:605, 1984.

Food and Drug Administration. Food additives permitted for direct addition to food for human consumption; aspartame. *Federal Register* 48:31376, 1983.

Hayes, A. H., Jr. Summary of Commissioner's Decision on Aspartame. Department of Health and Human Services, Public Health Service, Food and Drug Administration, Docket No. 75F-0355. July 15, 1981.

Lennon, H. D., et al. The biological properties of aspartame. IV. Effects on reproduction and lactation. *J. Environ. Pathol. Toxicol.* 3:375, 1980.

Opperman, J. A., Muldoon, E., and Ranney, R. E. The metabolism of aspartame in the monkey. *J. Nutr.* 103:1454, 1973.

Ranney, R. E., et al. The phenylalanine and tyrosine content of maternal and fetal body fluids from rabbits fed aspartame. *Toxicol. Appl. Pharmacol.* 32:339, 1975.

Steginsk, L. D., Filer, L. J., and Baker, G. L. Plasma, erythrocyte and human milk levels of free amino acids in lactating women administered aspartame or lactose. *J. Nutr.* 109:2173, 1979.

Atropine

Indications and Recommendations

During pregnancy, parenteral atropine should be limited to its use as a preanesthetic agent in surgical patients to reduce salivation and bronchial secretions. Concern has been raised when atropine is used as a premedication for cesarean section because it decreases the "barrier" pressure of the lower cardioesophageal sphincter and might predispose to aspiration in the newborn. This effect could be sustained after a single dose since transplacental passage is rapid, and recent data indicate that elimination of the drug is prolonged in children less than 2 years of age.

Atropine diminishes beat-to-beat heart rate variability and may mask the effects of vagal stimulation on the fetal heart. The intrapartum administration of atropine for the treatment of fetal bradycardia is controversial, but most perinatologists believe that it currently has no role in this setting.

Ophthalmic solutions for topical administration may be used to produce mydriasis and cycloplegia for refraction and in the treatment of inflammatory conditions of the uveal tract. Systemic absorption can be minimized by compressing the lacrimal sac during and for 1 minute following instillation of the drops.

The use of belladonna alkaloids in over-the-counter preparations is discussed under *Belladonna Alkaloids*.

Special Considerations in Pregnancy

Atropine crosses the placenta and is secreted in breast milk; 93% of the maternal serum concentration has been found in umbilical vein blood within 5 minutes of the time the drug was injected into the maternal circulation. Fetal lamb studies have shown that atropine inhibits fetal bradycardia and may increase carotid and cerebral blood flow. In the human fetus, atropine is known to diminish beat-to-beat variability and to mask early (type I) and mild variable fetal heart rate decelerations.

Dosage

The usual parenteral dose is 0.5–1.0 mg. The ophthalmic dose is 1–2 drops of a 0.5%, 1%, 2%, or 3% solution instilled 1 hour before refraction or up to 3 times a day for treatment of uveitis.

Adverse Effects

Annoying anticholinergic effects include dryness of mucous membranes, thirst, and constipation. In larger dosages slurred speech and blurred vision may occur. Overdosage may produce ataxia, excitement, disorientation, hallucinations, delirium, coma, high fever, and antidiuresis.

Mechanism of Action

The principal action of atropine occurs as a result of competitive antagonism of acetylcholine at muscarinic sites. It also has a direct effect on the medulla and higher cerebral centers.

Atropine-induced parasympathetic block may be preceded by a transient phase of mild stimulation. This is probably a result of central vagal stimulation by dosages too small to block peripheral muscarinic receptors. With average clinical dosages, the heart rate may be minimally slowed. Larger dosages, however, cause progressively increasing tachycardia by blocking vagal effects on the pacemaker in the sinoatrial node. Atropine decreases intestinal motility by blocking extrinsic parasympathetic nervous control as well as that of intramural nerve plexuses. Mydriasis and cycloplegia occur because atropine blocks the responses of the sphincter muscle of the iris and the ciliary muscle of the lens to cholinergic stimulation. In addition, the secretory activity of exocrine glands is decreased.

Absorption and Biotransformation

Atropine is usually administered parenterally, but it is well absorbed from all mucosal surfaces. Only limited absorption occurs from the eye, but any portion of a dose that traverses the nasolacrimal duct into the pharynx will be absorbed. Atropine is primarily hydrolyzed in the liver. Most of the drug is excreted in the urine within the first 12 hours, 13–50% being unchanged and the remainder appearing as metabolites.

Recommended Reading

Brand, E. Use of atropine to differentiate normoxic from hypoxic bradycardia (letter). *Am. J. Obstet. Gynecol.* 151:142, 1985.

Cohn, H. E., Piasecki, G. J., and Jackson, B. T. The effect of atropine blockade on the fetal cardiovascular response to hypoxemia. *Gynecol. Invest.* 7:57, 1976.

Gilman, A. G., Goodman, L. S., and Gilman, A. *The Pharmacological Basis of Therapeutics* (6th ed.). New York: Macmillan, 1980. Pp. 120–137.

Goodlin, R. C. Inappropriate fetal bradycardia. *Obstet. Gynecol.* 48:117, 1976.

Goodlin, R. C., and Haesslein, H. Fetal reacting bradycardia. *Am. J. Obstet. Gynecol.* 129:845, 1977.

Ikenoue, T., Quilligan, E. J., and Murata, Y. Circulatory response to atropine in sheep fetus. *Am. J. Obstet. Gynecol.* 126:253, 1976.

Kanto, J. New aspects in the use of atropine. *Int. J. Clin. Pharmacol. Ther. Toxicol.* 21:92, 1983.

Kivado, I., and Saari Roski, S. Placental transmission of atropine at full term pregnancy. *Br. J. Anaesth.* 49:1017, 1977.

Parer, J. T. The effect of atropine on heart rate and oxygen consumption of the hypoxic fetus. *Am. J. Obstet. Gynecol.* 148:1118, 1984.

Parer, J. T. Reply to Dr. Brand (letter). *Am. J. Obstet. Gynecol.* 151:142, 1985.

Azathioprine (Imuran®)

Indications and Recommendations

The administration of azathioprine to pregnant women should be limited to the treatment of serious, life-threatening conditions. This drug is an immunosuppressive agent approved for the treatment of transplant recipients (to prevent rejection) and adults with severe, active rheumatoid arthritis that has been shown to be unresponsive to conventional management. It has also been used for the treatment of other diseases presumed to have an autoimmune cause, including systemic lupus erythematosus and autoimmune thrombocytopenic purpura, when unresponsive to conventional therapy. Because of unresolved concerns about fetal effects, great caution should be taken in prescribing this drug during pregnancy.

Special Considerations in Pregnancy

Azathioprine and its metabolites, 6-mercaptopurine and thiouric acid, cross the placenta and appear in fetal blood, placenta, and amniotic fluid within 150 minutes of maternal oral administration in the late first and early second trimesters.

Azathioprine has been found to be teratogenic in some laboratory animals, but not in others. Many human pregnancies have occurred in renal transplant recipients, most of whom have been treated with both azathioprine and prednisone. Although reports of this experience have largely been anecdotal, most exposed infants have been free of structural anomalies. There is a single case report of preaxial polydactyly, as well as one of pulmonic stenosis. There has been an increased frequency of small-for-gestational-age infants born to mothers receiving azathioprine, but it has been impossible to distinguish the effects of the drug from the effects of the underlying maternal disease.

There is a report of a child with two apparent *de novo* chromosomal aberrations, born to a mother taking azathioprine and prednisone before and during pregnancy. An increased percentage of chromosomal abnormalities (gaps, breaks, deletions, fragments) has been noted in lymphocytes of renal transplant recipients treated with azathioprine and also in their offspring. These chromosomal aberrations have generally disappeared from the children's bloodstreams by the age of 2–3 years and have not been associated with clinical problems. Some studies have failed to verify these chromosomal abnormalities.

Normal immunoglobulin levels have been demonstrated in seven neonates whose mothers were treated with azathioprine throughout pregnancy, but transient immunosuppression has been observed in one such infant whose mother received both azathioprine and prednisone. Another infant, exposed to azathioprine and prednisone throughout pregnancy, was lymphopenic at birth, had reduced immunoglobulin (Ig) M and G levels, and an absent thymic shadow on x ray. This child had a cytomegalovirus (CMV) infection and persistently shed virus, but otherwise appeared immunologically normal at the age of 1 year. There is a second case report of a neonate with brain damage from intrauterine CMV infection whose mother took azathioprine and prednisone for lupus erythematosus.

The risks to infants of nursing mothers who take azathioprine are not clear at present. Normal IgA levels have been found in the milk of one such mother, and in another report two nursing infants whose mothers took azathioprine grew normally, had normal blood cell counts, and had no increased infection rate.

Two cases of pregnancy occurring in renal transplant recipients who used intrauterine devices while taking azathioprine and prednisone have raised the possibility that immunosuppressive therapy may interfere with the effectiveness of this form of contraception. No incidence figures are available.

Dosage

Azathioprine is available in 50-mg tablets and as a solution for intravenous injection (100 mg/20 ml). For transplant recipients, the drug is initiated at 3–5 mg/kg/day in a single intravenous or oral dose. It is usually possible to reduce the dose to 1–3 mg/kg/day. For severe, resistant adult rheumatoid arthritis, the drug is initiated at 1 mg/kg/day (50 or 100 mg), and increased after 6–8 weeks if necessary. The dosage should be increased no more frequently than every 4 weeks, in steps of 0.5 mg/kg/day. The maximum dose used is 2.5 mg/kg/day. Once a therapeutic response has been demonstrated, the dosage should be reduced if possible, in steps of 0.5 mg/kg/day every 4 weeks. The lowest possible dosage should be used for maintenance. Patients with renal dysfunction may require lower dosages.

Adverse Effects

Severe toxicities include leukopenia, thrombocytopenia, macrocytic anemia, and bone marrow depression. These problems are dose related. It is recommended that complete blood counts be obtained weekly during the first month of therapy, twice monthly for the next 2 months, and monthly thereafter. Evidence of significant bone marrow suppression dictates immediate reduction in dosage or discontinuation of the drug. Serious infections may occur in patients receiving immunosuppressive agents and may be fatal.

There is evidence for an increased risk of solid tumors and lymphomas in patients treated with azathioprine. This appears to be especially true for transplant recipients, but cases have also been reported among patients with rheumatoid arthritis.

Gastric disturbances, including nausea and vomiting, are common among patients treated with this drug, especially during the first few months of therapy. These side effects are often ameliorated by administering the drug in divided doses and after meals. Hypersensitivity pancreatitis, toxic hepatitis with biliary stasis, skin rashes, alopecia, fever, arthralgias, diarrhea, and steatorrhea have also been reported.

Mechanism of Action

Azathioprine is a derivative of 6-mercaptopurine, a purine analog. It was synthesized in order to act as a "prodrug," which slowly liberates 6-mercaptopurine. It is believed that the intracellular accumulation of purine analogs can produce major metabolic disruptions, with subsequent cytotoxicity. Lymphocytes appear to be especially sensitive to such effects.

This drug suppresses cell-mediated hypersensitivity and alters antibody production. Suppression of T-cell effects is dependent on the drug being administered before the antigenic stimulus has been presented. Although transplant recipients taking azathioprine have subnormal responses to vaccines, low numbers of T cells, and abnormal phagocytosis by peripheral blood cells, their serum immunoglobulin levels and secondary antibody responses are usually normal. The mechanism by which azathioprine acts against autoimmune diseases is poorly understood.

Absorption and Biotransformation

Azathioprine is rapidly absorbed after oral administration and is slowly converted to 6-mercaptopurine. Both compounds are rapidly eliminated from blood and are oxidized or methylated in erythrocytes and liver. Although renal clearance is not believed to be critical for these drugs, reduction in dosage is recommended for patients with reduced renal function. Tissue levels are not well correlated with blood levels, and the biologic effect appears to be much longer than the serum half-life of approximately 5 hours.

Recommended Reading

Cederqvist, L. L., Merkatz, I. R., and Litwin, S. D. Fetal immunoglobulin synthesis following maternal immunosuppression. *Am. J. Obstet. Gynecol.* 129:687, 1977.

Cote, C. J., Meuwissen, H. J., and Pickering, R. J. Effects on the neonate of prednisone and azathioprine administered to the mother during pregnancy. *J. Pediatr.* 85:324, 1974.

Coulam, C. B., et al. Breast-feeding after renal transplantation. *Transplant Proc.* 13:605, 1982.

Gebhardt, D. O. E. Azathioprine teratogenicity: Review of the literature and case report. *Obstet. Gynecol.* 61:270, 1983.

Gilman, A. G., Goodman, L. S., and Gilman, A. *The Pharmacological Basis of Therapeutics* (6th ed.). New York: Macmillan, 1980. Pp. 1282–1287.

Grekas, D. M., Vasiliou, S. S., and Lazarides, A. N. Immunosuppressive therapy and breast-feeding after renal transplantation. *Nephron* 37:68, 1984.

Hayes, K., Symington, G., and Mackay, I. R. Maternal immunosuppression and cytomegalovirus infection of the fetus. *Aust. N.Z. J. Med.* 9:430, 1979.

McGeown, M. G., and Nevin, N. C. Cytogenetic analysis on children born of parents treated with immunosuppressive drugs. *Proc. Eur. Dial. Transplant Assoc.* 15:384, 1978.

Ostrer, J., Stamberg, J., and Perinchief, P. Two chromosome aberrations in the child of a woman with systemic lupus erythematosus treated with azathioprine and prednisone. *Am. J. Med. Genet.* 17:627, 1984.

Physicians' Desk Reference. Oradell, N.J.: Medical Economics, 1985. Pp. 790–792.

Pirson, Y., et al. Retardation of fetal growth in patients receiving immunosuppressive therapy. *N. Engl. J. Med.* 313:328, 1985.

Price, H. V., et al. Immunosuppressive drugs and the foetus. *Transplantation* 21:294, 1976.

Rosenkrantz, J. G., et al. Azathioprine (Imuran) and pregnancy. *Am. J. Obstet. Gynecol.* 97:387, 1967.

Saarikoski, S., and Seppala, M. Immunosuppression during pregnancy: Transmission of azathioprine and its metabolites from the mother to the fetus. *Am. J. Obstet. Gynecol.* 115:1100, 1973.

Schmid, B. P. Monitoring of organ formation in rat embryos after in vitro exposure to azathioprine, mercaptopurine, methotrexate or cyclosporin A. *Toxicology* 31:9, 1984.

Scott, J. R. Fetal growth retardation associated with maternal administration of immunosuppressive drugs. *Am. J. Obstet. Gynecol.* 128:668, 1977.

Sharon, E., et al. Pregnancy and azathioprine in systemic lupus erythematosus. *Am. J. Obstet. Gynecol.* 118:25, 1974.

Williamson, R. A., and Karp, L. E. Azathioprine teratogenicity: Review of the literature and case report. *Obstet. Gynecol.* 58:247, 1981.

Zerner, J., et al. Intrauterine contraceptive device failures in renal transplant patients. *J. Reprod. Med.* 26:99, 1981.

Beclomethasone (Beclovent®, Vanceril®)

Indications and Recommendations

Beclomethasone may be used for the pregnant woman who needs steroids to control her bronchospasm and in whom systemic steroid therapy may not be necessary. It is an aerosol glucocorticoid compound that has been used in patients who have failed to respond to bronchodilators and cromolyn sodium. It should be appreciated that the effect of beclomethasone on the fetus is presently unknown.

Special Considerations in Pregnancy

Although no well-controlled studies of fetal risk with beclomethasone have been published, the authors of one survey of 45 pregnancies in 40 steroid-dependent asthmatics taking beclomethasone throughout pregnancy reported the incidence of congenital anomalies to be 2.3%. This rate is similar to what is seen in the general population. It is unknown if the drug crosses the human placenta or is secreted into breast milk. Animal studies involving systemic glucocorticosteroids have suggested an increase in early fetal loss, cleft palate, and other malformations.

Dosage

The recommended dose is two inhalations (50 µg per inhalation) every 6–8 hours, with the maximal recommended dose 1,000 µg/day. This dosage did not produce suppression of early-morning cortisol concentration in adult volunteers. If a patient is to be switched from chronic oral systemic corticosteroids to beclomethasone, the aerosol should be used along with the systemic steroid. After 2 weeks, the steroid dosage can be reduced by 2.5 mg prednisone or equivalent every 2 weeks.

Adverse Effects

Unlike systemic steroids, inhaled beclomethasone has minimal systemic effects. In conventional dosages, it produces little or no suppression of the pituitary-adrenal axis. Side effects include hoarseness, oral candidiasis, and an increased incidence of pulmonary infection.

Mechanism of Action

Although the mode of action of steroids in asthma remains unclear, their effects are probably multiple and are mediated mainly through their antiinflammatory effect. In controlled trials, inhaled beclomethasone has been shown to be as effective as oral prednisone in controlling the symptoms of mild to moderate asthma in those asthmatics who require long-term corticosteroid therapy. The drug is not useful in an acute asthmatic attack since bronchospasm may prevent its distribution to more distal airways.

Absorption and Biotransformation

Beclomethasone is administered by a metered-dose oral unit. The drug is deposited in the mouth, nasal mucosa, trachea, bronchi, and lung tissue; a significant amount is swallowed. Systemic absorption does occur. The principal route of elimination of the drug and its metabolites is via the feces. Hypersensitivity to the drug and its propellant (trichlorofluoromethane and dichlorofluoromethane) has been reported.

Recommended Reading

Choo-Kang, Y. F. J., et al. Beclomethasone dipropionate by inhalation in the treatment of airways obstruction. *Br. J. Dis. Chest* 66:101, 1972.

Clark, T. J. H. Effect of beclomethasone dipropionate delivered by aerosol in patients with asthma. *Lancet* 1:1361, 1972.

Greenberger, P. A., and Patterson, R. Beclomethasone dipropionate for severe asthma during pregnancy. *Ann. Intern. Med.* 98:478, 1983.

Lal, S., et al. Comparison of beclomethasone dipropionate aerosol and prednisone in reversible airway obstruction. *Br. Med. J.* 3:314, 1972.

Martin, L. E., et al. Absorption and metabolism of orally administered beclomethasone dipropionate. *Clin. Pharmacol. Ther.* 15:267, 1974.

Simon, G. The place of new aerosol steroid beclomethasone dipropionate in the management of childhood asthma. *Pediatr. Clin. North Am.* 22:147, 1975.

Belladonna Alkaloids (over-the-counter): Atropine, Homatropine, Scopolamine

Indications and Recommendations

Belladonna alkaloids and their quaternary ammonium derivatives are present in a variety of over-the-counter (OTC) antidiarrheal and sedative products. They are usually combined with adsorbents for the treatment of diarrhea and antihistamines and analgesics for use as sedatives. As the belladonna alkaloids are not present in recognized therapeutic doses in OTC antidiarrheal preparations and since other nonadsorbable agents are available, their use for this purpose during pregnancy is not necessary. Products containing scopolamine in therapeutic dosages appear to be safe when used in the treatment of insomnia in pregnancy before the onset of labor. The use of parenteral and ophthalmic solutions of atropine and of parenteral scopolamine is discussed in separate sections of this book.

Special Considerations in Pregnancy

The Collaborative Perinatal Project found no association between first-trimester exposure to atropine, homatropine, or scopolamine and congenital malformations. The use of both atropine and scopolamine near term has been associated with decreased beat-to-beat heart rate variability in the fetus. This phenomenon has been seen primarily with large-dose parenteral use. Small amounts of atropine are secreted in breast milk. When bromides are also contained in compounds, acneform rash, hypotonia and lethargy, irritability, high-pitched cry, and difficulty in feeding have been reported in the newborn.

Dosage

The usual dosages of the belladonna alkaloids available in OTC medications are quite small. Scopolamine is found in doses of 0.083–0.500 mg in combination with other ingredients in OTC sedatives. The total dose of all belladonna alkaloids in the usual antidiarrheal compound is about 0.13 mg/30 ml.

Adverse Effects

The most common side effect of these agents is dryness of the mouth and throat. Other anticholinergic effects such as blurred vision, photophobia, and urinary retention are uncommon at the dosage provided in OTC preparations. Scopolamine may disrupt the sleep cycle by decreasing rapid eye movement (REM) time. When it is discontinued after several days of use, a rebound in REM occurs, resulting in nightmares, insomnia, and the feeling of having slept badly. This effect is not usual at the doses present in most OTC preparations, but it may be experienced by patients who use these preparations chronically or who exceed recommended dosages.

   The belladonna alkaloids are rapidly absorbed into the bloodstream and are distributed throughout the body. Elimination varies with the individual agent. The majority of the compounds are metabolized, but 13–50% of atropine and 1% of scopolamine are excreted in the urine unchanged.

Mechanism of Action

These antimuscarinic agents competitively inhibit acetylcholine at the receptor site of the effector organ. When used in doses equivalent to 0.6–1.0 mg atropine sulfate, belladonna alkaloids are effective in the treatment of diarrhea due to increased intestinal tone and peristalsis. However, most OTC antidiarrheal agents containing belladonna alkaloids contain less than this recognized effective dose.

When a sedative effect is the primary one required, scopolamine is the agent used. It acts as a hypnotic by depressing the cerebral cortex. Therapeutic dosages produce drowsiness, euphoria, fatigue, and dreamless sleep.

Recommended Reading

Gilman, A. G., Goodman, L. S., and Gilman, A. *The Pharmacological Basis of Therapeutics* (6th ed.). New York: Macmillan, 1980. Pp. 120–137.

Heinonen, O. P., Slone, D., and Shapiro, S. *Birth Defects and Drugs in Pregnancy.* Littleton, Mass.: Publishing Sciences Group, 1977. Pp. 346–353, 439.

Nelson, M. M., and Forfar, J. O. Associations between drugs administered during pregnancy and congenital abnormalities of the fetus. *Br. Med. J.* 1:523, 1971.

Schenkel, B., and Vorherr, H. Non-prescription drugs during pregnancy: Potential teratogenic and toxic effects upon embryo and fetus. *J. Reprod. Med.* 12:27, 1974.

Benzodiazepines: Chlordiazepoxide (Librium®), Clonazepam (Clonopin®), Clorazepate (Tranxene®), Diazepam (Valium®), Lorazepam (Ativan®), Oxazepam (Serax®), Prazepam (Centrax®), and others

Indications and Recommendations

The use of benzodiazepines during pregnancy should be limited to the control of status epilepticus and the intermittent treatment of anxiety states. Diazepam is the most widely used of these agents, and so the greatest amount of information about usage in pregnancy is available for this drug. Benzodiazepines are widely used in nonpregnant patients as sedatives, as hypnotics in sleep disorders, for the anxiety associated with depressive disorders, as preanesthetic medications, and in the management of opiate or alcohol withdrawal. Diazepam (and perhaps lorazepam) is the drug of choice for the treatment of status epilepticus but is not useful in the chronic management of epilepsy. It has been used to control eclamptic seizures, although magnesium sulfate is the drug of choice prior to delivery. Clonazepam is used in the treatment of absence seizures and myoclonic seizures in children, but is rarely indicated in women of reproductive age. Chronic use of diazepam during pregnancy may be associated with significant adverse effects in the neonate and is therefore not recommended.

As diazepam is excreted into breast milk and may cause lethargy, weight loss, and sedation in the nursing infant, its use by the lactating mother is not recommended.

The newer benzopdiazepines have not been well studied in pregnancy. At least two studies of lorazepam used as a labor medication suggest that neonatal depression is likely to be associated with the use of this drug.

Special Considerations in Pregnancy

Diazepam (and presumably other benzodiazepines) rapidly crosses the placental barrier with fetal-maternal equilibrium being reached within 1 hour in humans. Benzodiazepine concentrations in cord blood have been reported to exceed the levels in maternal blood. This may be due to their marked lipid solubility and delayed metabolism by the immature fetal liver.

The intravenous injection of 5–10 mg diazepam into pregnant ewes has been associated with an immediate cessation of fetal breathing activity. In humans, loss of beat-to-beat fetal heart rate variability has been reported within 2 minutes of the intravenous administration of 20 mg diazepam. This effect lasts approximately 60 minutes and does not affect fetal pH or Apgar scores. In addition, intravenous diazepam has been associated with a decrease in the frequency (but not amplitude) of uterine contractions during labor.

In a study performed in the early 1960s, it was reported that major congenital anomalies occurred in 4 in 35 infants born to mothers taking chlordiazepoxide during the first 42 days of gestation (11.4%). In contrast, only 2 in 77 infants whose mothers were diagnosed as having minor psychoneurotic complaints but who were not medicated during this time period in pregnancy were found to have major congenital anomalies (2.6%). This finding has not been corroborated.

A number of epidemiologic studies have suggested a relationship between diazepam use and various birth defects. The strongest association appeared to be with cleft lip or palate. Most recently, parents of 611 infants with oral clefts and of 2,498 control infants with other birth defects were interviewed via a structured questionnaire about drug use in pregnancy. Parents of children with other birth defects were used as the control group in order to avoid recall bias, which is believed to reduce the memory of drug use during pregnancy when the outcome was normal. Among the controls, 2.2% recalled taking diazepam during the first 4 months of pregnancy. Similarly, 2.2% of parents with pregnancies producing a baby with cleft lip and 1.8% of those with pregnancies producing cleft palate recalled taking diazepam during the first 4 months. Thus, these authors believe that there is no association between diazepam use in early pregnancy and oral clefts. When prospective data on 32,395 pregnancies were analyzed by investigators at the National Institutes of Health, again no significant increase in relative risk for oral clefts was found among first-trimester users of diazepam. Disagreement regarding this issue continues, and it is probably best to avoid benzodiazepines during the first trimester unless the indications for their use are compelling.

Neonatal diazepam withdrawal symptoms have been reported after second- and third-trimester maternal ingestion, generally in doses of 15–20 mg/day for at least 12 weeks. It should be noted, however, that in one report only 10 mg every other day was taken for 16 weeks. The symptoms were similar to neonatal narcotic withdrawal symptoms. Severe neonatal respiratory depression can occur when diazepam is used in high dosages for control of eclampsia. Neonatal hypothermia is also commonly reported. In addition, hyperbilirubinemia in the neonate is believed to be potentiated by benzodiazepines, probably due to delayed bilirubin metabolism.

The benzodiazepines, and their metabolite N-demethyldiazepam, are secreted into human breast milk. Lethargy, sedation, and weight loss have been reported in nursing infants whose mothers took diazepam. Since N-demethyldiazepam has a long half-life and is metabolized in the liver, it is not unexpected that neonates might be susceptible to such effects.

Dosage

Chlordiazepoxide is available as tablets and capsules (5, 10, and 25 mg) and as ampules of 100 mg/2 ml. The usual daily oral dose is 15–60 mg in two to four divided doses. Intravenous or intramuscular doses of 50–100 mg are used for alcohol withdrawal, acute and severe anxiety disorders, and as preoperative medication. No more than 300 mg should be injected over a 24-hour period.

Diazepam is available as 2-, 5-, and 10-mg tablets and in an injectable form (5 mg/ml). The usual dosage range for chronic oral therapy is from 2 mg at bedtime for the treatment of mild anxiety associated with insomnia to as much as 20 mg tid for the management of alcohol withdrawal, severe anxiety, or muscle spasm. Intravenous dosages as high as 30 mg may be required to control status epilepticus.

Oxazepam is supplied as 10-, 15-, and 30-mg capsules and as 15-mg tablets. Dosage ranges from 10 mg tid to 30 mg qid, depending on symptoms. Clorazepate dipotassium is available as 3.75-, 7.5.0- and 15.00- mg tablets and capsules. The usual daily dose ranges from 15–30 mg in one to four divided doses. Lorazepam is available as 0.5-, 1.0-, and 2.0 mg tablets, and in injectable forms of 2 and 4 mg/ml. The usual oral dose is 2–6 mg/day in two to four divided doses. As a preoperative medication, a dose of 0.05 mg/kg up to a maximum of 4.0 mg is given intramuscularly; for intravenous sedation, the dose is 0.044 mg/kg up to a maximum of 2.0 mg. Prazepam comes in 5-, 10-, and 20-mg capsules. The usual daily dose is 20–40 mg in divided doses.

Adverse Effects

Side effects most commonly encountered are drowsiness, excessive somnolence, lethargy, impairment of intellectual function, ataxia, and memory impairment. Paradoxic effects such as increased hostility or anxiety have been reported. Excessive intravenous administration or intravenous therapy in the presence of other central nervous system depressants can produce significant respiratory depression. The therapeutic index is high, and fatal benzodiazepine overdosage in the absence of other drugs is distinctly uncommon. Chronic administration can lead to drug dependence, and true physiologic addiction has been documented.

Mechanism of Action

The presence of specific benzodiazepine receptors in the central nervous system has been well documented, and these drugs bind to their receptors with high affinity. The ultimate effect of the benzodiazepine-receptor interaction is to enhance the inhibitory neuronal properties of gamma-aminobutyric acid (GABA). The receptors are most abundant in the cortex and in limbic-forebrain areas. Although the presence of specific receptors suggests the existence of a corresponding natural neurotransmitter, such a compound has not yet been identified. Antagonists to benzodiazepines exist, and behavior reminiscent of fear and anxiety has been produced by their administration to animals.

Absorption and Biotransformation

The differences in the various compounds lie mainly in their lipid solubility. More lipid-soluble drugs cross the blood-brain barrier rapidly and thus have a rapid onset of action after a single intravenous dose, but their duration of action is limited by redistribution to lipid depots around the body. Conversely, less lipid-soluble forms have a slower onset of action but a longer duration. After oral dosing, gastrointestinal absorption is the rate-limiting factor. Diazepam is very rapidly absorbed, reaching peak concentrations in about 1 hour, as is its metabolite, N-demethyldiazepam. Some of the compounds with slower onset (i.e., prazepam) are limited by the rate of their conversion to N-demethyldiazepam, which is then immediately absorbed. Chlordiazepoxide and oxazepam are much more slowly absorbed, reaching peaks in several hours. The kinetics of these drugs are quite complex and a detailed discussion is beyond the scope of this book. Although absorption may be rapid, the elimination half-lives can be prolonged (more than 24 hours), and secondary peaks in blood levels may occur, presumably due to enterohepatic recirculation. Thus, the drugs may accumulate with increasing blood levels until a steady state is achieved, usually after the drug has been taken for 4–5 times the elimination half-life.

The benzodiazepines are cleared by the liver, either through oxidation or conjugation. Different compounds are differentially cleared by these two pathways. The clinical importance of this difference among compounds is not yet clearly established.

Recommended Reading

Cole, A. P., and Hailey, D. M. Diazepam and active metabolites in breast milk and their transfer to the neonate. *Arch. Dis. Child.* 50:741, 1975.

Erkkola, R., and Kanto, J. Diazepam and breast feeding. *Lancet* 1:1235, 1972.

Erkkola, R., Kangas, L., and Pekkarinen, A. The transfer of diazepam across the placenta during labor. *Acta Obstet. Gynecol. Scand.* 52:165, 1973.

Gilman, A. G., Goodman, L. S., and Gilman, A. *The Pharmacological Basis of Therapeutics* (6th ed.). New York: Macmillan, 1980. Pp. 437–442, 466–467.

Greenblatt, D. J., and Shader, R. I., and Abernethy, D. R. Current status of benzodiazepines, parts 1 and 2. *N. Engl. J. Med.* 309:354, 410, 1983.

Mazzi, E. Possible neonatal diazepam withdrawal: A case report. *Am. J. Obstet. Gynecol.* 129:586, 1977.

Mcauley, D. M., et al. Lorazepam premedication for labour. *Br. J. Obstet. Gynaecol.* 89:149, 1982.

Milkovich, L., and van den Berg, B. J. Effects of prenatal meprobamate and chlordiazepoxide hydrochloride on human embryonic and fetal development. *N. Engl. J. Med.* 291:1268, 1974.

Mofid, M., Brinkman, C. R., and Assali, N. S. Effects of diazepam on uteroplacental and fetal hemodynamic metabolism. *Obstet. Gynecol.* 41:364, 1973.

Patrick, M. J., Tilstone, W. J., and Reavey, P. Diazepam and breast feeding, *Lancet* 1:542, 1972.

Rosenberg, L., et al. Lack of relation of oral clefts to diazepam use during pregnancy. *N. Engl. J. Med.* 309:1282, 1983.

Shiono, P. H., and Mills, J. L. Oral clefts and diazepam use during pregnancy. *N. Engl. J. Med.* 311:919, 1984.

Whitelaw, A. G. L., Cummings, A. J., and McFadyen, I. R. Effect of maternal lorazepam on the neonate. *Br. Med. J.* 282:1106, 1981.

Beta-adrenergic Blocking Agents: Atenolol (Tenormin®), Metoprolol (Lopressor®), Nadolol (Corgard®), Pindolol (Visken®), Propranolol (Inderal®), Timolol (Blocadren®)

Indications and Recommendations

The use of beta blockers during pregnancy is indicated for treatment of specific life-threatening conditions. These include therapy of thyroid storm, reduction of afterload on the heart in patients at risk to dissect an aortic aneurysm, control of beta-adrenergic side effects of intravenous hydralazine therapy for an acute hypertensive episode, idiopathic hypertrophic subaortic stenosis, and any other potentially lethal condition that requires beta-adrenergic blockade. Their use in the treatment of hypertension during pregnancy is still controversial, although evidence is growing that the selective beta-1 blockers may be safely used for this purpose.

Special Considerations in Pregnancy

These drugs easily cross the placenta and are also secreted into breast milk, although in small amounts. There have been no reports of congenital malformations ascribed to the beta blockers.

Intravenous administration of propranolol during dysfunctional labor has been reported to increase coordinated contraction patterns without an appreciable concomitant elevation in resting tonus. More experimental work in this setting is needed, however, before the use of beta blockers for the treatment of dysfunctional labor can be recommended. Clinical trials in which beta blockers have been used for other indications do not reveal an increased risk of premature labor.

Experiments with pregnant sheep have demonstrated a significant reduction in umbilical flow when propranolol was given intravenously to the mother. Uterine blood flow, however, was not affected. Propranolol administered during pregnancy has been thought to cause intrauterine growth retardation (IUGR), but a definitive association has not been proved. Most of the studies involving propranolol in pregnant women have been retrospective and contain small numbers of patients. In a large, prospective controlled study using atenolol (a selective beta blocker) for the treatment of pregnancy-associated hypertension, no increase in the incidence of IUGR was found.

Neonatal bradycardia has been noted in association with the maternal use of beta blockers. Neonatal hypoglycemia has been reported with maternal propranolol administration, but not with atenolol. When beta blockers are administered during labor, both mother and fetus should have continuous cardiac monitoring, especially if general anesthesia is used. Neonates of mothers given intravenous propranolol immediately before cesarean section have had difficulty in establishing spontaneous respiratory activity. Propranolol can cause nonreactivity of nonstress tests, which become reactive once the drug is discontinued. However, no adverse effects on fetal heart rate patterns in labor have been reported with atenolol.

Dosage

The usual oral dose of propranolol ranges from 10–100 mg every 6 hours. Intravenous doses are given slowly, 1 mg at a time, with a range of 1–5 mg. Careful cardiac monitoring is necessary during intravenous administration.

Information regarding the other beta blockers may be found in Table 1.

Adverse Effects

Numerous side effects may occur with the use of beta blockers. These include sinus bradycardia in most patients and congestive heart failure in those with poor cardiac reserve who cannot tolerate a reduction in cardiac output. Bronchospasm occurs in 2–10% of patients who take nonselective beta blockers. A history of asthma is, therefore, a contraindication to the use of propranolol. Compromised peripheral circulation may be worsened, and Raynaud's phenomenon contraindicates the use of beta blockers. Central nervous system effects include insomnia, nightmares, hallucinations, depression, paresthesias, ataxia, and dizziness. Nausea, diarrhea, abdominal discomfort, constipation, and hyperglycemia are noted in some patients. Acute hypertensive episodes have been reported in patients with pheochromocytoma, or when propranolol is given with methyldopa. It is hypothesized that alpha-methylnorepinephrine, a metabolite of methyldopa, becomes a potent pressor agent in the presence of beta-adrenergic blockade.

Table 1. Pharmacology of beta-adrenergic blocking agents

Drug	Beta-blockade potency ratio (propranolol = 1.0)	Selectivity for beta-1 receptors	Half-life (h)	Absorption	Hepatic metabolism	Renal excretion (% excreted unchanged)	Recommended daily dose (range)
Propranolol (Inderal®)	1.0	0	3.5–6.0	>90%	Extensive	<1	40–320 mg (2 divided doses)
Atenolol (Tenormin®)	1.0	+	6–9	≅50%	Minimal	85–100	50–200 mg (1 dose)
Metoprolol (Lopressor®)	1.0	+	3–4	>95%	Extensive	<5	100–400 mg (2 divided doses)
Timolol (Blocadren®)	6.0	0	3–4	>90%	Extensive	13–20	20–60 mg (2 divided doses)
Nadolol (Corgard®)	1.0	0	12–24	≅30%	Minimal	70	40–320 mg (2 divided doses)
Pindolol (Visken®)	6.0	0	3–4	>90%	60%	40	15–60 mg (2 divided doses)

Mechanism of Action

The beta-adrenergic receptors of various tissues can be differentiated pharmacologically as being beta-1 (lipolysis and cardiostimulation) and beta-2 (bronchodilatation and vasodilatation) (Table 2). Blockers of these receptors are classified as being selective or nonselective according to their activity at relatively low dosage levels. When administered in usual therapeutic regimens, beta-1 selective blocking agents, such as atenolol, primarily inhibit cardiac beta-adrenergic receptors and have less of an effect on the beta-2 receptors in the bronchi and vasculature. In higher dosages, however, beta-1 selective agents will also block beta-2 receptors.

Beta-1 adrenergic blockade causes decreased cardiac output, slowing of the heart rate, and prolonged mechanical systole. Beta-2 blockade inhibits the release of renin by the kidney, and blood pressure is lowered further by direct action on the central nervous system.

Intravenous administration of nonselective beta blockers causes a rapid fall in heart rate and cardiac output by directly decreasing the force and frequency of myocardial contractions. Initially, there is a rise in peripheral vascular resistance and no change or a slight decrease in blood pressure. An antihypertensive effect begins several hours after administration, especially in patients with elevated plasma renin activity. This effect occurs because of the persistent decrease in cardiac output as well as a fall in peripheral resistance back to or below control levels. The latter may be due to the central action of the drugs or to their inhibition of the release of renal renin.

Respiratory airway resistance is consistently increased by nonselective beta blockers. Insulin release is mediated by beta-adrenergic mechanisms, and nonselective beta blockers blunt the normal response to an elevation in blood glucose. These drugs also block the adrenergic signs and symptoms of severe thyrotoxicosis.

Table 2. Effects of beta-adrenergic blocking agents

System	Receptor	Effect of blockade
Heart	Beta-1	Decreased rate of sinoatrial node discharge
	Beta-1	Decreased contractility
	Beta-1	Decreased conduction velocity in atria, atrioventricular node, and ventricles
	Beta-1	Decreased ventricular automaticity
Blood vessels	Beta-2	Constriction of arterioles, especially in skeletal muscle
Lungs	Beta-2	Bronchoconstriction
Fat cells	Beta-1	Inhibition of lipolysis
Pancreas	Beta-2	Decreased insulin release
Liver	Beta-2	Decreased glycogenolysis and gluconeogenesis
Kidney	Beta-2	Decreased renin release

Absorption and Biotransformation

Most beta blockers are readily absorbed from the gastrointestinal tract except for atenolol and nadolol, which are less lipid soluble. Propranolol is completely absorbed from the small intestine but much of it is rapidly metabolized by the liver. When given orally, propranolol appears in the plasma within 30 minutes, and peak levels are obtained 60–90 minutes after administration. When given as a single dose, the half-life is 2–3 hours, but this is increased to 3.5–6.0 hours when the drug is administered over a long period of time. Information regarding the other beta blockers may be found in Table 1 (see p. 45).

The beta blockers can be divided into two groups according to their route of elimination. Propranolol, metoprolol, and timolol are extensively metabolized by the liver, whereas others, such as atenolol and nadolol, are excreted largely unchanged by the kidneys.

Renal insufficiency has very little effect on the metabolism of propranolol and metoprolol, and their dosage regimen need not be changed in patients with compromised renal function. The less lipid-soluble beta blockers nadolol and atenolol achieve lower brain concentrations than do propranolol, metoprolol, and timolol, and therefore may result in less central nervous system side effects.

Phenobarbital increases the clearance and decreases the half-life of the drugs metabolized by the liver, so that higher dosages may be required if these agents are administered concurrently.

Recommended Reading

Dubois, D., et al. Beta blocker therapy in 125 cases of hypertension during pregnancy. *Clin. Exp. Hypertens.* 2:41, 1983.

Frishman, W. H. Atenolol and timolol, two new systemic β-adrenoceptor antagonists. *N. Engl. J. Med.* 306:1456, 1982.

Rubin, P. C. Beta-blockers in pregnancy. *N. Engl. J. Med.* 305:1323, 1981.

Rubin, P. C., et al. Obstetric aspects of the use in pregnancy-associated hypertension of the β-adrenoceptor antagonist atenolol. *Am. J. Obstet. Gynecol.* 150:389, 1984.

Rubin, P. C., et al. Placebo-controlled trial of atenolol in treatment of pregnancy associated hypertension. *Lancet* 1:431, 1983.

Thornley, K. J., McAinsh, J., and Cruckshank, J. M. Atenolol in the treatment of pregnancy-induced hypertension. *Br. J. Clin. Pharmacol.* 12:725, 1981.

Bromocriptine (Parlodel®)

Indications and Recommendations

Bromocriptine is safe to use during pregnancy when continued suppressive therapy of a prolactin-secreting pituitary adenoma is thought to be desirable. Although most women with amenorrhea-galactorrhea syndromes who undergo ovulation induction with bromocriptine are advised to discontinue the medication once conception has occurred, a number of clinicians continue therapy throughout pregnancy in order to prevent neurologic complications. Others use the drug selectively for pregnant women with macroadenomas or for those who develop neurologic complications during pregnancy. The efficacy of prophylactic bromocriptine use during pregnancy in women with prolactinomas has not been adequately tested with controlled studies. However, the reported experience with the use of this drug during pregnancy to date suggests that fetal risk is not appreciable.

Bromocriptine is commonly used as a lactation suppression agent post partum for women who choose not to nurse their babies.

Special Considerations in Pregnancy

Most patients who have taken bromocriptine during pregnancy have done so inadvertently, after successful ovulation induction. Sandoz, Inc., the company that markets the drug, surveyed patients in 30 countries who were treated during pregnancy between 1973 and 1980. There were reports on 1,410 pregnancies in 1,335 women. The daily dose ranged from 1–40 mg, with a mean of 5 mg. The mean duration of treatment after conception was 21 days. The spontaneous abortion rate was 11.1%, and the voluntary termination rate was 1.8%. There were 12 extrauterine pregnancies (0.9%) and 3 molar pregnancies (0.2%). There were 28 sets of twins and three sets of triplets. Of the 1,241 pregnancies proceeding past the twentieth week, there were 5 stillbirths, for an antenatal mortality of 4 : 1,000. Of these 1,241 live- and stillborn children, 43 (3.5%) had congenital anomalies. Twelve of the anomalies were major, 11 moderate, and 20 minor. The dosage and duration of exposure to bromocriptine did not differ between the pregnancies producing anomalous, stillborn, or normal babies. Neonatal mortality was not mentioned. This survey suggests that the stillbirth and anomaly rates observed in pregnant women exposed to bromocriptine in the first trimester did not differ from those seen in the general population.

In a series reported from Paris, eight women with grade II and III prolactinomas were treated with bromocriptine at a dose (5–20 mg/day) sufficient to suppress the prolactin level below 20 ng/ml continuously throughout pregnancy. None had tumor-related neurologic complications. Two additional patients, not known to be pregnant, had their bromocriptine discontinued after 2–3 weeks of treatment. Both developed bitemporal hemianopia during the second trimester (at serum prolactin levels around 50 ng/ml), and the symptoms responded to bromocriptine in both cases. The authors believe that bromocriptine treatment should be continued throughout pregnancy in patients with prolactinomas. It should be pointed out, however, that prolactin levels in normal women generally exceed 100 ng/ml during pregnancy, and so there is no evidence that maintaining tumor patients at levels below 20 ng/ml is appropriate. In addition, most authors report a lower rate of neurologic complications in pregnant women with prolactinomas than the 2 in 2 (100%) noted in the untreated patients in the above study. Thus, the prophylactic use of bromocriptine throughout pregnancy in such women remains controversial.

There are reports of pituitary macroadenomas responding to bromocriptine during pregnancy, and at least one patient with excessive breast enlargement (gigantomastia) has been successfully treated with this drug during pregnancy.

Dosage

Bromocriptine is available as a 2.5-mg tablet and a 5-mg capsule. For postpartum prevention of breast engorgement and lactation, the drug is started at least 4 hours post partum, and the dose is 2.5 mg bid with meals. This therapy is continued for 14–21 days. Approximately one-fourth of patients experience rebound engorgement or milk secretion once therapy has been discontinued; this is usually mild and self-limited. It should be noted that, even without suppressive therapy, postpartum breast engorgement is self-limited and not usually severe.

When bromocriptine is used to treat amenorrhea-galactorrhea, the starting dose is generally 2.5 mg at bedtime with a snack, increasing to bid over 1 week's time. The patient mentioned previously who was treated for a macroadenoma during pregnancy received 2.5 mg tid. Bromocriptine is also used, in much higher dosage, to treat Parkinson's disease. This diagnosis, however, is quite unusual among women in the reproductive age group.

Adverse Effects

Side effects occur in the majority of treated patients. Nausea has been reported in over 50%, with headaches, dizziness, fatigue, abdominal cramps, vomiting, nasal congestion, constipation, and diarrhea being somewhat less common. Faintness, believed to be due to orthostatic hypotension, is commonly reported. Rarely, neurologic symptoms, including hallucinations, occur. Much higher dosages have been used to treat patients with Parkinson's disease, with more severe side effects reported.

Mechanism of Action

Bromocriptine is a dopamine receptor agonist and an ergot derivative. It inhibits pituitary prolactin secretion just as prolactin inhibitory factor (thought to be dopamine) does. The side effects of bromocriptine are also ascribed to its dopamine-like action.

Absorption and Biotransformation

Approximately 28% of an oral dose is absorbed from the gastrointestinal tract, and peak plasma levels are reached within 2 hours. The drug is highly protein bound. It is completely metabolized, and excretion is in bile. Almost all of an orally administered dose is excreted in the feces over 120 hours.

Recommended Reading

Gilman, A. G., Goodman, L. S., and Gilman, A. *The Pharmacological Basis of Therapeutics* (6th ed.). New York: Macmillan, 1980. Pp. 483–484.

Hedberg, K., Karlsson, K., and Lindstedt, G. Gigantomastia during pregnancy: Effect of a dopamine agonist. *Am. J. Obstet. Gynecol.* 133:928, 1979.

Konopka, P., et al. Continuous administration of bromocriptine in the prevention of neurological complications in pregnant women with prolactinomas. *Am. J. Obstet. Gynecol.* 146:935, 1983.

Maeda, T., et al. Effective bromocriptine treatment of a pituitary macroadenoma during pregnancy. *Obstet. Gynecol.* 61:117, 1983.

Speroff, L., Glass, R. H., and Kase, N. G. *Clinical Gynecologic Endocrinology and Infertility* (3rd ed.). Baltimore: Williams & Wilkins, 1983. Pp. 167–168.

Turkalj, I., Braun, P., and Krupp, P. Surveillance of bromocriptine in pregnancy. *J.A.M.A.* 247:1589, 1982.

Bulk-forming Agents (over-the-counter): Agar, Bran, Methylcellulose, Psyllium, Tragacanth

Indications and Recommendations

Bulk-forming agents are safe to use during pregnancy. The over-the-counter (OTC) drugs listed above are used as stool softeners in people with constipation, hemorrhoids, anorectal disorders, hernias, and cardiovascular disease.

Special Considerations in Pregnancy

There are no maternal effects unique to pregnancy.

Dosage

Methylcellulose and carboxymethylcellulose are supplied as a 500-mg powder, tablet, or capsule. The dose is 1–6 g/day taken 1–4 times a day, each dose taken with one to two glasses of water. Onset of action is 1–2 days.

Psyllium preparations from the plantain seed are powders. One to 2 teaspoons of powder are mixed in water and taken 1–3 times a day.

Agar is usually mixed with psyllium or cathartics and 4–16 g is taken daily.

Tragacanth is available in many preparations in a variety of dosages.

Bran contains 20% indigestible cellulose and is generally taken with cereal.

Adverse Effects

With the exception of the psyllium preparations, none of these bulk-forming laxatives is significantly absorbed, and thus no systemic effects occur. Psyllium preparations are absorbed to some degree and have been shown to decrease plasma cholesterol levels by interfering with absorption of bile acids. Bulk-forming laxatives may increase flatulence, and if taken with inadequate water, intestinal obstruction may occur.

Mechanism of Action

These agents, which include methylcellulose and carboxymethylcellulose, psyllium preparations, agar, tragacanth, and bran, all swell when in contact with water, forming a mass that promotes peristalsis, decreases transit time, and keeps the feces soft.

Recommended Reading

Gilman, A. G., Goodman, L. S., and Gilman, A. *The Pharmacological Basis of Therapeutics* (6th ed.). New York: Macmillan, 1980. Pp. 1002–1005.

Nelson, M. M., and Forfar, J. O. Associations between drugs administered during pregnancy and congenital abnormalities of the fetus. *Br. Med. J.* 1:523, 1971.

Schenkel, B., and Vorherr, H. Non-prescription drugs during pregnancy: Potential teratogenic and toxic effects upon embryo and fetus. *J. Reprod. Med.* 12:27, 1974.

Calcium-channel Blockers: Diltiazem (Cardizem®), Nicardipine (Nicardipin®), Nifedipine (Procardia®), Verapamil (Calan®, Isoptin®)

Indications and Recommendations

The use of the calcium-channel blockers during pregnancy is indicated for the treatment of specific life-threatening cardiovascular conditions and as adjunctive therapy for the pharmacologic conversion of fetal supraventricular tachyarrhythmias. Despite the fact that these agents have been widely used in Europe and other parts of the world, experience with their use in pregnant women in the United States is extremely limited. Because other relatively effective drugs have been more extensively studied, the calcium-channel blockers cannot be recommended as tocolytic agents at this time. It should be noted, however, that these drugs may prove to be excellent pharmacologic agents for the arrest of premature labor.

At the present time, only diltiazem, nifedipine, and verapamil have been released by the FDA for use in the United States. These drugs have different degrees of selectivity in their effects on vascular smooth muscle, the myocardium, or conduction and pacemaker tissues within the heart, and have been used for a wide variety of conditions in nonpregnant patients. Their uses include the management of vasospastic and chronic stable angina pectoris, paroxysmal supraventricular tachycardia, essential hypertension, primary and secondary hypoxic pulmonary hypertension, hypertrophic cardiomyopathy, and Raynaud's phenomenon. The calcium-channel blockers have also been used to treat asthma, chronic obstructive lung disease, and esophageal motor disorders such as achalasia and diffuse esophageal spasm.

Special Considerations in Pregnancy

Nicardipine suppresses spontaneous in vitro uterine contractions in rabbit myometrium as well as contractions in postpartum rats. It has also been shown to be effective in abolishing the uterine response of gravid rats to intraamniotically administered oxytocin or prostaglandin F_2 alpha, and in delaying the delivery of subsequent fetuses when administered after the birth of the first pup of the litter. When this experimental model was used to compare the calcium blockers to ethanol, ritodrine, and albuterol, calcium blockers were found to be the most active of the compounds tested. In that study, nifedipine was found to be more effective than verapamil or diltiazem.

In a comparative study performed on isolated human term pregnant and nonpregnant myometrial preparations, nicardipine as well as nifedipine relaxed muscle strips contracted with hyperosmolar potassium, prostaglandin F_2 alpha, oxytocin, and vasopressin. Nicardipine had a slower onset of action but appeared to be significantly more potent than nifedipine in pregnant myometrium.

All of these drugs cross the placenta. During the first stage of labor, a single 80-mg oral dose of verapamil was given to six women when their cervical dilatation was 3–4 cm. In two patients who delivered at 49 and 109 minutes after maternal dosing, cord levels of this drug were 17 and 26% of those in maternal serum. The other women all delivered more than 170 minutes after maternal administration, and no verapamil could be detected in their infants' cord blood.

In instrumented pregnant ewes, verapamil administered intravenously to the mother at a dose of 0.2 mg/kg resulted in decreased maternal mean and diastolic blood pressures but no significant change in fetal systolic, diastolic, and mean blood pressures. Maternal and fetal heart rates were unchanged, but atrioventricular conduction was prolonged in both. In a study of six instrumented pregnant goats given bolus injections of nifedipine at doses of 2.5–45.0 mg/kg, no significant fall in uterine blood flow was noted despite transient maternal hypotension and tachycardia. When studies were performed on seven instrumented pregnant monkeys, however, a continuous infusion of nifedipine for 1 hour was associated with a decline in fetal PO_2 from 21.7 ± 2.1 to 14.2 ± 1.8 mm Hg, and a fall in fetal pH from 7.38 to 7.24. Mean fetal arterial pressure appeared to decline during the infusion, but this was not statistically significant.

In 10 selected Swedish patients who were in premature labor at 33 weeks or less, nifedipine successfully postponed labor for 3 days or more, during which time glucocorticoids were administered to accelerate fetal lung maturation. Delivery was performed 1–28 days after completed therapy, and all the infants had 5-minute Apgar scores of 7 or greater. Follow-up at 1 year showed all infants to be developing normally. In an American study, delivery was delayed for more than 48 hours in 9 in 13 women in premature labor who were treated with oral nifedipine in doses up to a maximum of 80 mg/day. Six of these women had had severe reactions to ritodrine, while the other seven had failed therapy with both ritodrine and magnesium sulfate. No untoward maternal or fetal side effects were attributed to the drug, and follow-up on 10 of the 13 neonates was normal at 1 year.

Verapamil, in addition to its tocolytic action, has been shown to be useful in reducing cardiovascular side effects associated with the beta agonists. With ritodrine infusions in excess of 200 µg/minute, the addition of verapamil at a dose of 80–120 µg/minute has been reported to diminish the incidence of maternal tachycardia and hypotension.

At the University of Mannheim, a combination of feneterol and

Table 3. Comparative adverse effects of calcium-channel blockers

	Verapamil	Nifedipine	Diltiazem
Hypotension	+ +	+ + +	+
Headaches	+	+ + +	0
Peripheral edema	+ +	+ + +	±
Constipation	+ +	0	0
Congestive heart failure	+	0	0
Use with beta blockers	Caution	Yes	Yes
AV block	+ +	0	+

verapamil has been used to treat premature labor for more than 15 years. At that institution, 31 newborns of women exposed to this drug regimen were compared to 19 neonatal control subjects whose mothers did not receive tocolytic therapy. Evaluation consisted of serial electrocardiograms and serum potassium, calcium, and magnesium levels at 24 hours and at 2 and 4 weeks of life. Creatine phosphokinase (CPK) and CPK-MB were measured at 24 and 96 hours and again at 2 and 5 weeks, and neonatal heart size was measured at 2 weeks. No pathologic cardiac effects of the tocolytic regimen were demonstrable in this study.

Verapamil has been used to successfully treat a supraventricular tachycardia in a digitalized hyperthyroid patient at 36 weeks. A single intravenous dose of 5 mg given over 5 minutes rapidly broke the arrhythmia, and the patient remained in sinus rhythm for the remaining 5 weeks of her pregnancy. No adverse maternal or fetal effects were noted, and the neonate had 1- and 5-minute Apgar scores of 8 and 9, respectively.

A case has been reported of a fetus at 34 weeks with a tachycardia between 240 and 280 beats/minute and ultrasonic signs of early congestive heart failure that were successfully treated with beta acetyldigoxin and verapamil in utero. The mother was maintained on 0.4 mg/day of the digitalis preparation and 80 mg of verapamil 3 times a day. During the 4 days after onset of treatment, the tachyarrhythmia slowed transiently to 180–196 beats/minute. Five days after the onset of therapy, the fetal heart rate was normal at 138–150 beats/minute, and this persisted until delivery 5 weeks later. The infant appeared to be healthy at birth, was in sinus rhythm with a rate of 160–170 beats/minute during the first day of life, had no signs of cardiac hypertrophy or disturbances in repolarization, and had a normal atrioventricular (AV) conduction time.

It has recently been hypothesized that the calcium-channel blockers may be ideal agents for treating preeclampsia because of their potential for controlling generalized vasospasm, hypertension, and eclamptic seizures. The author of this suggestion recognizes, however, that current methods of treating preeclampsia have proved to be reasonably effective and remarkably safe, and they should not be hastily abandoned in favor of unproved therapies. Until carefully performed, prospective controlled studies demonstrate the safety and efficacy of these agents, they cannot currently be recommended for the treatment of preeclampsia.

Dosage

Pharmacokinetic property	Verapamil†	Nifedipine*	Diltiazem*,†
Dose			
Oral (mg/8 h)	80–160	10–20	30–60
IV (μg/kg)	75–150		
Absorption	90% PO	90% PO	90% PO
	100% IV	90% SL	
Onset of action	2 min IV	3 min SL	30 min PO
	2 h PO	20 min PO	
Therapeutic serum level (μg/ml)	0.05–0.40	0.025–0.100	0.040–0.200
Peak effect	10–15 min IV	1–2 h PO	0.5–2.0 h PO
	5 h PO	10 min SL	
Plasma half-life			
Initial (distribution)	15–30 min	2.5–3.0 h	20 min
Beta (elimination)	2–5 h	5 h	4–7 h

Adverse Effects

In general, the calcium-channel blockers exhibit relatively minor and infrequent side effects. Most studies report the incidence of undesirable side effects to be less than 10%. Fatigue, headache, dizziness, skin rash, and peripheral edema are the adverse sequelae most commonly observed. In a comparison between three of these drugs, diltiazem had the overall best side-effect profile, verapamil was intermediate, and nifedipine was the worst. See Table 3 for comparative side effects.

These agents are relatively contraindicated in the sick sinus syndrome, second- or third-degree AV block, shock, and congestive heart failure. Both verapamil and nifedipine can increase serum levels of digoxin, and verapamil may also interact with beta-adrenergic blockers and the methylxanthines.

Mechanism of Action

The calcium-channel blockers inhibit the inward passage of calcium across myocardial, myometrial, and vascular smooth muscle cells and probably interfere with the intracellular release of calcium. The net effect of these actions is to uncouple the excitation-contraction process, causing smooth muscle relaxation. This results in a reduction in coronary artery and peripheral vascular resistance, as well as myometrial relaxation.

These agents constitute a heterogeneous group with different structural, electrophysiologic, and pharmacologic properties. Some of them depress myocardial contractility, while others affect the electrical conduction system of the heart.

Verapamil prolongs AV conduction in a dose-dependent fashion. It also decreases sinoatrial (SA) node automaticity, myocardial contractility, and peripheral vascular resistance. Its effect on heart

---

*Nifedipine and diltiazem are not available in injectable dosage forms.
†Verapamil and diltiazem are not administered sublingually (SL).

rate and cardiac output is variable. Intravenous verapamil is considered by some authorities to be the drug of choice for treatment of acute paroxysmal supraventricular tachyarrhythmias.

Nifedipine is a potent, long-acting vasodilator. It has mild myocardial depressant effects and no antiarrhythmic properties. This drug has proved to be very useful in relieving anginal symptoms caused by coronary vasospasm and has been used successfully in the treatment of essential hypertension.

Diltiazem reduces SA node automaticity, AV node conduction, myocardial contractility, and peripheral vascular resistance, but not to the same extent as verapamil. It has a variable effect on heart rate and cardiac output and increases vascular oxygen consumption. The chief use of this drug has been in the treatment of coronary artery spasm associated with variant angina. Because it can improve the balance between myocardial oxygen supply and demand and can reduce cellular injury secondary to ischemia, diltiazem is likely to be of benefit in the treatment of the acutely ischemic myocardium during cardiopulmonary bypass and possibly acute myocardial infarction as well.

Absorption and Biotransformation

Verapamil, nifedipine, and diltiazem are well absorbed after oral administration, but their absolute bioavailability is reduced substantially by a "first-pass" effect in the liver, where they are extensively metabolized. All of these drugs are highly bound to plasma proteins, but this only appears to be clinically significant for nifedipine.

Verapamil undergoes an 80–90% first-pass hepatic elimination after an oral dose. The major metabolite is norverapamil, which maintains 20% of the pharmacologic activity of the parent compound. Seventy-five percent of an oral dose is excreted in the urine.

Nifedipine is metabolized to inert products, 80% of which are excreted via the kidneys.

After oral administration, diltiazem undergoes a 60% first-pass metabolism. The major metabolite is desacetyldiltiazem, which maintains 40–50% of the pharmacologic activity of the parent compound. Approximately 35% of a dose of diltiazem undergoes renal excretion.

Recommended Reading

Andersson, K. E., and Ulmsten, U. Effects of nifedipine on myometrial activity and lower abdominal pain in women with primary dysmenorrhea. *Br. J. Obstet. Gynaecol.* 85:142, 1978.

Andersson, K. E., et al. Inhibition of prostaglandin-induced uterine activity by nifedipine. *Br. J. Obstet. Gynaecol.* 86:175, 1979.

Braunwald, E. Mechanism of disease: Mechanism of action of calcium-channel blocking agents. *N. Engl. J. Med.* 307:1618, 1982.

Council on Scientific Affairs. Calcium channel blocking agents. *J.A.M.A.* 250:2522, 1983.

Csapo, A. I., et al. Deactivation of the uterus during normal and premature labor by the calcium antagonist nicardipine. *Am. J. Obstet. Gynecol.* 142:483, 1982.

D'Alton, M. E., et al. Treatment of premature labor with the calcium antagonist nifedipine (abstract). Presented at the Society of Perinatal Obstetricians Annual Meeting. Las Vegas, Nev., 1985.

Ducsay, C. A., et al. Nifedipine tocolysis in pregnant rhesus monkeys: Maternal and fetal cardiorespiratory effects. Presented at the Society of Perinatal Obstetricians Annual Meeting. Las Vegas, Nev., 1985.

Forman, A., et al. Relaxant effects of nifedipine on isolated, human myometrium. *Acta Pharmacol. Toxicol.* 45:81, 1979.

Klein, V., and Repke, J. T. Supraventricular tachycardia in pregnancy: Cardioversion with verapamil. *Obstet. Gynecol.* 63(S):16s, 1984.

Lirette, M., Holbrook, R. H., and Katz, M. Effect of nicardipine HCl on prematurely induced uterine activity in the pregnant rabbit. *Obstet. Gynecol.* 65:31, 1985.

Miagaard, S., et al. Comparison of the effects of nicardipine and nifedipine on isolated human myometrium. *Gynecol. Obstet. Invest.* 16:354, 1983.

Murad, S. H. N., et al. Verapamil: Placental transfer and effects on maternal and fetal hemodynamics and atrioventricular conduction in the pregnant ewe. *Anesthesiology* 62:49, 1985.

Proceedings of a symposium. New directions in the use of calcium channel blockers. *Am. J. Med.* 78(Suppl.):1, 1985.

Review of calcium channel blockers. *Curr. Inf. Drugs* 16:2, 1984.

Rodriguez-Escudero, F. J., Aranguren, G., and Benito, J. A. Verapamil to inhibit the cardiovascular side effects of ritodrine. *Int. J. Gynaecol. Obstet.* 19:333, 1981.

Spelger, G., et al. Cardiac parameters of the newborn after tocolysis. *Klin. Paediatr.* 192:319, 1980.

Ulmsten, U., Andersson, K. E., and Forman, A. Relaxing effects of nifedipine on the nonpregnant human uterus: In vitro and in vivo. *Obstet. Gynecol.* 52:436, 1978.

Ulmsten, U., Andersson, K. E., and Wingerup, L. Treatment of premature labor with the calcium antagonist nifedipine. *Arch. Gynecol.* 229:1, 1980.

Veille, J. C., et al. The effect of a calcium channel blocker (nifedipine) on uterine blood flow in the pregnant goat. Presented at the Society of Perinatal Obstetricians Annual Meeting. Las Vegas, Nev., 1985.

Wolff, F., et al. Prenatal diagnosis and therapy of fetal heart rate anomalies: With a contribution on the placental transfer of verapamil. *J. Perinat. Med.* 8:203, 1980.

Zaret, G. M. Possible treatment of pre-eclampsia with calcium channel blocking agents. *Med. Hypotheses* 12:303, 1982.

Camphor (over-the-counter)

Indications and Recommendations

Camphor is safe to use during pregnancy. This drug is applied topically and produces local anesthetic and antipruritic effects. It is taken orally as an ingredient in paregoric and is used to relieve or prevent flatulence.

Special Considerations in Pregnancy

There are no maternal effects unique to pregnancy. It is theoretically possible for fetal convulsions to occur if large dosages are taken systemically.

Adverse Effects

Camphor is a rubefacient when rubbed on the skin. If not vigorously applied, however, it may cause a feeling of coolness.

When taken systemically, camphor may stimulate the central nervous system. It does not selectively stimulate respiration and has very little effect on the circulation. If children ingest large amounts of solid camphor, convulsions can occur. In small oral dosages, this drug produces a sensation of warmth and comfort in the stomach. It may, however, cause nausea and vomiting in larger dosages.

Recommended Reading

Gilman, A. G., Goodman, L. S., and Gilman, A. *The Pharmacological Basis of Therapeutics* (6th ed.). New York: Macmillan, 1980. Pp. 955–956.

Nelson, M. M., and Forfar, J. O. Associations between drugs administered during pregnancy and congenital abnormalities of the fetus. *Br. Med. J.* 1:523, 1971.

Schenkel, B., and Vorherr, H. Non-prescription drugs during pregnancy: Potential teratogenic and toxic effects upon embryo and fetus. *J. Reprod. Med.* 12:27, 1974.

Weiss, J., and Catalano, P. Camphorated oil intoxication during pregnancy. *Pediatrics* 52:713, 1973.

Candicidin (Candeptin®)

Indications and Recommendations

Candicidin vaginal ointment and tablets are safe to use during pregnancy for the treatment of candidal vaginitis. These preparations should not be applied vaginally when membranes are ruptured.

Special Considerations in Pregnancy

No teratogenic effects have been reported with intravaginal candicidin. Microbiologic cure rates between 59 and 100% have been reported. Pregnant patients appear to require a longer duration of therapy or multiple treatment courses for a complete clinical and microbiologic cure.

Dosage

Candicidin is available as a vaginal ointment and in vaginal tablet form. The recommended dose is the contents of one applicator or one tablet inserted high into the vagina, twice daily, for 14 days.

Mechanism of Action

Candicidin is a polyene antibiotic that alters yeast membrane permeability, allowing leakage of essential metabolic substrates.

Absorption and Biotransformation

Candicidin is not absorbed to a significant degree through the vaginal mucosa.

Recommended Reading

Bodey, G. P., Adachi, L., and Jones, V. Effects of candicidin on fungal flora of gastrointestinal tract. *Curr. Ther. Res.* 16:207, 1974.

Gilman, A. G., Goodman, L. S., and Gilman, A. *The Pharmacological Basis of Therapeutics* (6th ed.). New York: Macmillan, 1980. P. 984.

Hammond, G. M., and Kliger, B. N. Mode of action of polyene antibiotic candicidin: Binding factors in wall of *Candida albicans*. *Antimicrob. Agents Chemother.* 9:561, 1976.

Melges, F. J. A new antifungal antibiotic? *Obstet. Gynecol.* 24:921, 1964.

Morese, K. N. Candicidin tablets and ointment in treatment of candidal vaginitis. *N.Y. State J. Med.* 75:1443, 1975.

Vartiainen, E., and Tervila, L. Use of Candeptin® for treatment of moniliasis. *Acta Obstet. Gynecol. Scand.* 49(Suppl):21, 1970.

Captopril (Capoten®)

Indications and Recommendations

Captopril is contraindicated during pregnancy. It is an orally active inhibitor of angiotensin-converting enzyme, which is the enzyme responsible for conversion of inactive angiotensin I to the potent pressor peptide angiotensin II. In nonpregnant patients, this drug is primarily used for the treatment of severe or resistant hypertension.

Captopril has been associated with a statistically significant increase in stillborn rates in several species of pregnant animals. In addition, there are several case reports of intrauterine growth retardation, oligohydramnios, patent ductus arteriosus, and neonatal hypotension associated with the use of captopril during human pregnancies. Only one report has suggested an association between the use of this drug and the delivery of a malformed infant.

Captopril crosses the placenta and inhibits angiotensin-converting enzyme activity in the human fetus. Small amounts of this drug are excreted in the breast milk of lactating mothers.

While some of these adverse neonatal effects may have been due to the hypertensive disorder being treated, a direct or indirect consequence of captopril therapy cannot be ruled out. Furthermore, the animal data are worrisome. Since better-studied antihypertensive agents are effective in controlling maternal blood pressure in the overwhelming majority of cases, captopril cannot be recommended for use during pregnancy.

Recommended Reading

Boughton-Pipkin, F., Symonds, E. M., and Turner, S. R. The effect of captopril (SQ14225) upon mother and fetus in the chronically cannulated ewe and in the pregnant rabbit. *J. Physiol.* 323:415, 1982.

Boughton-Pipkin, F., Turner, S. R., and Symonds, E. M. Possible risk with captopril in pregnancy: Some animal data (letter). *Lancet* 1:1256, 1980.

Boutroy, M. J., et al. Captopril administration in pregnancy impairs fetal angiotensin converting enzyme activity and neonatal adaptation. *Lancet* 2:935, 1984.

Devlin, R. G., and Fleiss, P. M. Selective resistance to the passage of captopril into human milk. *Clin. Pharmacol. Ther.* 27:250, 1980.

Duminy, P. C., and Burger, P. D. Fetal abnormality associated with the use of captopril during pregnancy (letter). *S. Afr. Med. J.* 60:805, 1981.

Ferris, T. F., and Weir, E. K. Effect of captopril on uterine blood flow and prostaglandin E synthesis in the pregnant rabbit. *J. Clin. Invest.* 71:809, 1983.

Fiocchi, R., et al. Captopril during pregnancy. *Lancet* 2:1153, 1984.

Millar, J. A., Wilson, P. D., and Morrison, N. Management of severe hypertension in pregnancy by a combined drug regimen including captopril. *N.Z. Med. J.* 96:796, 1983.

Vidt, D. G., Braud, E. L., and Fouad, F. M. Drug therapy: Captopril. *N. Engl. J. Med.* 306:214, 1982.

Carbamazepine (Tegretol®)

Indications and Recommendations

The use of carbamazepine during pregnancy should be limited to the treatment of trigeminal neuralgia and seizures refractory to therapy with more established agents. It may be used alone or in combination with other agents in the treatment of simple and complex partial seizures and generalized tonic-clonic seizures. The risk of taking carbamazepine in pregnancy is unknown. If this drug is administered, it is imperative that plasma levels be monitored and hematologic and hepatic parameters be closely followed.

The following recommendations were made in a bulletin published in 1979 by the American Academy of Pediatrics Committee on Drugs in collaboration with the American College of Obstetrics and Gynecology (ACOG) Committee on Obstetrics: Maternal and Fetal Medicine.

> No woman should receive anticonvulsant medication unnecessarily. When possible, a woman who has been seizure free for many years should be withdrawn from her medication prior to pregnancy. When a woman who has epilepsy and requires medication asks about pregnancy, she should be advised that she has a 90% chance of having a normal child, but that the risk of congenital malformations and mental retardation is two to three times greater than average because of her disease or its treatment.*

Special Considerations in Pregnancy

Teratogenesis has not been documented in humans, although this has not been extensively studied. In general, dosage adjustments are not necessary during pregnancy but serum levels should be monitored.

Carbamazepine crosses the placenta and is present in fetal serum at levels equal to those in maternal serum. It is also excreted in

Pediatrics 63:331, summary 333, February 1979. Copyright © 1979 by American Academy of Pediatrics.

breast milk, with milk-plasma ratios of 0.4–0.6. No clinically significant effects have been described in breast-fed infants.

Dosage

The initial dose is 100 mg PO bid; dosage may be increased to as high as 1,200 mg/day to achieve seizure control. The therapeutic plasma level has been proposed as 6–8 μg/ml.

Adverse Effects

The most common side effects include diplopia, ataxia, drowsiness, blurred vision, paresthesias, gastrointestinal disturbances, and headache. Often these occur at the beginning of therapy and are transient, but they may necessitate an adjustment of dosage. A number of cases of bone marrow suppression occasionally resulting in death have been reported, but this seems to be age related, as most of the patients were elderly. Nevertheless, hematologic parameters should be followed during therapy. A transient rise in hepatic enzymes may occur and at least one case of fatal hepatitis has been reported. Rarely, a variety of different dermatologic reactions may develop. Drug interactions with coumarin (increased metabolism) and phenytoin (decreased serum levels) have been described.

Mechanism of Action

Carbamazepine blocks posttetanic potentiation and appears to act selectively on areas of the brain frequently involved in epileptogenesis. Its therapeutic effect in trigeminal neuralgia is particularly related to the blockade of afferent synaptic transmission in the trigeminal nerve.

Absorption and Biotransformation

Carbamazepine has a variable oral absorption, is highly protein bound, and is metabolized in the liver. The initial plasma half-life is 25–65 hours, but this decreases to 10–20 hours with repeated doses. Its major active metabolite, the 10,11-epoxide, has a half-life of 5–8 hours.

Recommended Reading

Gilman, A. G., Goodman, L. S., and Gilman, A. *The Pharmacological Basis of Therapeutics* (6th ed.). New York: Macmillan, 1980. Pp. 459–460.

Med. Lett. Drugs Ther. 25:81, 1983.

Pynnonen, S., et al. Carbamazepine: Placental transport, tissue concentrations in foetus and newborn, and levels in milk. *Acta Pharmacol. Toxicol.* 41:244, 1977.

Wilder, B. J., and Bruni, J. *Seizure Disorder: A Pharmacological Approach to Treatment.* New York: Raven, 1981.

Woodbury, D. M., Penry, J. K., and Peppenger, C. E. *Antiepileptic Drugs.* New York: Raven, 1982.

Cathartics, Contact (over-the-counter)

ANTHRACENE CATHARTICS: ALOE, CASCARA, DANTHRON, SENNA

Indications and Recommendations

With the exception of aloe, anthracene cathartics are safe to use during pregnancy. Despite their safety, however, attention to proper diet and exercise is preferable to dependence on these agents. The anthracene cathartics include senna, cascara sagrada, and danthron. Aloe is contraindicated in pregnancy because it can cross the placenta and stimulate the fetal intestine, leading to the passage of meconium.

The presence of anthracene derivatives in breast milk and the incidence of diarrhea among nursing infants whose mothers ingest these substances are controversial. In his book on drugs in breast milk, Wilson notes that the standard recommendation is for nursing mothers to avoid these medications, but that documentation of risk is lacking.

Special Considerations in Pregnancy

Aloe should not be used in pregnancy because of the possible increased likelihood of meconium passage. Although data from the Collaborative Perinatal Project suggest an increase in the relative risk for birth defects among infants exposed to cascara derivatives in the first 16 weeks of pregnancy, this was not statistically significant and no confirmatory reports have appeared.

Dosage

Senna is taken in a 2-g dose with results in 6 hours. Fluid extract of cascara sagrada, 2.5 ml, will give results in 8 hours. Danthron causes stool softening 6–8 hours after a 25–150-mg dose.

Adverse Effects

Side effects include intestinal melanosis with prolonged use. This is reversible when the drug is discontinued.

Mechanism of Action

The anthracene cathartics act directly on the bowel wall to stimulate intestinal motility, which is primarily a large bowel effect. They are hydrolyzed by colonic bacteria with release of the active agent.

CASTOR OIL

Indications and Recommendations

Castor oil is safe to use during pregnancy. It is used as a cathartic agent, most commonly when patients are to have x rays of the kidney or colon, or both.

Special Considerations in Pregnancy

Although abdominal x rays are relatively contraindicated during pregnancy, the use of castor oil in preparation for x rays poses no special problems to the obstetric patient.

Dosage

The usual dose is 15–30 ml PO on demand.

Adverse Effects

The major problem with castor oil is its very unpleasant taste. There is also some evidence of potential cytotoxic effects on the small intestine.

Mechanism of Action

Castor oil is hydrolyzed in the small intestine to glycerol and ricinoleic acid, the latter of which stimulates motility of the small intestine.

DIPHENYLMETHANES: BISACODYL, PHENOLPHTHALEIN

Indications and Recommendations

Diphenylmethanes are safe to use during pregnancy. Despite their safety, however, attention to proper diet and exercise is preferable to dependence on these agents. The diphenylmethanes include phenolphthalein and bisacodyl and are widely used in over-the-counter (OTC) cathartic preparations.

Special Considerations in Pregnancy

There are no special considerations in pregnancy.

Dosage

Phenolphthalein is taken in a dose of 60–200 mg and acts in 6–8 hours. Bisacodyl is taken in a dose of 10–15 mg orally, acting in 6–8 hours, or as a 10-mg rectal suppository acting within 15–60 minutes.

Adverse Effects

Side effects include cramps, mucous stools, and excessive fluid loss in the stools. Allergic skin reactions have been reported with phenolphthalein. Proctitis has been reported with bisacodyl.

Mechanism of Action

Diphenylmethanes act mainly on the large intestine, stimulating peristalsis.

Absorption and Biotransformation

Although phenolphthalein is mainly excreted in the feces, up to 15% may be absorbed, conjugated, and excreted in the urine. Some is excreted in bowel. The urine or stools, or both, will be pink to red in color if the pH is alkaline.

Up to 5% of bisacodyl is absorbed and conjugated as a glucuronide appearing in the urine.

Recommended Reading

Gilman, A. G., Goodman, L. S., and Gilman, A. *The Pharmacological Basis of Therapeutics* (6th ed.). New York: Macmillan, 1980. Pp. 1005–1009.

Heinonen, O. P., Slone, D., and Shapiro, S. *Birth Defects and Drugs in Pregnancy.* Boston: John Wright PSG, 1977. Pp. 385, 442.

Nelson, M. M., and Forfar, J. O. Associations between drugs administered during pregnancy and congenital abnormalities of the fetus. *Br. Med. J.* 1:523, 1971.

Schenkel, B., and Vorherr, H. Non-prescription drugs during pregnancy: Potential teratogenic and toxic effects upon embryo and fetus. *J. Reprod. Med.* 12:27, 1974.

Wilson, J. T. *Drugs in Breast Milk.* Lancaster, Engl.: MTP, 1981. Pp. 67–68.

Cathartics, Saline (over-the-counter): Magnesium Salts, Including Milk of Magnesia and Epsom Salt; Sodium and Potassium Salts

Indications and Recommendations

Saline cathartics, which include magnesium, sodium, and potassium salts, are safe to use during pregnancy. Their use, however, should be avoided in patients with significant cardiovascular disease or impairment of renal function. They are used for cathartic cleaning of the bowel before surgery and radiologic or proctologic examination, in patients with functional constipation, and in those with constipation due to inadequate fluid intake or exercise.

Special Considerations in Pregnancy

There are no special considerations in pregnancy.

Dosage

Of the magnesium salts, magnesium sulfate (epsom salt) is given in doses of 15–30 g. It should be dissolved in fruit juice to overcome the objectionable taste. Magnesium citrate is available in a 10-ounce bottle of effervescent solution. The usual dose is 5–10 ounces. Some patients are nauseated by this preparation, and its action may be quite violent. Magnesium hydroxide is available in an 8% aqueous solution (milk of magnesia), and the usual dose is 8–30 ml. It also acts as an antacid.

The usual cathartic dose of the phosphate salts of sodium and potassium is from 4–20 g. The onset of action for these preparations is 3–6 hours or less.

Adverse Effects

There is little systemic effect except for the possibility of dehydration resulting from fluid loss in the feces; this occurs because they are so slowly absorbed that they retain water in the gastrointestinal tract and may even draw fluid into it. Congestive heart failure because of the salt load could occur in patients predisposed to this condition. Magnesium intoxication may occur in patients with impaired renal function.

Recommended Reading

Gilman, A. G., Goodman, L. S., and Gilman, A. *The Pharmacological Basis of Therapeutics* (6th ed.). New York: Macmillan, 1980. P. 1005.

Nelson, M. M., and Forfar, J. O. Associations between drugs administered during pregnancy and congenital abnormalities of the fetus. *Br. Med. J.* 1:523, 1971.

Schenkel, B., and Vorherr, H. Non-prescription drugs during pregnancy: Potential teratogenic and toxic effects upon embryo and fetus. *J. Reprod. Med.* 12:27, 1974.

Cephalosporins: Cefaclor (Ceclor®), Cefadroxil (Duricef®, Ultracef®), Cefamandole (Mandol®), Cefazolin (Ancef®, Kefzol®), Cefonicid (Monocid®), Cefoperazone (Cefobid®), Ceforanide (Precef®), Cefotaxime (Claforan®), Cefoxitin (Mefoxin®), Ceftizoxime (Cefizox®), Ceftriaxone (Rocephin®), Cefuroxime (Zinacef®), Cephalexin (Keflex®), Cephalothin (Keflin®), Cephapirin (Cefadyl®), Cephradine (Anspor®, Velosef®), Moxalactam (Moxam®)

Indications and Recommendations

The first- and second-generation cephalosporins are safe to use during pregnancy. These drugs are broad-spectrum antibiotics that have been extensively used during pregnancy because of their low potential for toxicity and clinical effectiveness. They are effective against infections caused by streptococci, *Staphylococcus aureus, Proteus, Salmonella,* and *Shigella* species. The following bacteria are relatively resistant to the first-generation agents: enterococci, *Bacteroides fragilis, Enterobacter aerogenes, Serratia marcescens,* and *Pseudomonas aeruginosa.* The second-generation agents provide enhanced activity against Enterobacteriaceae, while cefoxitin is also effective against *Bacteroides* species.

The third-generation cephalosporins have broader spectra and different pharmacokinetic properties than the first- and second-generation agents. Until more experience is accumulated in pregnant women, these agents should be reserved for use when no other safer antibiotic is available.

Special Considerations in Pregnancy

Pharmacokinetic studies of several cephalosporins have demonstrated that, as with penicillins, mean serum levels are lower in pregnant than in nonpregnant patients receiving equivalent dosages. The half-lives tend to be shorter and the volumes of distribution and clearances larger.

The cephalosporins cross the placenta and are found in fetal serum and urine as well as in amniotic fluid. No teratogenic effects have been associated with the use of cephalosporins; the third-generation agents, however, have yet to be extensively used during pregnancy.

Dosage

Drug	Route	Usual daily dose*	Interval
First-generation agents			
Cefadroxil	PO	1–2 g	q12–24h
Cephalexin	PO	1–4 g	q6h
Cephradine	PO	1–2 g	q12h
	IM/IV	2–4 g	q6h
Cephapirin	IM/IV	2–6 g	q4–6h
Cephalothin	IM/IV	2–6 g	q4–6h
Cefazolin	IM/IV	0.75–6.00 g	q6–8h
Second-generation agents			
Cefaclor	PO	0.75–4.00 g	q8h
Cefamandole	IM/IV	1.5–6.0 g	q4–8h
Cefoxitin	IM/IV	3–8 g	q6–8h
Cefuroxime	IM/IV	2.4–4.5 g	q8h
Cefonicid	IM/IV	1–2 g	q24h
Ceforanide	IM/IV	1–2 g	q12h
Third-generation agents			
Cefotaxime	IM/IV	3–4 g	q6–8h
Ceftizoxime	IM/IV	2–6 g	q8–12h
Ceftriaxone	IM/IV	1–2 g	qd
Cefoperazone	IM/IV	2–4 g	q12h
Moxalactam	IM/IV	2–6 g	q8h

Adverse Effects

Side effects include thrombophlebitis with intravenous use and a serum sickness–like reaction with prolonged parenteral administration. Allergic reactions and gastrointestinal disturbances may occur. The incidence of hypersensitivity reactions to the cephalo-

*Dosages must be adjusted in the face of renal impairment.

sporins is higher in patients who have shown an allergic reaction to penicillin. This is apparently related to sensitization to the beta-lactam ring common to both drugs. Controversy exists as to the incidence of cross sensitivity to this drug. With the exception of patients who have had anaphylactic reactions to penicillin, however, cephalosporins are not contraindicated in patients with penicillin allergy.

Rarely, hemolytic anemia, hepatic dysfunction, blood dyscrasias, and renal damage (especially with cephaloridine) may occur. Toxic renal damage may be potentiated by the concurrent use of aminoglycosides, probenecid, or potent diuretics such as furosemide or ethacrynic acid.

Mechanism of Action

These drugs inhibit bacterial cell wall synthesis and are consequently bactericidal. The cephalosporins, like penicillin, contain a beta-lactam ring. They also have a dihydrothiazine ring with attached side chains that give the various compounds their individual properties.

Absorption and Biotransformation

Drug	Oral absorption	Protein bound (%)	Unchanged in urine (%)	Half-life (h)
First-generation agents				
Cefadroxil	+	20	90	1–2
Cephalexin	+	10–15	85–95	0.5–1.0
Cephradine	+	10–15	80–95	0.7–1.0
Cephapirin	−	50	60	0.3–0.7
Cephalothin	−	60–80	60–70	0.50–0.85
Cefazolin	−	80	85–95	1.5–2.0
Second-generation agents				
Cefaclor	+	25	60–85	0.5–1.0
Cefamandole	−	67–74	65–85	0.7–1.2
Cefoxitin	−	65–80	85–90	0.7–1.0
Cefuroxime	−	33	85–95	1.0–1.5
Cefonicid	−	98	98	3.5–4.5
Third-generation agents				
Cefotaxime	−	30	20–36	0.8–1.2
Ceftizoxime	−	28	85–95	1.7–1.8
Ceftriaxone	−	83–96	60–65	6.5–8.6
Cefoperazone	−	85–95	15–30	1.6–2.1
Moxalactam	−	50	60–80	2–3

Recommended Reading

Bernard, B., et al. Maternal-fetal transfer of cefazolin in the first twenty weeks of pregnancy. *J. Infect. Dis.* 136:377, 1977.

Giamarellou, H., et al. A study of cefoxitin, moxalactam, and ceftazidime kinetics in pregnancy. *Am. J. Obstet. Gynecol.* 147:914, 1983.

Landers, D. V., Green, J. R., and Sweet, R. L. Antibiotic use during pregnancy and the postpartum period. *Clin. Obstet. Gynecol.* 26:391, 1983.

Thompson, R. L., and Wright, A. J. Cephalosporin antibiotics. *Mayo Clin. Proc.* 58:79, 1983.

Chloral Hydrate (Noctec®)

Indications and Recommendations

The use of chloral hydrate during pregnancy is relatively contraindicated because other therapeutic agents are preferable. It has sedative and hypnotic actions similar to those of paraldehyde, alcohol, and the barbiturates, and it is used primarily as a hypnotic in the treatment of simple insomnia. Chloral hydrate and its active metabolite, trichloroethanol, are known to cross the placental barrier rapidly after maternal administration. The effects of its use during pregnancy have not been adequately studied. A British study of the pharmacokinetics of a single antepartum dose of chloral hydrate in 52 pregnant women and their offspring has been published. The authors report that no deleterious effects were noted in either mothers or neonates.

No sedative has been found to be absolutely safe during pregnancy, as most cross the placenta and produce sedation and withdrawal symptoms in the newborn. Should such therapy be required during pregnancy, phenobarbital may be used in the lowest dosage and frequency possible.

Chloral hydrate appears in breast milk, with a milk-plasma ratio of less than 0.5. No adverse effects of chloral hydrate have been reported in nursing mothers.

Recommended Reading

Berstine, J. B., Meyer, A. E., and Berstine, R. L. Maternal blood and breast milk estimation following the administration of chloral hydrate during the puerperium. *J. Obstet. Gynaecol. Br. Emp.* 63:228, 1956.

Berstine, J. B., Meyer, A. E., and Hayman, H. B. Maternal and foetal blood estimation following the administration of chloral hydrate during labor. *J. Obstet. Gynaecol. Br. Emp.* 61:683, 1954.

Gilman, A. G., Goodman, L. S., and Gilman, A. *The Pharmacological Basis of Therapeutics* (6th ed.). New York: Macmillan, 1980. Pp. 361–363.

Wilson, J. T. *Drugs in Breast Milk*. Lancaster, Engl.: MTP, 1981. P. 79.

Chloramphenicol (Chloromycetin®)

Indications and Recommendations

Chloramphenicol should be avoided in late pregnancy and during labor because of the potential for the "gray syndrome" in the newborn infant. It should be used during pregnancy only for serious infections with organisms known to be sensitive to the drug. Because of the potential for life-threatening toxicity and hypersensitivity reactions, chloramphenicol should be used only when other antibiotics cannot be substituted. It may be necessary to use chloramphenicol to treat serious anaerobic infections, *Salmonella* infections, and rickettsial diseases. It is also often used against *Haemophilus influenzae* meningitis and brain abscesses.

Special Considerations in Pregnancy

The gray syndrome may be seen in chloramphenicol-treated newborns, especially those born prematurely. The syndrome usually begins 2–9 days after therapy is begun. It consists of vomiting, refusal to suck, rapid irregular respiration, and abdominal distention, followed in 24–48 hours by flaccidity, an ashen-gray color, and hypothermia. About 40% of these neonates die from circulatory collapse, usually on about the fifth day. It has been determined that newborns are unable to conjugate and excrete chloramphenicol, and the gray syndrome is related to toxic blood levels of the drug. Although toxic effects have not been observed in newborns whose mothers received as much as 1 g of chloramphenicol every 2 hours during labor, it is probably best to avoid this drug just prior to delivery. Chloramphenicol does cross the placenta.

Because chloramphenicol appears in breast milk, it is best for nursing mothers not to use this drug.

Dosage

Chloramphenicol may be given orally, intramuscularly, or intravenously. The usual oral dose is 500 mg q4h. The drug comes in capsules of 125 and 250 mg.

Intravenous dosage is the same as oral dosage, except for typhoid when a 2 g loading dose is recommended.

Patients with renal disease should receive the usual dosage of chloramphenicol, although anemia is more likely to occur. Patients with hepatic disease should receive reduced dosages and have serum levels monitored.

Adverse Effects

HYPERSENSITIVITY REACTIONS

Chloramphenicol is the most common drug cause of pancytopenia. This effect is not dosage-related, but is usually associated with prolonged oral therapy, especially with multiple exposures. The incidence is 1 in 40,000 courses of therapy. The longer the interval between the last dosage of drug and the appearance of the first sign of blood dyscrasia, the greater the likelihood of fatality. When total aplasia of the bone marrow occurs, the fatality rate is almost 100%. Other hypersensitivity reactions include a macular or vesicular skin rash, hemorrhage from skin and mucous membranes, fever, and atrophic glossitis.

TOXIC EFFECTS

Anemia occurs in patients having plasma concentrations of chloramphenicol above 25 μg/ml. It is seen most often with parenteral therapy, is dose-related, and usually disappears completely about 12 days after discontinuance of therapy. The drug inhibits the uptake and incorporation of iron into heme, resulting in anemia, reticulocytopenia, and elevated plasma iron levels.

Chloramphenicol can also cause nausea, vomiting, diarrhea, and perineal irritation. The drug has a bitter taste when taken orally. This bitterness is also noted with rapid intravenous administration. Optic neuritis has been reported with chloramphenicol. Large oral dosages may prolong the prothrombin time, presumably by altering the bacterial flora of the gastrointestinal tract.

Because of these relatively serious toxic and hypersensitivity effects, chloramphenicol should not be used for mild or self-limited infections, and should be considered contraindicated in pregnancy except in serious situations where other alternatives are not available.

Mechanism of Action

Chloramphenicol inhibits protein synthesis in bacteria and rickettsiae, primarily by preventing peptide-bond synthesis in ribosomes.

Absorption and Biotransformation

Chloramphenicol is rapidly absorbed after oral ingestion, with significant plasma concentrations present at 30 minutes and peak levels attained in 2 hours. The half-life is 1.5–3.0 hours. Intramuscular administration gives lower plasma levels than intravenous or oral dosing, and it is probably most efficient to avoid this route or monitor serum levels if it is used.

The drug is inactivated in the liver by conjugation in a step mediated by glucuronyl transferase. The inactive metabolite is rapidly excreted in the urine. Over 80% of an oral dosage can be recovered from the urine.

Recommended Reading

Gilman, A. G., Goodman, L. S., and Gilman, A. *The Pharmacological Basis of Therapeutics* (6th ed.). New York: Macmillan, 1980. Pp. 1191–1196.

Kucers, A., and Bennett, N. McK. *The Use of Antibiotics* (2nd ed.). London: William Heinemann, 1975. Pp. 244–270.

Chloroquine (Aralen®)

Indications and Recommendations

The use of chloroquine during pregnancy should be limited to suppressive therapy in women entering areas with endemic malaria and to treatment of acute attacks of malaria. This drug should not be used for the treatment of inflammatory disease states in pregnancy.

Special Considerations in Pregnancy

Because malaria poses a distinct threat to the pregnant woman and her unborn child, prophylaxis is desirable. No studies have demonstrated untoward fetal effects when chloroquine is given in antimalarial dosages. Larger, antiinflammatory dosages taken during pregnancy, however, have resulted in spontaneous abortion and fetal vestibular and retinal damage.

Dosage

When necessary for suppressive therapy of malaria, chloroquine phosphate, 500 mg (300-mg base), should be given weekly beginning 1 week before arrival, throughout the stay, and for 3 weeks after leaving the malarious area.

An initial loading dose of 1 g is administered for the treatment of an acute attack of vivax or falciparum malaria. This dose is followed by an additional 500 mg after 6–8 hours and 500 mg again on the next 2 consecutive days. A total dose of 2.5 g is given over the 3-day treatment period.

Antiinflammatory doses range from 250–750 mg daily for prolonged periods.

Adverse Effects

When used in antimalarial dosages, side effects of chloroquine are mild and include transient headache, visual disturbances, gastrointestinal upset, and pruritus. Long-term therapy with antiinflammatory dosages may be associated with development of retinopathy, and irreversible vision loss may be sustained. Other side effects include dose-dependent myelosuppression, skin rashes, neuromyopathy, tinnitus and deafness, and electrocardiographic changes.

Mechanism of Action

The exact mechanism of chloroquine's activity is uncertain. Its antimalarial activity is thought to result from its interaction with DNA and its effect on malarial pigment in the host erythrocyte. Chloroquine exerts no significant activity against exoerythrocytic stages of plasmodia.

Chloroquine rapidly controls the parasitemia and clinical symptoms of acute malarial attacks. Fever is controlled within 24–48 hours after administration of therapeutic dosages. With the exception of certain strains, chloroquine completely cures falciparum malaria. Relapses of vivax malaria, however, are not prevented, although the intervals between relapses are substantially increased.

Absorption and Biotransformation

Chloroquine is rapidly and almost completely absorbed from the gastrointestinal tract. Much of the drug is bound to plasma proteins and to tissues; approximately 30% is metabolized. Chloroquine is cleared by the kidneys at a very slow rate, which may be increased by acidification of the urine. With single or weekly doses, the plasma half-life is approximately 3 days.

Recommended Reading

Gilman, A. G., Goodman, L. S., and Gilman, A. *The Pharmacological Basis of Therapeutics* (6th ed.). New York: Macmillan, 1980. Pp. 1042–1045.

Heinonen, O. P., Slone, D., and Shapiro, S. *Birth Defects and Drugs in Pregnancy.* Littleton, Mass.: Publishing Sciences Group, 1977. P. 229.

Main, E. K., Main, D. M., and Krogstad, D. J. Treatment of chloroquine-resistant malaria during pregnancy. *J.A.M.A.* 249:3207, 1983.

Malaria prophylaxis. *Br. Med. J.* 286:787, 1983.

Chlorpheniramine (Chlor-Trimeton®)

Indications and Recommendations

The use of chlorpheniramine during pregnancy should be limited to the provision of symptomatic relief of allergic symptoms caused by histamine release. These include urticaria, rhinitis, and pruritus. Because chlorpheniramine is an antihistamine that merely provides palliative therapy, the avoidance of allergens should be the primary treatment for these symptoms whenever possible. Chlorpheniramine does not appear to have teratogenic effects at recommended dosages; however, no prospective studies are available. This drug is not recommended for use by lactating women.

Special Considerations in Pregnancy

No prospective studies that evaluate the safety of chlorpheniramine use during pregnancy have been conducted. One large retrospective study, however, found no evidence incriminating this drug as a teratogenic agent.

Due to its anticholinergic properties, chlorpheniramine may inhibit lactation. In addition, small amounts may be secreted into breast milk. This drug and all antihistamines, therefore, should be avoided by the lactating mother.

Dosage

The usual oral dose of chlorpheniramine is 2–4 mg 3–4 times a day. It is available in an extended-release formulation, 8–12 mg, that may be given 2–3 times a day.

Adverse Effects

Anticholinergic side effects are most common. These include dry mouth and eyes and, rarely, blurred vision. Drowsiness, anorexia, nausea, epigastric distress, and dizziness may also be seen.

Mechanism of Action

Chlorpheniramine is a competitive antagonist of histamine that decreases edema formation by diminishing capillary dilatation and permeability. It has anticholinergic activity, produces drowsiness, and possesses local anesthetic activity when applied topically.

Absorption and Biotransformation

The drug is primarily metabolized in the liver, probably by hydroxylation followed by glucuronidation. Excretion is via the kidney.

Recommended Reading

Gilman, A. G., Goodman, L. S., and Gilman, A. *The Pharmacological Basis of Therapeutics* (6th ed.). New York: Macmillan, 1980. P. 627.

Greenberger, P., and Patterson, R. Safety of therapy for allergic symptoms during pregnancy. *Ann. Intern. Med.* 89:234, 1978.

Heinonen, O. P., Slone, D., and Shapiro, S. *Birth Defects and Drugs in Pregnancy*. Littleton, Mass.: Publishing Sciences Group, 1977. Pp. 322–334.

Nishimura, H., and Tanimura, T. *Aspects of the Teratogenicity of Drugs*. Amsterdam: Excerpta Medica, 1976.

Cholestyramine (Cuemid®, Questran®)

Indications and Recommendations

Cholestyramine is safe to use for symptomatic relief of pruritus secondary to cholestasis of pregnancy. The patient's prothrombin time should be monitored and fat-soluble vitamins supplemented when this drug is administered.

Special Considerations in Pregnancy

Since cholestyramine is not absorbed, any problems associated with its administration would be related to fat-soluble vitamin deficiency or interactions with other drugs.

Cholestyramine is often prescribed for symptomatic relief of the pruritus associated with cholestasis of pregnancy. At least one study has failed to demonstrate any sustained fall in serum bile acids or improvement in symptoms with cholestyramine treatment. Studies in rats have shown that the fall in cholesterol and bile acid synthesis observed in cholestyramine-treated nonpregnant animals did not occur when pregnant animals were given this resin.

Dosage

Cholestyramine is given as 10–12 g in an oral suspension in three divided (3–4 g) doses before meals. Steatorrhea and malabsorption of fat-soluble vitamins do not occur with doses below 20–30 g/day. Pruritus often recurs 1–2 days after withdrawal of the drug.

Adverse Effects

Because cholestyramine is not absorbed from the gastrointestinal tract, most side effects are digestive. These include constipation, abdominal discomfort and distention, flatulence, nausea, vomiting, diarrhea, heartburn, anorexia, and steatorrhea. Deficiencies of fat-soluble vitamins (vitamins K, A) can occur. Cholestyramine also is described by most patients as having an unpleasant taste.

Mechanism of Action

Cholestyramine is a resin that combines with bile acids in the intestine to form an insoluble complex that is excreted in the feces. As a result, bile acids are partially removed from the enterohepatic circulation, which may reduce the systemic circulating bile acid concentration, thereby reducing skin levels of bile acids and decreasing pruritus.

Recommended Reading

Burrow, G. N., and Ferris, T. F. (eds.). *Medical Complications During Pregnancy* (2nd ed.). Philadelphia: Saunders, 1982. P. 284.

Gilman, A. G., Goodman, L. S., and Gilman, A. *The Pharmacological Basis of Therapeutics* (6th ed.). New York: Macmillan, 1980. Pp. 842–843.

Innis, S. M. Altered effect of 3% dietary cholestyramine on plasma lipids and biliary bile acid output in the pregnant rat. *Am. J. Obstet. Gynecol.* 150:742, 1984.

Shaw, D., et al. A prospective study of 18 patients with cholestasis of pregnancy. *Am. J. Obstet. Gynecol.* 142:621, 1982.

Cimetidine (Tagamet®)

Indications and Recommendations

Cimetidine, a histamine (H_2) receptor antagonist, is safe to use during pregnancy. Cimetidine inhibits gastric acid secretion. It is clinically used to treat duodenal ulcer disease, as well as gastric hypersecretory states. This drug is commonly used for preanesthetic prophylaxis against gastric acid aspiration pneumonitis, and widespread experience in this setting has revealed no adverse consequences for mother or neonate. Data concerning its use in early human pregnancy are currently nonexistent, but animal studies have failed to reveal any evidence of teratogenicity.

Special Considerations in Pregnancy

When cimetidine was administered during organogenesis to rats, rabbits, and mice, in dosages far exceeding the usual recommendations for humans, no adverse fetal effects were found. Human teratology data are lacking.

Cimetidine has been shown to cross the placenta in animal models. In humans given this drug just before delivery, cord cimetidine levels averaged 50% of those in the mother. There is a single case report of transient impaired hepatic excretory function in a neonate whose mother took 1,200 mg daily for treatment of an ulcer during the month prior to delivery. Another woman, who took 1,000 mg daily from the sixteenth to the twentieth week of gestation, gave birth to an apparently normal 2,500-g child, although no neonatal liver function test results are described in the case report.

There is one report that three preeclamptic patients with thrombocytopenia, elevated liver enzymes, and epigastric pain responded to cimetidine, 300 mg IV every 6 hours, with marked improvement in blood pressure, no longer requiring hydralazine therapy. The authors speculate that the drug may have blocked the action of a histamine-like pressor agent derived from the ischemic placenta.

Cimetidine appears in the breast milk in greater concentration than in maternal serum, and some authorities have recommended against its use in lactating mothers. However, adverse effects in nursing human infants have not been reported.

Dosage

Cimetidine is available for oral use as 200-, 300-, and 400-mg tablets, and as an aqueous solution containing 300 mg/5 ml. It may also be given intravenously and intramuscularly and is available in vials containing 150 mg/ml. The usual oral dose is 300 mg with or immediately after each meal and at bedtime (i.e., 1,200 mg/day) for 4–6 weeks. It has also been given in lower doses (200 mg with each meal and 400 mg at bedtime) with apparently good results. Rectal administration has also been used. Hospitalized patients unable to take the medication orally may be given 300 mg IM every 6 hours, or 300 mg (diluted in 100 ml IV solution) infused intravenously over 15–20 minutes every 6 hours. Overdosages up to 10 g have not been associated with any untoward effects.

The use of cimetidine as preanesthetic prophylaxis against gastric acid aspiration (Mendelson's syndrome) at cesarean section has been controversial. Various oral, intramuscular, and intravenous dosing regimens have been used and compared with either no prophylaxis or with other antacids. Because Mendelson's syndrome is relatively rare, the standard used for evaluating effectiveness has been gastric fluid volume and pH, with a pH above 2.5 considered a treatment success.

Most reports suggest that 50–60% of unmedicated patients undergoing cesarean section have a gastric pH below 2.5. In studies of cimetidine prophylaxis, timing seems to be a critical factor. A scheduled elective cesarean section, performed before labor, allows the dose-delivery interval to be planned. Here, prophylactic cimetidine appears to have been highly successful, as long as induction of anesthesia occurred within 90–150 minutes after cimetidine administration. However, the success of cimetidine prophylaxis given to laboring women who then underwent emergency cesarean section has been less uniform. The major problems encountered seem to be the unpredictable timing of cesarean section, along with changes in gastrointestinal absorption engendered by labor. Usually, one does not have the luxury of waiting 90 minutes between the administration of cimetidine and the induction of anesthesia when emergency cesarean section is necessary. Thus, most prophylaxis regimens have involved a primary 400-mg dose, followed by repeated dosing with 200 mg cimetidine every 2 hours in all patients during labor. Failures have usually been ascribed to lapses in adherence to this regimen. However, poor gastrointestinal motility with decreased drug absorption during labor may also have been a contributing factor. Intramuscular injection of cimetidine may circumvent the absorption issue, but 2-hourly injections are unlikely to be popular among laboring women. Another alternative is to use cimetidine prior to scheduled or semielective cesarean sections, where a 90-minute interval between dosing and induction of anesthesia is practical, but to use liquid oral antacids, such as sodium citrate or magnesium trisilicate, when immediate intervention is necessary.

Adverse Effects

Side effects are uncommon and usually minor. Headache, dizziness, fatigue, muscle pains, constipation, diarrhea, and skin rashes have been reported. Increases in serum creatinine and in liver enzymes have occurred. In elderly patients and those with impaired renal function, neurologic effects including confusion, slurred speech, delirium, hallucinations, and coma have occurred. Fever has occasionally been reported. Gynecomastia in men and galactorrhea in women have been reported when high dosages were given for long periods of time.

Mechanism of Action

Cimetidine acts as a reversible competitive antagonist at H_2 (histamine) receptors. There appears to be no action against H_1 receptors. The major H_2 receptor effect that is inhibited by cimetidine is gastric acid secretion, which is diminished in a dose-dependent manner. Gastrin and pentagastrin-invoked acid secretion are also effectively blocked, while the acid-secretion stimulating effects of acetylcholine and muscarinic drugs are only partially blocked. All phases of gastric secretion (basal, food-induced, gastric distention–induced, and hormonally induced) are inhibited. The volume and hydrogen ion concentration of gastric juice are both diminished.

Absorption and Biotransformation

About 60% of orally administered cimetidine is absorbed. Blood levels are maximal at 1.0–1.5 hours, and a single oral dose produces effective concentrations for about 4 hours. The presence of food delays the absorption, so that giving the drug with or shortly after meals yields a more prolonged action. Most of an oral dose is excreted unchanged in the urine within 24 hours.

Recommended Reading

Gilman, A. G., Goodman, L. S., and Gilman, A. *The Pharmacological Basis of Therapeutics* (6th ed.). New York: Macmillan, 1980. Pp. 629–632.

Glade, G., Saccar, C. L., and Pereira, G. R. Cimetidine in pregnancy: Apparent transient liver impairment in the newborn. *Am. J. Dis. Child.* 134:87, 1980.

Goodlin, R., Woods, R., and Williams, N. Cimetidine and the epigastric pain of preeclampsia. *Am. J. Obstet. Gynecol.* 145:645, 1983.

Hodgkinson, P., et al. Comparison of cimetidine with antacid for safety and effectiveness in reducing gastric acidity before elective cesarean section. *Anesthesiology* 59:86, 1983.

Husemeyer, R. P., and Davenport, H. T. Prophylaxis for Mendelson's syndrome before elective cesarean section. A comparison of cimetidine and magnesium trisilicate mixture regimens. *Br. J. Obstet. Gynaecol.* 87:565, 1980.

Johnston, J. R., et al. Use of cimetidine as an oral antacid in obstetric anesthesia. *Anesth. Analg.* 62:720, 1983.

McCaughey, W., et al. Cimetidine in elective caesarean section. Effect on gastric acidity. *Anaesthesia* 36:167, 1981.

McGowan, W. A. W. Safety of cimetidine in obstetric patients. *J. R. Soc. Med.* 72:902, 1979.

Qvist, N., and Storm, K. Cimetidine pre-anesthetic. *Acta Obstet. Gynecol. Scand.* 62:157, 1983.

Somogyi, A., and Gugler, R. Cimetidine excretion into breast milk. *Br. J. Clin. Pharmacol.* 7:627, 1979.

Zulli, P., and DiNisio, Q. Cimetidine treatment during pregnancy. *Lancet* 2:945, 1978.

Clindamycin (Cleocin®)

Indications and Recommendations

The use of clindamycin during pregnancy should be limited to the treatment of infections suspected to be caused by strains of *Bacteroides fragilis* that are not sensitive to safer antibiotic therapies (e.g., penicillin G) or that occur late in pregnancy, thereby precluding the use of chloramphenicol.

Clindamycin has an antibacterial spectrum similar to that of lincomycin and erythromycin, although it is slightly more effective against anaerobic bacteria, especially *B. fragilis*. If diarrhea develops during the administration of this drug, proctoscopy should be performed. Therapy may be continued if proctoscopic findings are normal but should be stopped if pseudomembranous plaques are observed.

Special Considerations in Pregnancy

There are no unusual maternal effects during pregnancy. The drug rapidly crosses the placenta and is 90% bound to serum protein. Cord concentrations of the drug are approximately 50% of those found in the maternal circulation. There are no reports of adverse fetal reactions to clindamycin administration.

Clindamycin is excreted in small amounts in breast milk. It is not known if these doses may induce pseudomembranous colitis in the infant. Prescribing the drug to nursing mothers is, therefore, best avoided when possible.

Dosage

The oral dose of clindamycin is 150–450 mg every 6 hours. The intramuscular or intravenous dose is 300–600 mg every 6 hours. A topical preparation used in the treatment of acne is applied twice daily.

Adverse Effects

Frequent side effects include diarrhea and allergic reactions. Pseudomembranous colitis, sometimes fatal, has been reported in 2–10% of patients receiving clindamycin. This condition can occur both during treatment and up to 3–4 weeks after completion of therapy. It occurs with both oral and parenteral therapy.

Mechanism of Action

Clindamycin inhibits bacterial protein synthesis by binding to the 50S ribosomal subunit.

Absorption and Biotransformation

Clindamycin is nearly completely absorbed after oral administration. Approximately 4–5% of a topical dose is systemically absorbed, but this amount may be increased in certain individuals. The drug is widely distributed throughout the body, but does not gain access to the cerebrospinal fluid. Most of the drug is metabolized in the liver to products excreted in the urine and bile. Only 10% of the drug is excreted unchanged in the urine. Little adjustment of dosage is required for patients with renal failure, but the dosage may need adjustment in patients with hepatic decompensation.

Recommended Reading

Dhawan, V. K., and Haragopal, T. Clindamycin: A review of fifty years of experience. *Rev. Infect. Dis.* 4:1133, 1982.

Gilman, A. G., Goodman, L. S., and Gilman A. *The Pharmacological Basis of Therapeutics* (6th ed.). New York: Macmillan, 1980. Pp. 1226–1227.

Steen, B., and Rane, A. Clindamycin passage into human milk. *Br. J. Clin. Pharmacol.* 13:661, 1982.

Weinstein, A. J., Gibbs, R. S., and Gallagher, M. Placental transfer of clindamycin and gentamicin in term pregnancy. *Am. J. Obstet. Gynecol.* 124:688, 1976.

Clofibrate (Atromid-S®)

Indications and Recommendations

Clofibrate is not recommended for use during pregnancy. This drug is an antilipemic agent of unproved efficacy that is used in the treatment of some forms of hyperlipidemia that do not respond to diet alone.

The use of this drug in nonpregnant patients is controversial because many serious side effects were reported in two large clinical trials, and no substantial evidence of beneficial effects on cardiovascular mortality were evident. One of these placebo-controlled studies showed a significantly higher mortality due to noncardiovascular causes in the clofibrate-treated group. Half of this difference was due to malignancy. Other causes of death included postcholecystectomy complications and pancreatitis. Clofibrate users have been shown to have twice the risk of developing cholelithiasis and cholecystitis requiring surgery as nonusers. In addition, administration in high dosages to rodents has resulted in a higher incidence of benign and malignant liver tumors than in controls.

There are no data regarding the effects of clofibrate on the human fetus. It has been demonstrated, however, that the drug crosses the rat placenta and causes decreased fetal weight. In this species, clofibrate has also been found to appear in breast milk. In rabbits, fetal serum concentrations of the drug have been shown to be higher than those in the maternal serum.

Recommended Reading

Chhabra, S., and Kurup, C. K. R. Maternal transport of chlorophenoxyisobutyrate at the foetal and neonatal stages of development. *Biochem. Pharmacol.* 27:2063, 1978.

Gilman, A. G., Goodman, L. S., and Gilman, A. *The Pharmacological Basis of Therapeutics* (6th ed.). New York: Macmillan, 1980. Pp. 840–842.

Sanfeliu, C., Zapatero, J., and Bruseghini, L. Toxicological studies of plafibride. *Arzneimittelforsch.* 31:1831, 1981.

Clomiphene Citrate (Clomid®)

Indications and Recommendations

Clomiphene is contraindicated during pregnancy. There is no indication for its use during pregnancy since it is utilized to induce ovulation. Some women, however, not knowing that they are pregnant, may inadvertently continue to take clomiphene citrate during the first trimester.

Clomiphene works on the central nervous system at the hypothalamic level to block estrogen uptake. This results in increased follicle-stimulating hormone (FSH) production by the pituitary with a consequent increase in follicular estradiol production. The elevated estradiol level stimulates a luteinizing hormone (LH) surge during midcycle, which in turn causes ovulation to occur. Clomiphene is taken approximately 7–12 days before ovulation, and studies have shown most of it to be cleared at the time of conception.

Maternal side effects when this drug is taken during the first trimester include scotomas, nausea, and abdominal pain. Effects on the fetus are unknown. Exposure of pregnant rats to a single dose of clomiphene was associated with abnormalities in the reproductive tract reminiscent of diethylstilbestrol (DES) exposure. There have been case reports in humans of neural tube defects, cleft lip and palate, Down's syndrome, congenital heart defects, and other anomalies. However, when large series were reviewed, there did not appear to be a significant difference from the general population with regard to malformation rates. In one large retrospective series from Sweden, the incidence of malformations when ovulation was induced with clomiphene was similar to that observed in a series of pregnancies induced with gonadotropin therapy and, at 5.4%, was slightly higher than the 3.2% observed in the general population. It may be that this represents an expression of the subfertility that made ovulation induction necessary.

Clomiphene should not be administered during pregnancy. If it is inadvertently taken for a short course, however, the patient can be reassured that this drug will probably have no adverse effect on the fetus.

Recommended Reading

Ahlgren, M., Kallen, B., and Rannevik, G. Outcome of pregnancy after clomiphene therapy. *Acta Obstet. Gynecol. Scand.* 55:371, 1976.

Asch, R. H., and Greenblatt, R. B. Update on the safety and efficacy of clomiphene citrate as a therapeutic agent. *J. Reprod. Med.* 17:175, 1976.

Goldfarb, A. F., et al. Critical review of 160 clomiphene-related pregnancies. *Obstet. Gynecol.* 31:342, 1968.

Huppert, L. C., and Wallach, E. C. Induction of ovulation with clomiphene citrate. *J. Reprod. Med.* 18:201, 1977.

McCormack, S., and Clark, J. H. Clomid administration to pregnant rats causes abnormalities of the reproductive tract in offspring and mothers. *Science* 204:629, 1979.

Clonidine (Catapres®)

Indications and Recommendations

Clonidine is relatively contraindicated during pregnancy because other therapeutic agents are preferable. It is an imidazoline derivative that can be used as an antihypertensive agent. Clonidine reduces blood pressure primarily by stimulating alpha-adrenergic receptor sites in the hypothalamus and other vasomotor centers in the central nervous system. It also suppresses the release of renal renin.

Side effects include postural hypotension, fluid and sodium retention, drowsiness, and bowel disturbances. Occasionally a weakly positive Coombs' test will result, and an acute hypertensive crisis may accompany abrupt withdrawal of the drug after prolonged therapy.

Despite one report of its successful use in five Australian obstetric patients, the drug has been insufficiently evaluated to recommend its use during pregnancy. Other agents currently available can achieve the same objectives and have been more thoroughly studied. A case has been reported of a neonate born with Roberts' syndrome to a hypertensive mother who was treated with clonidine, 0.3 mg/day, throughout her pregnancy. This syndrome, which includes tetraphocomelia, cleft lip and palate, and dysmorphia, could be due to a disturbance in development before the seventh week of gestation. While the syndrome may be a genetic disorder transmitted in an autosomal recessive pattern, the question of a relationship between this infant's abnormalities and the mother's use of clonidine during the early first trimester should be considered.

Recommended Reading

Frohlich, E. D. The sympathetic depressant anti-hypertensives. *Drug Ther.* 5:24, 1975.

Johnson, C. I., and Aickin, D. R. The control of high blood pressure during labour with clonidine (Catapres). *Med. J. Aust.* 2:132, 1971.

Kelly, J. V. Drugs used in the management of toxemia of pregnancy. *Clin. Obstet. Gynecol.* 20:395, 1977.

Martin, J. D. A critical survey of drugs used in the treatment of hypertensive crises of pregnancy. *Med. J. Aust.* 2:252, 1974.

Stoll, C., Levy, J. M., and Beshara, D. Robert's syndrome and clonidine. *J. Med. Genet.* 16:486, 1979.

Yudkin, J. S. Withdrawal of clonidine. *Lancet* 1:546, 1977.

Clotrimazole (Gyne-Lotrimin®, Lotrimin®)

Indications and Recommendations

The use of clotrimazole during pregnancy should be limited to the topical treatment of vaginal and skin infections caused by susceptible yeast and fungi. These include *Candida albicans* and *Trichophyton* species. At this time, there are no data implicating clotrimazole as a teratogen. This medication should not be applied vaginally after membranes have ruptured.

Special Considerations in Pregnancy

The use of clotrimazole for the treatment of vaginal candidiasis during pregnancy has been extensively studied. Although reports disagree as to this drug's efficacy relative to other antifungal agents, none of the studies implicate it as a teratogen.

Dosage

For the treatment of vaginal candidiasis, one vaginal tablet or one applicator dose of the vaginal cream should be inserted high into the vagina for 7 consecutive nights.

Adverse Effects

Untoward effects of clotrimazole therapy are uncommon and may include erythema, burning, stinging, edema, pruritus, urticaria, and general irritation of the skin or vagina. Rarely, patients complain of lower abdominal cramps and slight urinary frequency.

Mechanism of Action

Clotrimazole is structurally unrelated to the other antifungal agents and appears to act by interfering with the phospholipid layer of the fungal membrane. It has broad-spectrum antifungal activity. Clotrimazole therapy is effective in the treatment of vulvovaginal candidiasis, tinea pedis, tinea cruris, tinea corporis, and tinea versicolor.

Absorption and Biotransformation

Clotrimazole has been found to be only slightly absorbed from skin and vaginal mucosa. Only 0.15% of the dose was recovered in the urine after it had been applied to inflamed skin. Serum levels of 0.05 μg/ml were achieved after administration of a single intravaginal 100-mg tablet.

Recommended Reading

Frerich, W., and Gad, A. The frequency of *Candida* infections in pregnancy and their treatment with clotrimazole. *Curr. Med. Res. Opin.* 4:640, 1977.

Gilman, A. G., Goodman, L. S., and Gilman A. *The Pharmacological Basis of Therapeutics* (6th ed.). New York: Macmillan, 1980. P. 983.

Haran, K., and Digranes, A. Vulvovaginal candidiasis in pregnancy treated with clotrimazole. *Acta Obstet. Gynecol. Scand.* 57:453, 1978.

Lindeque, B. G., and Niekirk, W. A. Treatment of vaginal candidiasis in pregnancy with a single clotrimazole 500 mg vaginal pessary. *S. Afr. Med. J.* 65:123, 1984.

Tan, C. G. A comparative trial of six day therapy with clotrimazole and nystatin in pregnant patients with vaginal candidiasis. *Postgrad. Med.* 50(Suppl. 1):102, 1974.

Cocaine

Indications and Recommendations

Cocaine is contraindicated during pregnancy. This drug is a local anesthetic and has no other indications. Other local anesthetic agents have now replaced cocaine. It is most widely used as a social drug, taken intranasally, intravenously, or orally (chewing coca leaves or smoking coca paste), because it brings about a feeling of well-being and euphoria. Such uses are illegal. In addition, a withdrawal syndrome has been described for cocaine, which consists of craving for the drug, fatigue, hyperphagia, and depression, as well as suppression of rapid eye movement (REM) sleep. Whether this represents physiologic addiction is controversial, since tolerance to the effects of the drug has not been clearly documented. Acute intoxication with cocaine may include convulsions and cardiac arrhythmias, as with other local anesthetics, as well as vasoconstriction, hypertension, and respiratory arrest.

Cocaine has not been shown to be teratogenic in animal studies or human reports. However, its effects on the pregnant woman and her fetus have not been thoroughly investigated. There is one report of two cases of hypertension and abruptio placentae that were believed to be related to recent cocaine use. In another study, women who used cocaine at the time of conception and during most of pregnancy had a significantly higher incidence of previous spontaneous abortion, and the offspring of the pregnancies under study had significant depression of interactive behavior and a poor organizational response to environmental stimuli. Four in 14 women continuing cocaine use throughout pregnancy had abruptio placentae in the third trimester immediately after intravenously injecting cocaine. Since this drug has no therapeutic value, it is clearly contraindicated in pregnancy.

Recommended Reading

Acker, D., et al. Abruptio placentae associated with cocaine use. *Am. J. Obstet. Gynecol.* 146:220, 1983.

Chasnoff, I. J., et al. Cocaine use in pregnancy. *N. Engl. J. Med.* 313:666, 1985.

Fantel, A. G., and MacPhail, B. J. The teratogenicity of cocaine. *Teratology* 26:17, 1982.

Gilman, A. G., Goodman, L. S., and Gilman, A. *The Pharmacological Basis of Therapeutics* (6th ed.). New York: Macmillan, 1980. Pp. 307–308, 553–557.

Colchicine

Indications and Recommendations

Colchicine is contraindicated during pregnancy. It is used to relieve the pain of attacks of acute gouty arthritis and in the prophylactic treatment of recurrent gout attacks.

Colchicine reduces the inflammatory response to deposition of monosodium urate crystals in joint tissue, in part by inhibiting polymorphonuclear leukocyte metabolism, mobility, and chemotaxis. It also inhibits cell division in metaphase by interfering with the mitotic spindle.

Colchicine is embryocidal in mice and rabbits. The risk of teratogenesis in humans is unknown. While receiving daily maintenance colchicine therapy for prevention of familial Mediterranean fever, five patients became pregnant and were followed through delivery. One of these women continued the drug throughout pregnancy and gave birth to a normal child. Of the four who stopped colchicine after pregnancy was detected, one had a spontaneous abortion in the second month and three gave birth to healthy infants.

There is concern that colchicine given around conception will result in an increased frequency of Down's syndrome in the offspring by causing chromosomal nondisjunction. One study of lymphocyte cultures from three gouty patients on colchicine showed a significant increase in cells with abnormal numbers of chromosomes, both tetraploid and peridiploid, when compared to matched controls. In this report, 2 in 54 parents of 27 children with Down's syndrome were found to be receiving colchicine therapy.

Gout is uncommon in women and is rarely seen before menopause. If treatment of an acute attack becomes necessary, a short course of phenylbutazone may be required. An elevated serum uric acid is common in toxemia but rarely requires therapy. Probenecid has been safely used and is indicated for treatment of significant hyperuricemia in pregnancy.

For the couple planning to have a child, it is recommended that colchicine ingestion by *either* parent be discontinued 3 months before conception.

Recommended Reading

American Hospital Formulatory Service. *Monograph for Colchicine.* Washington, D.C.: American Society of Hospital Pharmacists, 1973.

Ferrcira, N. R., and Breoniconti, A. Trisomy after colchicine therapy (letter). *Lancet* 2:1304, 1968.

Gilman, A. G., Goodman, L. S., and Gilman, A. *The Pharmacological Basis of Therapeutics* (6th ed.). New York: Macmillan, 1980. Pp. 718–720.

Santhanogopalas, T. Serum uric acid levels and transaminase activities in toxemias of pregnancy. *J. Obstet. Gynecol. India* 15:561, 1965.

Zemer, D., et al. Colchicine in familial Mediterranean fever (letter). *N. Engl. J. Med.* 294:170, 1976.

Contraceptives, Oral

Indications and Recommendations

The use of oral contraceptives is contraindicated during pregnancy since there is no reason for their use. Some patients, however, not knowing that they have conceived, may inadvertently continue to take oral contraceptives early in the first trimester.

Combination oral contraceptive pills in the United States contain a 19-nortestosterone progestin and a synthetic estrogen. When taken during pregnancy, these drugs may increase maternal nausea and vomiting and cause cholestatic jaundice.

The ingestion of large dosages of synthetic estrogens during the first trimester (e.g., diethylstilbestrol [DES]) has been associated with vaginal adenosis and adenocarcinoma of the vagina, as well as reproductive problems, in female offspring. Testicular cysts, oligospermia, and hypospadias have been reported in male offspring. Although these disturbances have not been associated with oral contraceptives inadvertently taken during the first trimester, extrapolation from DES data suggests the theoretic possibility of such a risk.

Presumably because of the weak androgenic effect of many of the 19-nortestosterone derivatives used as progestational agents, masculinization of exposed female fetuses has been reported, particularly with older high-dosage formulations.

There are inconclusive data to link early-pregnancy oral contraceptive exposure with neural tube defects, limb defects, cardiac abnormalities, and cleft palate. More recent large-scale case-control studies (including the report from the Finnish Register of Congenital Malformations containing 3,002 mothers of infants with malformations) have failed to confirm any strong association. Interestingly, one large study suggested that the combination of maternal smoking and oral contraceptive use during early pregnancy may be a risk factor for malformations. There is a single provocative case report of an infant with transposition of the great vessels born to a mother who attempted to induce abortion by the ingestion of 120–150 oral contraceptive pills early in the first trimester.

Other effects of oral contraceptives taken within 2 months of conception may include a doubling of the dizygous twinning rate, as reported in one study.

The steroid hormones in oral contraceptives pass into the breast milk in measurable amounts. Oral contraceptive pill ingestion during lactation has been associated with a measurable diminution in the milk supply, but not with clinically significant problems in the nursing infant.

The oral contraceptives are contraindicated in pregnancy because of potential adverse effects on the fetus. It goes without saying that they have no therapeutic value in pregnant women. Although there may be an association between congenital anomalies and oral contraceptives taken during the first trimester, the preponderance of current evidence suggests that the risk, if any, is small when compared to the background risk for birth defects.

Recommended Reading

Bracken, M. B. Oral contraception and twinning: An epidemiologic study. *Am. J. Obstet. Gynecol.* 133:432, 1979.

Bracken, M. B., et al. Role of oral contraception in congenital malformations of offspring. *Int. J. Epidemiol.* 7:309, 1978.

Bracken, M. B., and Srisuphan, W. Oral contraception as a risk factor for preeclampsia. *Am. J. Obstet. Gynecol.* 142:191, 1982.

Chez, R. A. Proceedings of the symposium: Progesterone, progestins, and fetal development. *Fertil. Steril.* 30:16, 1978.

Heinonen, O. P., et al. Cardiovascular birth defects and antenatal exposure to female sex hormones. *N. Engl. J. Med.* 296:67, 1977.

Janerich, D. T., Piper, J. M., and Glebatis, D. M. Oral contraceptives and congenital limb-reduction defects. *N. Engl. J. Med.* 291:697, 1974.

Keith, L., and Berger, S. L. The relationship between congenital defects and the use of exogenous progestational (contraceptive) hormones during pregnancy: A 20 year review. *Int. J. Gynecol. Obstet.* 15:115, 1977.

Linn, S., et al. Lack of association between contraceptive usage and congenital malformations in offspring. *Am. J. Obstet. Gynecol.* 147: 923, 1983.

Nilsson, S., Nygren, K., and Johansson, E. D. B. D-Norgestrel concentrations in maternal plasma, milk and child plasma during administration of oral contraceptives to nursing women. *Am. J. Obstet. Gynecol.* 129:178, 1977.

Redline, R. W., and Abramowsky, C. R. Transportation of the great vessels in an infant exposed to massive doses of oral contraceptives. *Am. J. Obstet. Gynecol.* 141:468, 1981.

Rothman, K. J., and Louik, C. Oral contraceptives and birth defects. *N. Engl. J. Med.* 299:522, 1978.

Savolainen, E., Saksela, E., and Saxen, L. Teratogenic hazards of oral contraceptives analyzed in a national malformation register. *Am. J. Obstet. Gynecol.* 140:521, 1981.

Corticosteroids: Betamethasone (Celestone®), Dexamethasone (Decadron®), Hydrocortisone (Cortef®, Solu-Cortef®), Methylprednisolone (Medrol®, Solu-Medrol®), Prednisone (Deltasone®)

Indications and Recommendations

Corticosteroid therapy may be administered during pregnancy and lactation if it is medically indicated. These agents are used as replacement therapy for acute or chronic adrenal insufficiency, as suppressive therapy for congenital adrenal hyperplasia, and in the treatment of a large number of pathologic states as antiinflammatory agents. They are also commonly used in obstetrics for the prevention of respiratory distress syndrome (RDS) in the neonate in situations in which premature delivery of the infant is likely.

When administered for maternal indications, it is recommended that prednisone be used in preference to other steroids whenever possible since it has the poorest transport across the placenta. Neonates should be observed for transient adrenocortical insufficiency if their mothers had chronic steroid therapy during pregnancy.

Exogenous corticosteroid therapy to mothers with impending premature delivery is best administered within these guidelines.

1. They should not be given to patients who are likely to deliver within 24 hours after initiation of therapy.
2. After 34 weeks' gestation, measurable efficacy has not been demonstrated.
3. The safety and efficacy of their use in the presence of ruptured membranes are currently controversial.

Special Considerations in Pregnancy

Chronic maternal steroid ingestion during the first trimester of pregnancy has been associated with approximately a 1% incidence of cleft palate in human offspring. Animal studies have suggested an effect on neurologic and pulmonary development in fetuses exposed to steroids in utero, but no such effects have been demonstrated in humans exposed to steroids for short or long periods of time. In a case-control study, children exposed to both short- and long-term steroid therapy in utero were evaluated for in vitro cell-mediated immunocompetence at age 3–4 years and were not found to be different from nonexposed control subjects. Numerous reports document apparent normalcy in infants whose mothers had Cushing's syndrome or were treated with steroids for other conditions throughout the pregnancy. Sporadic cases of transient adrenocortical insufficiency in newborns have been reported. Well-controlled prospective studies have not been performed.

High-dose maternal glucocorticoid therapy has been shown to decrease the incidence of RDS in the offspring of women who are delivered of their infants before 34 weeks. Initial reports from investigators in New Zealand suggested that this relationship may not hold true when the mother is hypertensive, but subsequent studies have failed to confirm this. Numerous controlled studies have confirmed the efficacy of steroids in preventing respiratory complications in the newborn delivered prior to 34 weeks, with the prospective trial of dexamethasone by the Collaborative Group on Antenatal Steroid Therapy being the largest (696 subjects). In the latter trial, steroids were found to be significantly more efficacious among female and black fetuses than among males or whites. Follow-up studies at 6 years of age on 259 children participating in the original New Zealand randomized study of betamethasone therapy in utero have not shown any disadvantage in cognitive development among steroid-exposed children. There have, however, been reports suggesting hypercholesterolemia and leukocytosis in newborns exposed to high-dose steroids just before delivery, and many unanswered questions of safety remain.

Large amounts of corticosteroids (75 mg/day cortisol) may suppress fetal adrenal production of estrogen precursor, with subsequent lowering of plasma and urinary estriol values. In one series of 21 patients who received steroids during 29 pregnancies, however, there was no evidence of fetal adrenocortical insufficiency despite total doses of 11,000 mg cortisone in one case and 6,250 mg prednisone in another.

Female fetuses with 21-hydroxylase deficiency tend to be masculinized in utero, with the effect presumably occurring between the tenth and sixteenth week. Unfortunately, prenatal diagnosis of this inborn error of metabolism is currently not possible before the sixteenth week of gestation. Theoretically, it may be possible to prevent masculinization by suppressing the fetal adrenal gland with corticosteroid therapy if begun prior to the tenth week. There has now been at least one report of successful prevention of virilization of a female fetus with 21-hydroxylase deficiency by adrenal suppression with dexamethasone, 0.5 mg bid, given to the mother from the fifth week of pregnancy until term. A second case was reported in which hydrocortisone administration to the mother partially suppressed fetal adrenal function.

Corticosteroids cross the placenta with varying success; dexamethasone and betamethasone cross efficiently while prednisone crosses poorly. Prednisolone crosses to a greater extent than does prednisone. Little human data exist regarding the concentrations of corticosteroids appearing in breast milk. Small amounts of prednisone and prednisolone have been detected, but the dosage absorbed by a nursing infant would probably be negligible.

Dosage

The dosage of glucocorticoids varies depending on the condition being treated. Table 4 lists the equivalent amounts for some of the available forms. For acute adrenal insufficiency, the dose of hydrocortisone is 100 mg IV every 8 hours, then 25 mg IM every 6–8 hours. The usual dose for the treatment of chronic adrenal insufficiency is 5–15 mg hydrocortisone or its equivalent tid, guided by the patient's blood pressure and sense of well-being. Depending on the form of steroid given and the patient's electrolyte picture, mineralocorticoids may need to be added.

For anteropituitary insufficiency, 25 mg cortisone given on arising and 12.5 mg in the late afternoon are adequate replacement and somewhat mimic the normal diurnal cycle. Higher-than-physiologic dosages are employed in the treatment of rheumatoid arthritis, systemic lupus erythematosus nephritis, autoimmune hemolytic anemia, renal transplantation, and other situations in which the immune response is to be depressed. For suppression of cerebral edema, the conventional dose is 100 mg prednisone per day in divided doses (equivalent to 400 mg hydrocortisone).

Asthmatics requiring steroid therapy for an acute attack are generally started at 100 mg cortisol (Solu-Cortef®) IV every 8 hours, then placed on oral prednisone, 20–40 mg/day, after which the dosage is tapered rapidly. Steroids are used in retention enemas for refractory ulcerative colitis, as eye drops for nonbacterial and nonviral inflammatory conditions, and as creams and lotions for various dermatologic conditions. These topical forms are systemically absorbed, especially through inflamed hyperemic tissues.

In the study by the Collaborative Group on Antenatal Steroid

Table 4. Equivalent amounts for some available forms of corticosteroids

Equivalent doses	Mg	Route of administration
Cortisone	25	IM, PO
Hydrocortisone	20	IV, IM, PO
Prednisone	5	PO
Methylprednisolone	4	IV, IM, PO
Triamcinolone	4	IM, PO
Paramethasone	2	PO
Betamethasone	0.75	IV, IM, PO
Dexamethasone	0.75	IV, IM, PO

Data derived from G. W. Thorne, et al. (eds.). *Harrison's Principles of Internal Medicine* (8th ed.). New York: McGraw-Hill, 1977. P. 554.

Therapy, the dose of dexamethasone administered for the antenatal prevention of RDS was 5 mg IM every 6 hours 4 times. In earlier studies, a mixture of betamethasone phosphate and acetate at a dose of 12 mg IM every 24 hours 2 times was utilized.

Adverse Effects

Side effects include fluid and electrolyte imbalance, hyperglycemia, peptic ulcers (that may bleed or perforate), susceptibility to infections (including tuberculosis), osteoporosis, psychosis, myopathy, striae, ecchymoses, acne, and fat deposition characteristic of Cushing's syndrome.

Mechanism of Action

Corticosteroids are a family of 21-carbon compounds. Their action is dependent on specific cytoplasmic receptors that, when combined with the steroid, migrate to the cell nucleus, after which enzyme

Table 5. Antiinflammatory and sodium-retaining potencies of various corticosteroid compounds

Compound	Relative anti-inflammatory potency	Relative sodium-retaining potency
Hydrocortisone (cortisol)	1	1
Tetrahydrocortisol	0	0
Prednisone (Δ^1-cortisone)	4	0.8
Prednisolone (Δ^1-cortisol)	4	0.8
6α-Methylprednisolone	5	0.5
9α-Fluorocortisol	10	125
11-Desoxycortisol	0	0
Cortisone	0.8	0.8
Corticosterone	0.35	15
11-Desoxycorticosterone	0	100
Aldosterone	?	3,000
Triamcinolone (9α-fluoro-16α-hydroxyprednisolone)	5	0
Paramethasone (6α-fluoro-16α-methylprednisolone)	10	0
Betamethasone (9α-fluoro-16β-methylprednisolone)	25	0
Dexamethasone (9α-fluoro-16α-methylprednisolone)	25	0

Adapted from A. G. Gilman, L. S. Goodman, and A. Gilman. *The Pharmacological Basis of Therapeutics* (6th ed.). New York: Macmillan, 1980. P. 1482.

synthesis is influenced. Their physiologic effects are widespread. They stabilize lysosomal membranes, inhibiting the production and release of inflammatory mediators and decreasing chemotaxis. They also decrease mast cell activity and lymphocyte lysis, which consequently disturbs cell-mediated immunity.

Hematologic effects include granulocytosis (due to demargination of white blood cells), increased platelets, and decreased eosinophils.

Metabolic effects include increased peripheral gluconeogenesis, hepatic glycogenolysis, and hepatic gluconeogenesis. In the presence of growth hormone, corticosteroids promote lipolysis. Electrolyte changes include sodium and water retention, along with potassium loss in the urine (Table 5).

Absorption and Biotransformation

Some of the available corticosteroid compounds are well absorbed orally while others must be given parenterally (see Table 4). All biologically active adrenocortical steroids and their synthetic congeners have a double bond in the 4–5 position. Reduction of this bond can occur at hepatic or extrahepatic sites to yield an inactive compound. Conversion occurs, primarily in the liver, to sulfate esters or glucuronides; excretion is then via the kidneys.

Recommended Reading

Andersen, G. E., and Friis-Hansen, B. Hypercholesterolemia in the newborn: Occurrence after antepartum treatment with betamethasone-phenobarbital-ritodrine for the prevention of the respiratory distress syndrome. *Pediatrics* 62:8, 1978.

Baden, M., et al. A controlled trial of hydrocortisone therapy in infants with respiratory distress syndrome. *Pediatrics* 50:526, 1972.

Beck, J. C., et al. Betamethasone and the rhesus fetus: Effect on lung-morphometry and connective tissue. *Pediatr. Res.* 15:235, 1981.

Challis, J. R., Kendall, J. Z., and Robinson, J. S. The regulation of corticosteroids during late pregnancy and their role in parturition. *Biol. Reprod.* 16:57, 1977.

Collaborative Group on Antenatal Steroid Therapy. Effect of antenatal dexamethasone administration on the prevention of respiratory distress syndrome. *Am. J. Obstet. Gynecol.* 141:276, 1981.

David, M., and Forest, M. G. Prenatal treatment of congenital adrenal hyperplasia resulting from 21-hydroxylase deficiency. *J. Pediatr.* 105:799, 1984.

Fitzhardinge, P. M., et al. Sequelae of early steroid administration to the newborn infant. *Pediatrics* 53:877, 1974.

Gilman, A. G., Goodman, L. S., and Gilman, A. *The Pharmacological Basis of Therapeutics* (6th ed.). New York: Macmillan, 1980. Pp. 1470–1492.

Katz, F. H., and Duncan, B. R. Entry of prednisone into human milk. *N. Engl. J. Med.* 293:1154, 1975.

Kauppila, A., et al. Cell-mediated immunocompetence of children exposed in utero to short- or long-term action of glucocorticoids. *Gynecol. Obstet. Invest.* 15:41, 1983.

Liggins, G. C., and Howie, R. N. A controlled trial of antepartum glucocorticoid treatment for prevention of the respiratory distress syndrome in premature infants. *Pediatrics* 50:515, 1972.

MacArthur, B. A., et al. School progress and cognitive development of 6-

year-old children whose mothers were treated antenatally with betamethasone. *Pediatrics* 70:99, 1982.

Murphy, B. E. P., Patrick, J., and Denton, R. L. Cortisol in amniotic fluid during human gestation. *J. Clin. Endocrinol. Metab.* 40:164, 1975.

Otero, L., et al. Neonatal leukocytosis associated with prenatal administration of dexamethasone. *Pediatrics* 68:778, 1981.

Ricke, P. S., Elliott, J. P., and Freeman, R. K. Use of corticosteroids in pregnancy-induced hypertension. *Obstet. Gynecol.* 55:206, 1980.

Schapiro, S. Some physiologic biochemical and behavioral consequences of neonatal hormone administration: Cortisol and thyroxin. *Gen. Comp. Endocrinol.* 10:214, 1968.

Thorne, G. W., et al. (eds.). *Harrison's Principles of Internal Medicine* (8th ed.). New York: McGraw-Hill, 1977. P. 554.

Update: Drugs in breast milk. *Med. Lett. Drugs Ther.* 21:21, 1979.

Yackel, D. B., Kempers, R. D., and McConahey, W. M. Adrenocorticosteroid therapy in pregnancy. *Am. J. Obstet. Gynecol.* 96:985, 1966.

Co-trimoxazole:
Trimethoprim-Sulfamethoxazole (Bactrim®, Septra®)

Indications and Recommendations

The use of co-trimoxazole during pregnancy is relatively contraindicated since, for most of its indications, other more desirable alternatives exist. Its use should be limited to treatment of life-threatening infections, such as those caused by *Pneumocystis carinii*, which are not amenable to treatment with less hazardous antibiotics. It should not be administered in the third trimester because of the danger of kernicterus to the neonate.

Special Considerations in Pregnancy

Despite favorable outcomes in a few limited studies that used co-trimoxazole to treat bacteriuria during various stages of pregnancy, the use of this agent should be avoided whenever possible.

Both trimethoprim and sulfamethoxazole cross the placenta and appear in measurable amounts in fetal blood. Although no instances have been documented, there is a theoretic possibility that trimethoprim will inhibit the reduction of dihydrofolate to tetrahydrofolate in the fetus, thereby causing congenital anomalies. In addition, the use of sulfonamides in the last 3 months of pregnancy is contraindicated because of the danger of kernicterus in the neonate (see *Sulfonamides*).

Dosage

The usual adult dose is 800 mg sulfamethoxazole plus 160 mg trimethoprim every 12 hours for 10–14 days. Larger dosages have been used in special circumstances in patients with serious or life-threatening diseases. The dosages must be reduced in patients with renal disease.

Adverse Effects

Sulfonamide use is often associated with skin reactions, and the same spectrum of reactions is seen with co-trimoxazole therapy. Nausea and vomiting are common side effects, as are glossitis and stomatitis. While there is no evidence that co-trimoxazole causes folate deficiency in normal people at recommended dosages, megaloblastosis may be seen in those who are folate deficient. Additional hematologic reactions include other types of anemia and coagulation disorders.

Mechanism of Action

The antimicrobial activity of the trimethoprim-sulfamethoxazole combination results from their individual and synergistic actions on the tetrahydrofolate synthesis pathway. Sulfonamides inhibit the incorporation of para-aminobenzoic acid (PABA) into folic acid, and trimethoprim prevents the reduction of dihydrofolate to tetrahydrofolate. The toxicity is selective for microorganisms, as mammalian cells do not utilize PABA and trimethoprim is a highly selective inhibitor of enzyme activity in lower organisms.

Because of this unique mechanism of action, co-trimoxazole has a broad spectrum of action against gram-positive and gram-negative organisms and is effective in the treatment of *P. carinii* infections in impaired hosts.

Absorption and Biotransformation

The individual ingredients of co-trimoxazole have been selected to achieve optimal blood and tissue concentration ratios of 20:1. While trimethoprim is absorbed more quickly than sulfamethoxazole, their half-lives are well matched at approximately 10 and 9 hours, respectively.

Trimethoprim is rapidly distributed and concentrated in tissues. It enters the cerebrospinal fluid and sputum readily. Up to 60% is excreted in the urine in 24 hours. Metabolites of trimethoprim are also excreted. The rate of excretion is significantly decreased in uremia.

Sulfamethoxazole is approximately 65% bound to plasma proteins. In 24 hours, 25–50% is excreted in the urine, approximately one-third as conjugates. The rate of excretion is significantly decreased in uremia.

Recommended Reading

Bailey, R. R., Bishop, V., and Peddie, B. A. Comparison of single dose with a five day course of co-trimoxazole for asymptomatic (covert) bacteriuria of pregnancy. *Aust. N.Z. J. Obstet. Gynecol.* 23:139, 1983.

Gilman, A. G., Goodman, L. S., and Gilman, A. *The Pharmacological Basis of Therapeutics* (6th ed.). New York: Macmillan, 1980. Pp. 1116–1119.

Williams, J. D., et al. The treatment of bacteriuria in pregnant women with sulfamethoxazole and trimethoprim. *Postgrad. Med. J.* 45 (Suppl.):75, 1969.

Ylikorkala, O., et al. Trimethoprim-sulfonamide combination administered orally and intravaginally in the first trimester of pregnancy: Its
absorption into serum and transfer to amniotic fluid. *Acta Obstet.
Gynecol. Scand.* 52:229, 1973.

Coumarin Anticoagulants: Warfarin (Coumadin®, Panwarfin®)

Indications and Recommendations

The use of oral anticoagulants in the warfarin family is contraindicated during pregnancy. During the first trimester, these compounds have the potential for causing warfarin embryopathy. During the second and third trimesters, their use can result in the
development of central nervous system and ocular anomalies. In
addition, since these drugs readily cross the placental barrier they
anticoagulate the fetus. Deaths from fetal hemorrhage occurring
before and during labor have been reported.

Fetal abnormalities associated with maternal ingestion of
Coumadin® include nasal hypoplasia, stippling of bone, hydro-
cephalus, microcephaly, ophthalmologic abnormalities, intrauterine growth retardation, and developmental delays.

Some authors have advocated the use of warfarin anticoagulants
during the second trimester and up to 3 weeks before the estimated
date of delivery. The rationale for this regimen is that it avoids first-
trimester exposure and also reduces the risk of fetal hemorrhage at
the time of labor and delivery at term. It has been found, however,
that while the warfarin embryopathy syndrome results from exposure in the first trimester, central nervous system abnormalities
may develop at any gestational age. In addition, the onset of premature labor cannot be anticipated, and consequently, the infant could
be fully anticoagulated at the time of an early delivery. We therefore recommend that heparin be used as the drug of choice in any
patient who requires anticoagulation throughout pregnancy.

Postpartum administration of warfarin poses no hazard to the
nursing infant since only an inactive form of the drug appears in
human milk.

Recommended Reading

Hall, J. G., Pauli, R. M., and Wilson, K. M. Maternal and fetal sequelae
of anticoagulation during pregnancy. *Am. J. Med.* 68:122, 1980.

Hirsh, J., Cade, J. F., and O'Sullivan, E. F. Clinical experience with
anticoagulant therapy during pregnancy. *Br. Med. J.* 1:270, 1970.

Shaul, W. L., Emery, H., and Hall, J. G. Chondroplasia puncta and
maternal warfarin use during pregnancy. *Am. J. Dis. Child.* 129:360,
1975.

Villasanta, U. Thromboembolic disease in pregnancy. *Am. J. Obstet.
Gynecol.* 93:142, 1965.

Wessler, S., and Gitel, S. N. Warfarin from bedside to bench. *N. Engl. J.
Med.* 311:645, 1984.

Cromolyn Sodium (Aarane®, Intal®)

Indications and Recommendations

Cromolyn sodium may be administered to pregnant asthmatics before unavoidable exposure to allergens that have been proved to cause severe bronchospasm and to prevent exercise-induced bronchospasm. This drug seems to be well tolerated in pregnancy, and its systemic absorption is minimal. Cromolyn sodium has no role in the treatment of acute asthmatic attacks.

Special Considerations in Pregnancy

No unusual maternal effects are reported. No information is available regarding the passage of cromolyn sodium across the placenta.

Teratogenicity has not been reported in humans. In one series of 296 pregnant asthmatics treated with cromolyn sodium, malformations were observed in only 4 newborns (1.4%), an incidence similar to, if not significantly lower than, the usual 2–3% seen in the general population. Studies in animals have failed to produce teratogenesis after prolonged intravenous administration of the drug. Decreased fetal weight, however, has been reported in association with dosages close to those that produce maternal toxicity in animals.

Dosage

The usual dose is 20 mg inhaled every 6 hours prn. A clinical response to this drug is often seen within 3–5 days but may take as long as a month.

Cromolyn sodium is only effective in exercise-induced bronchospasm if taken 1–20 minutes before exercise. This drug should not be given during an acute asthmatic attack because it can aggravate the existing bronchial irritation.

Adverse Effects

Side effects include mild sore throat, nasal congestion, cough, transient wheezing, urticaria, and maculopapular rash. Occasionally, angioedema, fever, nausea, vomiting, pulmonary infiltrates, muscular weakness, pericarditis, and anaphylaxis may occur.

Mechanism of Action

Cromolyn sodium inhibits the release of histamine and slow-reacting substance of anaphylaxis by mast cells. These are the chemical mediators of a bronchospastic response after either immunologic or nonimmunologic stimulation. This drug does not have direct bronchodilator, antihistaminic, or antiinflammatory effects. The amount of drug absorbed into the circulation following inhalation of therapeutic dosages does not appear to exert any generalized pharmacologic action.

Absorption and Biotransformation

The drug is marketed as a crystallized powder, with lactose as an inert propellant, in a gelatin capsule. It is administered via a special inhaler. Only 1–2 mg of the 20-mg dose reaches the alveoli. The remainder is retained in the trachea and oropharynx and is swallowed later. Eight percent of the drug is absorbed systemically in the lung and gastrointestinal tract. Eighty percent of the cromolyn sodium is eliminated in the feces. The absorbed drug is excreted unchanged in the urine. The plasma half-life is 60–90 minutes.

Recommended Reading

Berstein, I. L., et al. A controlled study of cromolyn sodium sponsored by the Drug Committee of the American Academy of Allergy. *J. Allergy Clin. Immunol.* 50:235, 1972.

Block, S. H. Nasal congestion as a side effect of cromolyn sodium. *J. Allergy Clin. Immunol.* 53:243, 1974.

Falliers, C. J. Cromolyn sodium (editorial). *J. Allergy* 47:298, 1971.

Falliers, C. J. Cromolyn sodium prophylaxis. *Pediatr. Clin. North Am.* 22:141, 1975.

Gwin, E., Kerby, G., and Ruth, W. Cromolyn sodium in the treatment of asthma associated with aspirin hypersensitivity and nasal polyps. *Chest* 72:148, 1977.

Khurana, S., and Hyde, J. S. Cromolyn sodium, five to six years later. *Ann. Allergy* 39:94, 1977.

Sheffer, A., Rocklin, R., and Goetzl, E. Immunologic components of hypersensitivity reactions to cromolyn sodium. *N. Engl. J. Med.* 293:1220, 1975.

Silverman, M., and Andrea, T. Time course of effect of disodium cromoglycate on exercise-induced asthma. *Arch. Dis. Child.* 47:419, 1972.

Wilson, J. Utilisation du cromoglycate de sodium au cours de la grossesse. *Acta Therapeutica* 8(Suppl.):45, 1982.

Cyclizine (Marezine®)

Indications and Recommendations

Cyclizine is safe to use during pregnancy for the prevention of nausea, vomiting, and dizziness associated with motion sickness. This drug is probably effective for control of postoperative nausea and vomiting when used parenterally or rectally. Although cyclizine has been shown to be teratogenic in rodents, this effect has not been demonstrated in humans when recommended dosages are used.

Special Considerations in Pregnancy

Cyclizine crosses the placenta and has been shown to be teratogenic in rodents. However, large-scale studies in humans show that the rate of severe congenital anomalies in children of mothers who took cyclizine during pregnancy is not significantly different than in the offspring of mothers who did not receive antinauseants.

Dosage

The dose for prevention of motion sickness is 50 mg a half-hour before departure, repeated every 4–6 hours prn. Dose should not exceed 200 mg/day.

For prevention of postoperative vomiting, the dose is 50 mg IM every 4–6 hours or 100 mg rectally every 4–6 hours.

Adverse Effects

The more common side effects of cyclizine include drowsiness, dry mouth, and rarely, blurred vision.

Mechanism of Action

Cyclizine is a piperazine antihistamine that depresses labyrinth excitability and vestibular-cerebellar pathway conduction. It inhibits the effects of histamine on capillary permeability and on smooth muscle by competitive inhibition at H_1 receptors. Either stimulation or depression of the central nervous system may occur through an unknown mechanism. It has anticholinergic activity, although no significant effects on the cardiovascular system occur at normal therapeutic dosages.

Absorption and Biotransformation

Cyclizine is readily absorbed from the gastrointestinal tract and is widely distributed to body tissues. The exact nature of elimination in humans is unknown, but it appears to be extensively metabolized in the liver and excreted in the urine.

Recommended Reading

Biggs, J. S. G. Vomiting in pregnancy: Causes and management. *Drugs* 9:299, 1975.

Gilman, A. G., Goodman, L. S., and Gilman, A. *The Pharmacological Basis of Therapeutics* (6th ed.). New York: Macmillan, 1980. P. 628.

Heinonen, D., Slone, D., and Shapiro, S. *Birth Defects and Drugs in Pregnancy*. Littleton, Mass.: Publishing Sciences Group, 1977. Pp. 323–333.

Long, J. W. *The Essential Guide to Prescription Drugs* (1st ed.). New York: Harper & Row, 1977. Pp. 206–208.

Milkovich, L., and Van den Berg, B. J. An evaluation of the teratogenicity of certain antinauseant drugs. *Am. J. Obstet. Gynecol.* 125:244, 1976.

Nishimura, H., and Tanimura. T. *Clinical Aspects of the Teratogenicity of Drugs*. Amsterdam: Excerpta Medica, 1976.

Cyclosporine (Sandimmune®)

Indications and Recommendations

The use of cyclosporine in pregnant women should be limited to clinical situations in which immunosuppression is critical to maternal survival. Indications currently are limited to prophylaxis against rejection in allogenic organ transplant recipients. The use of this drug should be limited to centers experienced in its use and equipped to deal with potential complications.

Special Considerations in Pregnancy

In studies on rats and rabbits, embryotoxicity occurred when cyclosporine doses high enough to be toxic to the mother (greater than 17 mg/kg/day) were administered. However, at dosages that were well tolerated by the mother, no embryotoxicity was demonstrated. Maintenance doses in the human average 5–10 mg/kg/day (see Dosage). When organ culture studies were performed using rat embryos, cyclosporine did not induce malformations, whereas azathioprine did so.

In one human case report, cord blood cyclosporine levels were similar to maternal levels, while amniotic fluid and placental extracts contained higher concentrations than did maternal blood. Neonatal cyclosporine levels had fallen by more than 50% at 48 hours of age and were undetectable at 1 week. In another report, no cyclosporine could be detected in amniotic fluid, while cord blood levels were approximately 60% of maternal levels at delivery. Of three case reports in which the mother took cyclosporine throughout pregnancy at doses of 325–550 mg/day, two babies were small-for-dates, while the third weighed 2,980 g at 38 weeks. Whether this high incidence of growth retardation is related to the cyclosporine or to the underlying disease states of the patients is impossible to ascertain. In addition, the manufacturer is said to have four additional reports of successful pregnancies as of July 1983 (Klintmalm et al.). As yet, there is no evidence for human teratogenicity with this drug.

Transient neonatal thrombocytopenia, as well as immunosuppression (demonstrated by suppression of third-party lymphocyte culture growth), has occurred in infants of mothers taking this drug. In addition, breast milk cyclosporine levels were in the same range as maternal serum levels, and the manufacturer advises against breast-feeding while taking this drug.

Dosage

Cyclosporine is available as an oral solution (100 mg/ml) and as an intravenous preparation (250 mg/5 ml). The initial dose is given 4–12 hours before transplantation. The drug is started at a single oral dose of 14–18 mg/kg/day; this dosage is continued for 1–2 weeks after surgery, then gradually tapered (5% per week) to a maintenance dose of 5–10 mg/kg/day. When facilities exist for monitoring plasma or whole blood levels of cyclosporine, dosage is adjusted to maintain trough plasma levels of 50–150 ng/ml once maintenance dosages are desired.

Intravenous administration of cyclosporine has been associated with anaphylaxis, so the use of this route should be limited to patients unable to take the drug orally. When used intravenously, the dosage of cyclosporine is one-third the oral dosage.

Corticosteroid therapy is generally used as an adjunct to cyclosporine, with initial high doses (as much as 200 mg/day prednisone in some series) but slow tapering to maintenance doses, often as low as 10–20 mg prednisone each day. Adjustments in dosage of cyclosporine and corticosteroids should be the responsibility of individuals experienced in the use of these drugs and in the care of transplant recipients.

Adverse Effects

Dose-related nephrotoxicity is seen in one-fourth to one-third of transplant recipients treated with cyclosporine. If it does not improve with adjustment in dosage, it may be necessary to switch to other forms of immunosuppressive therapy. Hypertension was reported in 26% of 227 renal transplant recipients receiving this drug in a randomized trial, as opposed to 18% of 228 receiving azathioprine. Hepatotoxicity, consisting of elevated liver enzymes and bilirubin, was reported in 4–7% of treated patients and usually responded to reduction in dosage. Hirsutism, tremors, paresthesias, gum dysplasia, nausea, and vomiting have all been reported. Anaphylaxis was reported in approximately 1 in 1,000 patients receiving cyclosporine intravenously, and for this reason, all such patients should be closely observed for at least 30 minutes after beginning the infusion. Anaphylactic reactions have not been reported with the oral route of administration.

Mechanism of Action

Cyclosporine (cyclosporin A) is a polypeptide containing 11 amino acids. It is a product of the fungus, Tolypocladium inflatum Gams. This drug inhibits cell-mediated immunity, such as allograft rejection, presumably by suppressing the generation of T lymphocytes, particularly helper T cells. It must be administered before these T lymphocytes have undergone proliferation in response to exposure to a specific antigen. B-cell function is not altered.

Absorption and Biotransformation

Gastrointestinal absorption of cyclosporine is incomplete and variable. Peak concentrations are achieved at 3–4 hours, and bioavailability is approximately 30% compared to intravenous dosing. Only about 40% is distributed in plasma, with the remainder being taken up by erythrocytes, granulocytes, and lymphocytes. Approximately 90% of plasma cyclosporine is protein bound. Elimination is mainly via the biliary system, with a half-life of approximately 19 hours.

Recommended Reading

AMA Drug Evaluations (5th ed.). Chicago: American Medical Association, 1983. P. 1448.

Deeg, H. J., et al. Successful pregnancy after marrow transplantation for severe aplastic anemia and immunosuppression with cyclosporine. *J.A.M.A.* 250:647, 1983.

Flechner, S. M., et al. The presence of cyclosporine in body tissues and fluids during pregnancy. *Am. J. Kidney Dis.* 5:60, 1985.

Klintmalm, G., et al. Renal function in a newborn baby delivered of a renal transplant patient taking cyclosporine. *Transplantation* 38:198, 1984.

Lewis, G. J., et al. Successful pregnancy in a renal transplant recipient taking cyclosporin A. *Br. Med. J.* 286:603, 1983.

Mason, R. J., et al. Cyclosporine-induced fetotoxicity in the rat. *Transplantation* 39:9, 1985.

Ryffel, B., et al. Toxicological evaluation of cyclosporin A. *Arch. Toxicol.* 53:107, 1983.

Sandimmune®. *Physicians' Desk Reference* (40th ed.). Oradell, N.J.: Medical Economics, 1986. Pp. 1592–1594.

Schmid, B. P. Monitoring of organ formation in rat embryos after in vitro exposure to azathioprine, mercaptopurine, methotrexate or cyclosporin A. *Toxicology* 31:9, 1984.

Cyproheptadine (Periactin®)

Indications and Recommendations

Cyproheptadine, an antihistamine and serotonin antagonist, is teratogenic at relatively high dosages in some laboratory animals. It has no clear advantages over other antihistamines when used to treat allergic reactions such as rhinitis, urticaria, and angioedema, but its serotonin antagonism is useful in treating postgastrectomy dumping syndrome and the intestinal hypermotility of carcinoid. Therefore, its use in pregnancy should be limited to the latter indications.

Special Considerations in Pregnancy

While some studies of cyproheptadine given to rats show no teratogenic or embryotoxic effects at subcutaneous doses up to 5 mg/kg/day (the usual human oral dose is approximately 0.2 mg/kg/day), others show teratogenic effects with single intraperitoneal doses of 10–50 mg/kg on day 7, 10, 13, or 15 of a 22-day gestation. Chronic intraperitoneal dosing at 2 mg/kg/day throughout pregnancy resulted in increased perinatal mortality. Finally, rats given cyproheptadine by gastric intubation on days 6–15 of pregnancy manifested increased anomalies among their offspring when doses of 15 mg/kg/day were exceeded. In a recent study, rats were given cyproheptadine orally (11 mg/kg/day) on days 13 to 20. When the offspring were tested at 50 days of age, they manifested glucose intolerance, higher insulin levels in the pancreas, and an exaggeration of the insulin-lowering effect of cyproheptadine on the pancreas. For these reasons, it seems prudent to avoid this drug in pregnancy when other equally effective alternatives exist.

There is a single case report of a patient treated with cyproheptadine throughout pregnancy for Cushing's syndrome (since adrenocorticotropic hormone [ACTH] secretion may be dependent on serotonergic neurons) who delivered a normal baby at term. The baby died of gastroenteritis at age 4 months. In another case, the drug was discontinued at the end of the first trimester. The pregnancy outcome was normal.

Sadovsky and colleagues have reported the use of cyproheptadine to prevent recurrent abortion, but appropriate control groups were not described. Interestingly, when 29 women were given 4–16 mg/day during the first and second trimesters, no teratogenic effects were seen in the 23 term and 5 premature infants. Unfortunately, follow-up information on these neonates is not available. Although the rationale for this application was the ability of cyproheptadine to block serotonin-induced abortion in rats, this drug appears to be incapable of prolonging normal pregnancy in laboratory animals.

No data on breast-feeding by women taking cyproheptadine are currently available.

Dosage

Cyproheptadine is available as a 4 mg-tablet and as a syrup (2 mg/5 ml). The usual dose is 12–16 mg/day. Doses should not exceed 0.5 mg/kg/day.

Adverse Effects

Atropine-like effects include drowsiness, dry mouth, blurred vision, palpitations, tachycardia, thickening of bronchial secretions, and urinary retention. Hypotension may occur. Allergic manifestations, including anaphylactic shock, have also been reported.

Mechanism of Action

Cyproheptadine blocks both H_1 receptors and serotonin (5-hydroxytryptamine) receptors. Of particular value is its ability to block serotonin receptors in vascular smooth muscle and in the gastrointestinal tract. It also has anticholinergic and sedative effects.

Absorption and Biotransformation

This drug is only administered orally. Much of its elimination is urinary and is diminished in the presence of renal insufficiency.

Recommended Reading

Chow, S. A., and Fischer, L. J. Alterations in rat pancreatic B-cell function induced by prenatal exposure to cyproheptadine. *Diabetes* 33:572, 1984.

De la Fuente, M., and Alia, M. The teratogenicity of cyproheptadine in two generations of Wistar rats. *Arch. Int. Pharmacodyn. Ther.* 257:168, 1982.

Gilman, A. G., Goodman, L. S., and Gilman, A. *The Pharmacological Basis of Therapeutics* (6th ed.). New York: Macmillan, 1980. P. 639.

Kasperlik-Zaluska, A., et al. Two pregnancies in a woman with Cushing's syndrome treated with cyproheptadine. *Br. J. Obstet. Gynaecol.* 87:1171, 1980.

Khir, A. S. M., How, J., and Bewsher, P. D. Successful pregnancy after cyproheptadine treatment for Cushing's disease. *Eur. J. Obstet. Gynecol. Reprod. Biol.* 13:343, 1982.

Rodriguez Gonzalez, M. D., Lima Perez, M. T., and Sanabria Negrin, J. G. The effect of cyproheptadine chlorhydrate on rat embryonic development. *Teratogenesis Carcinog. Mutagen.* 3:439, 1983.

Sadovsky, E., et al. Attempts to delay labor in rats by a serotonin antagonist, cyproheptadine. *Isr. J. Med. Sci.* 9:1590, 1974.

Sadovsky, E., et al. The use of antiserotonin-cyproheptadine HCl in pregnancy: An experimental and clinical study. *Adv. Exp. Med. Biol.* 27:399, 1972.

Weinstein, D., et al. Teratogenicity of cyproheptadine in pregnant rats. *Arch. Int. Pharmacodyn. Ther.* 215:345, 1975.

Danazol (Danocrine®)

Indications and Recommendations

Danazol is contraindicated in pregnancy. This drug is a testosterone derivative and a weak androgen. As of 1984, 10 in 15 female fetuses exposed to danazol (800 mg/day) in utero and reported to the FDA had virilization of the external genitalia. All had fused labia, and 7 in 10 had clitoral hypertrophy. In each of these cases, it is presumed that the pregnancies were established at the time danazol exposure was commenced. No case of virilization was reported in which danazol had been discontinued before the eighth week of embryogenesis. Another case has been reported in which danazol was started in a dose of 400 mg/day at the time of the last menstrual period prior to conception. The fetus was exposed to danazol until the eighteenth week of pregnancy (documented by ultrasound), at which time the medication was discontinued. The female neonate had fused, scrotalized labia, clitoromegaly, and a well-defined median raphe. Internal genitalia have been female in all of these cases. Unfortunately, no satisfactory denominator figures are available for danazol exposure during pregnancy. Reports of urogenital sinus formation in danazol-exposed pregnancies have recently appeared, and the possibility exists that this anomaly may be induced by the drug.

Danazol was originally developed as a drug for the treatment of endometriosis. Pregnancy also has a suppressive effect on endometriosis, and therefore, it is unlikely that a pregnant woman would be taking danazol for this indication. Furthermore, when this drug is administered, ovulation is usually suppressed. Nevertheless, in at least one of the previously mentioned cases, ovulation presumably occurred while the patient was taking danazol.

Recently, reports have appeared suggesting that danazol may be useful in the treatment of immune thrombocytopenic purpura, classic hemophilia, and Christmas disease, and alpha-1 antitrypsin deficiency. It may be expected that, if these become legitimate indications for danazol therapy, more and more patients will be encountered who are started on this drug while unknowingly pregnant.

Recommended Reading

Ahn, Y. S., et al. Danazol for the treatment of idiopathic thrombocytopenic purpura. N. Engl. J. Med. 308:1396, 1983.

Garewal, H. S., et al. Effect of danazol on coagulation parameters and bleeding in hemophilia. J.A.M.A. 253:1154, 1985.

Gralnick, H. R., et al. Benefits of danazol treatment in patients with hemophilia A (classic hemophilia). J.A.M.A. 253:1151, 1985.

Marwick, C. . . . danazol for severe disease. J.A.M.A. 249:3279, 1983.

Peress, M. R., et al. Female pseudohermaphroditism with somatic chromosomal anomaly in association with in utero exposure to danazol. Am. J. Obstet. Gynecol. 142:708, 1982.

Quagliarello, J., and Greco, M. A. Danazol and urogenital sinus formation in pregnancy. Fertil. Steril. 43:939, 1985.

Rosa, F. W. Virilization of the female fetus with maternal danazol exposure. Am. J. Obstet. Gynecol. 149:99, 1984.

Shaw, R. W. Female pseudohermaphroditism associated with danazol exposure in utero. Case report. Br. J. Obstet. Gynaecol. 91:386, 1984.

Dextran: Dextran-40 (Rheomacrodex®), Dextran-70 (Macrodex®)

Indications and Recommendations

Dextran is relatively contraindicated during pregnancy because other therapeutic agents, for example, heparin, are preferable. This compound has been used in thromboembolism prophylaxis and as a plasma expander.

The antithrombotic actions of dextran include reduced platelet adhesiveness, platelet factor III depression, altered fibrin clot structure, and hemodilution of clotting factors. Factors V, VII, IX, and fibrinogen are decreased more than might be expected by hemodilution.

Dextran is available in a high molecular weight form (mol wt 70,000, Macrodex®) and a low molecular weight form (mol wt 40,000, Rheomacrodex®). Most of the former is sequestered by the reticuloendothelial system and slowly metabolized over days to weeks. The latter is readily filtered by the kidney with little reabsorption. While most authors have not found significant differences in the effectiveness of the two forms, some have reported better results with the dextran-70. This may be due to its prolonged clearance or a failure to infuse dextran-40 for a sufficiently long period.

Adverse effects include severe anaphylactic reactions as well as minor allergic responses such as rash, urticaria, nausea, and vomiting. Some bacterial polysaccharides demonstrate cross sensitivity to dextrans. These include group H streptococci, pneumococci, and types II, XII, and XX *Salmonella typhosa.* Plasma expansion may precipitate congestive heart failure in a borderline-compensated cardiac patient. Finally, the following laboratory tests may be artificially altered: blood glucose, bilirubin, total serum protein, and cross matches.

No information is available regarding adverse fetal effects.

Dextran is an effective plasma expander, and it reduces the incidence of thromboembolic disease when administered prophylactically. However, in patients with hypovolemia secondary to blood loss, clotting problems may be aggravated; in patients with infection caused by streptococci, pneumococci, and *Salmonella,* the risk of anaphylaxis may increase. There may also be interference created with blood cross matching at a time when this is critical. It is therefore recommended that heparin be used for the prophylaxis and therapy of thromboembolic disorders during pregnancy and that more physiologic plasma expanders be used preferentially.

Recommended Reading

Atik, M. Dextran 40 and dextran 70, a review. *Arch. Surg.* 94:664, 1967.

Data, J. L., and Nies, A. S. Dextran 40. *Ann. Intern. Med.* 81:500, 1974.

Gilman, A. G., Goodman, L. S., and Gilman, A. *The Pharmacological Basis of Therapeutics* (6th ed.). New York: Macmillan, 1980. Pp. 859–862.

Dextromethorphan (over-the-counter)

Indications and Recommendations

Dextromethorphan is safe to use during pregnancy. It is used for its antitussive properties.

Special Considerations in Pregnancy

Respiratory depression in the fetus is a theoretic possibility if a pregnant woman with severely impaired renal function takes the drug chronically up to the time of delivery.

Dosage

The usual dose is 10–20 mg 3 or 4 times a day. It is generally administered in syrup form, with 5 ml containing 10–15 mg dextromethorphan. It is also available as a lozenge. An effect is usually observed within 30 minutes.

Adverse Effects

Unlike codeine, dextromethorphan rarely produces drowsiness or gastrointestinal disturbances. Its toxicity is low, but in very high dosages, it may produce central nervous system depression.

Mechanism of Action

Dextromethorphan is the d-isomer of the codeine analog of levorphanol, but it has no analgesic or addictive properties. The drug acts centrally, raising the threshold for coughing.

Absorption and Biotransformation

Metabolism is believed to occur in the liver with excretion in the kidney.

Recommended Reading

Gilman, A. G., Goodman, L. S., and Gilman, A. *The Pharmacological Basis of Therapeutics* (6th ed.). New York: Macmillan, 1980. Pp. 529–530.

Nelson, M. M., and Forfar, J. O. Association between drugs administered during pregnancy and congenital abnormalities of the fetus. *Br. Med. J.* 1:523, 1971.

Schenkel, B., and Vorherr, H. Non-prescription drugs during pregnancy: Potential teratogenic and toxic effects upon embryo and fetus. *J. Reprod. Med.* 12:27, 1974.

Diazoxide (Hyperstat®)

Indications and Recommendations

The use of diazoxide during pregnancy is controversial, and if used at all, it should be reserved for patients with *severe* acute hypertensive episodes. This drug is a potent and rapidly acting antihypertensive agent and is marketed for the intravenous therapy of hypertensive emergencies. An oral preparation is available for the treatment of hypoglycemia, but this should not be used during pregnancy.

Diazoxide is rarely the drug of choice for the treatment of hypertension during pregnancy. When it is administered, the patient should have an intravenous infusion running and ideally should have been given sufficient fluid therapy before its use to raise the central venous pressure to measurable levels. Concurrently, the fetal heart rate should be monitored electronically. The mother's blood sugars should be monitored regularly and a cord blood glucose obtained from the neonate immediately after delivery. Recent studies suggest that during pregnancy, minibolus therapy is as effective as standard administration schedules and is far less likely to cause significant side effects. Whenever possible, this drug should not be used in combination with either hydralazine or methyldopa.

Hypotensive episodes following diazoxide administration should be treated with the rapid infusion of 1 or more liters of 5% dextrose in normal saline. The use of sympathomimetic agents such as norepinephrine to restore the blood pressure should be avoided unless there is no response to the infusion of fluid. This should almost never be necessary.

Special Considerations in Pregnancy

The most serious potential side effect after the intravenous administration of a 150- or 300-mg bolus of diazoxide to a toxemic patient is significant hypotension. Several series have shown some diastolic pressure drops to 50–60 mm Hg in patients with initial readings of 100 mm Hg or higher. In a number of these patients, there was also concomitant fetal bradycardia. Severe hypotensive responses have been specifically related to the potentiating effects of other vasodilators (e.g., hydralazine) or catecholamine-depleting drugs (e.g., methyldopa or reserpine) given either before or subsequent to the administration of diazoxide.

Because sodium and water are retained when diazoxide is used, the concomitant use of furosemide has been advised for the medical patient. The use of potent diuretics, however, is probably ill advised in toxemic patients with significant hypovolemia.

Since diazoxide stops uterine contractions and termination of the pregnancy is an integral part of the management of severely hypertensive, toxemic patients, intravenous oxytocin to induce labor must be given if vaginal delivery is to be accomplished. Hyperglycemia must be looked for in both mother and neonate.

Diazoxide crosses the placenta, but when it is given intravenously, it seems to have little effect on the fetus. Fetal hyperglycemia may be produced, but there are very few circulatory alterations. Several cases of prolonged neonatal hyperglycemia have been reported in premature infants of women treated with standard bolus doses. The term fetus seems to rapidly clear the drug. The authors of one animal study in which the diazoxide dosage was several-fold higher than that used in humans described necrosis of the fetal pancreas.

When diazoxide is given orally to pregnant women for several weeks, newborn alopecia, lanuginous hypertrichosis, and decreased bone age have been reported.

Dosage

The standard recommendation is to rapidly inject a bolus of 300 mg or 5 mg/kg body weight of diazoxide within a period of 10–30 seconds. The dependence of the hypotensive effect on the injection rate is related to the rapidity with which the drug is bound by serum albumin. The hypotensive effect will be noted within 5 minutes; thereafter, blood pressure increases gradually and returns to pretreatment levels within 3–15 hours. If the initial response is unsatisfactory, the dose may be repeated in 30 minutes.

Recent studies have indicated that low or minibolus diazoxide therapy in severely hypertensive pregnant women can be as efficacious as standard bolus treatment while significantly reducing maternal and fetal morbidity. In one study, 11 gravid hypertensive patients with diastolic blood pressures of 110 mm Hg or greater were given 60-mg boluses of diazoxide and compared with 10 matched patients who were given 150-mg boluses at similar intervals. Only one patient in the first group, but three in the second, became hypotensive and had associated fetal heart rate decelerations. Another investigation utilized 30-mg boluses given over 30–60 seconds in 34 gravid women with blood pressures in excess of 160/115 mm Hg. These boluses were administered every 1–2 minutes until the diastolic blood pressure fell below 90 mm Hg. The average dose required to achieve this goal was 120 mg, and all 34 patients responded within 5–10 minutes. Each of these women was delivered within 6 hours of initiating therapy. No hypotensive episodes were noted, and no neonatal hyperglycemia was observed. Maternal hyperglycemia and sodium and water retention were also minimal with this regimen.

It may be that the decrease in maternal protein concentration that occurs during pregnancy results in higher levels of free drug and proportionally lower amounts of the protein-bound fraction when small boluses of diazoxide are injected. This could be the reason why smaller dosages can be given more slowly to pregnant patients, yet lower their blood pressure effectively while minimizing significant side effects.

Adverse Effects

Since cardiovascular reflexes and the sympathetic nervous system function normally, diazoxide rarely causes postural hypotension. Sodium and water retention usually occur because of the drug's direct tubular antinatriuretic effect. Hyperglycemia may occur because of reduced insulin secretion by the pancreatic beta cells as well as a direct effect on the liver to increase its rate of glucose release. Mild hyperuricemia may be noted. A direct relaxation of uterine musculature can cause labor to stop. Finally, symptoms associated with the sympathetic reflex response to vasodilatation may occur.

Mechanism of Action

Diazoxide primarily relaxes arteriolar smooth muscle in all circulatory beds, which results in a reduction of vascular resistance. In association with this reduction in arterial pressure, there is a reflex increase in heart rate, stroke volume, and cardiac output, which may partially counteract the hypotensive effect of the vascular dilatation. Blood flow through all circulatory beds is generally well maintained, and renal blood flow and glomerular filtration rate are usually unchanged or increased.

Absorption and Biotransformation

The drug is primarily eliminated from the body by glomerular filtration. The serum half-life is normally 20–30 hours, but 90% of the drug is rapidly bound to albumin after intravenous administration. Since only the free drug is active, diazoxide must be administered every 4–12 hours, despite the long half-life in serum.

Recommended Reading

Boulous, M. M., et al. Placental transfer of diazoxide and its hazardous effect on the newborn. *J. Clin. Pharmacol.* 11:206, 1971.

Davey, M., Moodley, J., and Soutter, P. Adverse effects of a combination of diazoxide and hydralazine therapy. *S. Afr. Med. J.* 59:496, 1981.

DiOrio, J., Jr., and Brauner, R. E. Adult respiratory distress syndrome occurring after therapy with diazoxide and betamethasone for premature labor: A case report. *R.I. Med. J.* 65:275, 1982.

Dudley, D. K. L. Minibolus diazoxide in the management of severe hypertension in pregnancy. *Am. J. Obstet. Gynecol.* 151:196, 1985.

Henrich, W. L., et al. Hypotensive sequelae of diazoxide and hydralazine therapy. *J.A.M.A.* 237:264, 1977.

Kelly, J. V. Drugs used in the management of toxemia of pregnancy. *Clin. Obstet. Gynecol* 20:395, 1977.

Koch-Weser, J. Diazoxide. *N. Engl. J. Med.* 294:1271, 1976.

Michael, C. A. Intravenous diazoxide in the treatment of severe preeclamptic toxaemia and eclampsia. *Aust. N.Z. J. Obstet. Gynaecol.* 13:143, 1973.

Milsap, R. L., and Auld, P. A. Neonatal hyperglycemia following maternal diazoxide administration. *J.A.M.A.* 243:144, 1980.

Morris, J. A., et al. The management of severe pre-eclampsia and eclampsia with intravenous diazoxide. *Obstet. Gynecol.* 49:675, 1977.

Neurman, J., et al. Diazoxide for the acute control of severe hypertension complicating pregnancy: A pilot study. *Obstet. Gynecol.* 53(Suppl.):50S, 1979.

Redman, C. W. G. The use of antihypertensive drugs in hypertension in pregnancy. *Clin. Obstet. Gynecol.* 4:685, 1977.

Smith, M. J., Aynsley-Green, A., and Redman, C. W. Neonatal hyperglycemia after prolonged maternal treatment with diazoxide. *Br. Med. J. Clin. Res.* 284:1234, 1982.

Diethylpropion (Tenuate®, Tepanil®)

Indications and Recommendations

Weight reduction is not indicated during pregnancy. For this reason, diethylpropion, a sympathomimetic anorectic agent, is contraindicated during pregnancy. There are no reports linking this drug with congenital malformations. There is a retrospective case-control study comparing 1,232 women who took the drug during pregnancy with an equal number of control subjects, in which no increased incidence of malformations was demonstrated. Therefore, a history of having taken the drug during pregnancy should not be considered an indication for pregnancy termination.

Recommended Reading

Bunde, C. A., and Leyland, H. M. A controlled retrospective survey in evaluation of teratogenicity. *J. New Drugs* 5:193, 1965.

Gilman, A. G., Goodman, L. S., and Gilman, A. *The Pharmacological Basis of Therapeutics* (6th ed.). New York: Macmillan, 1980. Pp. 171–172.

Silverman, M., and Okun, R. The use of an appetite suppressant (diethylpropion hydrochloride) during pregnancy. *Curr. Ther. Res.* 13:648, 1971.

Digoxin (Lanoxin®)

Indications and Recommendations

Digoxin is safe to use during pregnancy if the mother's blood levels are monitored frequently to avoid toxicity and to ensure adequate digitalization. Digoxin is the most frequently prescribed of the digitalis glycosides, a group of drugs used in the treatment of congestive heart failure and atrial fibrillation and in the prevention of paroxysmal atrial tachycardia.

Special Considerations in Pregnancy

Serum levels should be monitored in pregnant women near term to ensure maintenance of therapeutic levels. Digoxin levels in the mother at term are usually significantly lower than levels taken several weeks post partum on the same maintenance dosage.

The digitalis glycosides readily cross the placenta. They seem to be preferentially concentrated in the fetal heart during the second half of pregnancy. Amniotic fluid levels of digoxin have been used to monitor fetal levels. Levels of the drug in the amniotic fluid slightly exceed those in fetal serum. In a study of 11 mothers who received digoxin throughout pregnancy for rheumatic heart disease, paired cord and maternal blood samples obtained at parturition showed lower digoxin levels in cord blood than that of the mother. The total tissue-bound digoxin level in the placenta, however, correlated closely with maternal digoxin levels. Neonates and presumably the fetus seem to tolerate high serum levels of digoxin (2–4 ng/ml) much better than adults.

Digoxin has been used to treat a variety of fetal arrhythmias. When used for this indication, the mother should be fully digitalized and then followed with determination of serum digitalis and potassium levels. The therapeutic effect on the fetus can be followed with serial fetal echocardiograms.

Digoxin is excreted in maternal milk. Digoxin milk-plasma ratios vary from 0.6–0.9 in several pharmacokinetic studies. The total daily amount excreted, however, is far below the usual therapeutic dosage for a newborn.

Dosage

The usual initial digitalizing dose is approximately 1.0 mg. This may be given orally or parenterally in several divided doses. The usual maintenance dose is approximately 0.25 mg/day. Serum levels must be monitored carefully to avoid toxicity. The therapeutic plasma levels are 0.5–2.0 ng/ml in adults. In some patients with atrial fibrillation, levels of 2.5–4.0 ng/ml may be required to slow the ventricular rate.

Adverse Effects

Side effects of digoxin, which are rare when the drug is given in therapeutic dosages, include skin rashes, eosinophilia, and gynecomastia. Toxic effects of the digitalis derivatives include gastrointestinal symptoms of anorexia, nausea, and vomiting; visual changes; and alterations of cardiac rate and rhythm, especially extrasystoles and heart block. These toxic effects may be seen in patients with digoxin levels greater than 3 ng/ml. Digitalis toxicity can be potentiated by hypokalemia.

Mechanism of Action

The exact mechanism of action of digoxin is not known. The main pharmacologic action of all digitalis glycosides is to increase the force and velocity of the myocardial contraction. They have a direct action on both the failing and nonfailing heart. When given to patients in congestive heart failure, cardiac output is increased, systolic emptying is more complete, and end-diastolic volumes and pressures are reduced. Sympathetic tone is reduced, and in edematous patients, diuresis results. Digitalis glycosides also decrease conduction velocity through the atrioventricular node. This effect is most apparent in patients with supraventricular tachyarrhythmias.

Absorption and Biotransformation

Approximately 65–80% of an oral digoxin dose is absorbed. Only about 25% is bound to plasma proteins, and it is primarily excreted unchanged in the urine. The half-life of digoxin is approximately 36 hours and increases as renal function diminishes.

Recommended Reading

Allonen, H., Kanto, J., and Iisalo, E. The foeto-maternal distribution of digoxin in early human pregnancy. *Acta Pharmacol. Toxicol.* 39:477, 1976.

Chan, V., Tse, T. F., and Wong, V. Transfer of digoxin across the placenta and into breast milk. *Br. J. Obstet. Gynaecol.* 85:605, 1978.

Finley, J. P., et al. Digoxin excretion in human milk (letter). *J. Pediatr.* 94:339, 1979.

Levy, M., Granit, L, and Laufer, N. Excretion of drugs in human milk. *N. Engl. J. Med.* 297:789, 1977.

Loughnan, P. M. Digoxin excretion in human breast milk. *J. Pediatr.* 92:1019, 1978.

Rasmussen, R., Nawaz, M., and Steiness. E. Mammary excretion of digoxin in goats. *Acta Pharmacol. Toxicol.* 36:377, 1975.

Rogers, M. C., et al. Serum digoxin concentrations in the human fetus, neonate and infant. *N. Engl. J. Med.* 287:1010, 1972.

Saarikoski, S. Placental transfer and fetal uptake of ^{3}H digoxin in humans. *Br. J. Obstet. Gynaecol.* 83:879, 884, 1976.

Seyka, L. F. Digoxin: Placental transfer, effects on the fetus, and therapeutic use in the newborn. *Clin. Perinatol.* 2:23, 1975.

Dimenhydrinate (Dramamine®)

Indications and Recommendations

Dimenhydrinate is contraindicated during pregnancy. It is an antihistamine used in the prevention and treatment of nausea and vomiting associated with motion sickness. In one placebo-controlled study, the intravenous injection of dimenhydrinate was associated with a significantly increased level of uterine activity (as documented by internal pressure monitoring); this drug has also been anecdotally implicated with an increased incidence of premature labor. Meclizine is therefore preferable for the treatment of motion sickness during pregnancy.

Recommended Reading

American Hospital Formulary Service. *Monograph for Dimenhydrinate.* Washington, D.C.: American Society of Hospital Pharmacists, May, 1977.

Gilman, A. G., Goodman, L. S., and Gilman, A. *The Pharmacological Basis of Therapeutics* (6th ed.). New York: Macmillan, 1980. P. 628.

Long, J. W. *The Essential Guide to Prescription Drugs.* New York: Harper & Row, 1977. Pp. 250–251.

Shephard, B., Cruz, A., and Spellacy, W. The acute effects of Dramamine on uterine contractility during labor. *J. Reprod. Med.* 16:27, 1976.

Diphenhydramine (Benadryl®)

Indications and Recommendations

Diphenhydramine may be administered during pregnancy for the treatment of allergic disorders characterized by urticaria, pruritus, and rhinitis. It is the drug of choice for treatment of the oculogyric crisis resulting from phenothiazine administration and is useful in controlling other drug and blood transfusion reactions. Because of its possible association with an increased incidence of oral clefts, diphenhydramine should not be used in the first trimester for reducing self-limited symptoms or the discomfort of allergies. This drug is not recommended for use by nursing mothers since it may inhibit lactation; small amounts may be excreted in breast milk.

Special Considerations in Pregnancy

No prospective studies have been conducted that evaluate the safety of diphenhydramine's use during pregnancy. One large retrospective study, however, found no evidence incriminating this drug as a teratogen. In contrast with these findings, another, smaller, case-controlled study comparing groups of children with and without oral clefts found that the intake of diphenhydramine was significantly more frequent among the mothers of children with clefts. This was not true for mothers who had taken cyclizine. A presumed withdrawal syndrome has been reported in a single newborn exposed to large doses (150 mg/day, duration of therapy not stated) in utero.

Dosage

The usual oral dose is 50 mg taken 3 or 4 times a day. If parenteral administration is required, 10–50 mg may be given intravenously or by deep intramuscular injection. The maximum daily dose is 400 mg.

Adverse Effects

Anticholinergic side effects are most common; these include drowsiness, dry mouth and eyes, and rarely, blurred vision. Anorexia, nausea, epigastric distress, and dizziness can also occur.

Mechanism of Action

Diphenhydramine is a competitive antagonist of histamine that decreases edema formation by diminishing capillary dilatation and permeability. It has anticholinergic activity and therefore reduces the tremor and rigidity of parkinsonism. It produces drowsiness and possesses local anesthetic ability when used topically.

Absorption and Biotransformation

Diphenhydramine is rapidly absorbed when taken orally or from sites of parenteral administration. When taken orally, the maximum effects are noted within 1 hour, and the duration of action is 4–6 hours; that is, it reaches peak tissue concentrations in about 1 hour, and the tissues are almost depleted of the drug in about 6 hours. The main site of metabolic transformation is the liver, and excretion occurs via the kidney.

Recommended Reading

Gilman, A. G., Goodman, L. S., and Gilman, A. *The Pharmacological Basis of Therapeutics* (6th ed.). New York: Macmillan, 1980. Pp. 623–628.

Greenberger, P., and Patterson, R. Safety of therapy for allergic symptoms during pregnancy. *Ann. Intern. Med.* 89:234, 1978.

Heinonen, O. P., Slone, D., and Shapiro, S. *Birth Defects and Drugs in Pregnancy*. Littleton, Mass.: Publishing Sciences Group, 1977. Pp. 323–334.

Nashimura, H., and Tanimura, T. *Aspects of the Teratogenicity of Drugs*. Amsterdam: Excerpta Medica, 1976.

Parkin, D. E. Probable Benadryl withdrawal manifestations in a newborn infant. *J. Pediatr.* 85:580, 1974.

Saxen, I. Cleft palate and maternal diphenhydramine intake. *Lancet* 1:407, 1974.

Diphenoxylate (Lomotil®, When Combined with Atropine)

Indications and Recommendations

Diphenoxylate, a narcotic structurally related to meperidine, is safe to use during pregnancy. It is combined with atropine (to prevent abuse) and used as an antidiarrheal agent.

Special Considerations in Pregnancy

Only one case report of congenital malformations in an infant exposed to diphenoxylate in utero was found. That infant was exposed to the drug on days 104–110 of gestation, long after the cleft palate, cardiac defect, absent tibiae, and polydactyly had occurred. In addition, the infant was exposed to at least five other drugs (excluding vitamins) in utero. In the Collaborative Perinatal Project, seven infants were exposed to diphenoxylate in utero during the first 4 months, and no congenital malformations were found. Despite this paucity of data, the similarity of diphenoxylate to meperidine suggests that the drug is probably safe for pregnant women. Because this drug is excreted in breast milk and because diphenoxylate is considered to be contraindicated in children up to 2 years of age (severe toxic reactions may occur at presumably therapeutic dosages), breast-feeding mothers should not take the drug.

Dosage

Diphenoxylate is available as a tablet containing 2.5 mg combined with 0.025 mg atropine, and as a liquid containing the same dose in 5 ml. The usual adult dose is two tablets or 10 ml of liquid 4 times/day until diarrhea is controlled, usually within 48 hours.

Adverse Effects

Allergic reactions have been reported. In addition, some patients have reported abdominal distention, drowsiness, dizziness, depression, restlessness, nausea, headache, and blurred vision. Intestinal obstruction and toxic megacolon have occurred in patients with inflammatory bowel disease or parasitic colitis. Overdosage can lead to morphinelike symptoms.

The atropine added to this compound can give rise to typical atropinic side effects, especially when overdosage occurs.

Mechanism of Action

Diphenoxylate, a congener of meperidine, has a constipating effect similar to that of other opiates. This effect occurs at dosages considerably lower than those necessary to cause euphoria or physical dependence.

Absorption and Biotransformation

Diphenoxylate is rapidly absorbed after oral dosing, reaching peak plasma levels at approximately 2 hours. The half-life is approximately 12 hours. The drug is rapidly hydrolyzed to its active metabolite, which is diphenoxylic acid. Approximately 15% of diphenoxylate is excreted in the urine, and 50% is excreted in the stools.

A unique feature of diphenoxylate is the insolubility of the drug or its salts in aqueous solution, thus making parenteral drug abuse virtually impossible.

Recommended Reading

AMA Drug Evaluations (5th ed.). Chicago: American Medical Association, 1983. Pp. 1287–1288.

Gilman, A. G., Goodman, L. S., and Gilman, A. *The Pharmacological Basis of Therapeutics* (6th ed.). New York: Macmillan, 1980. P. 517.

Heinonen, O. P., Slone, D., and Shapiro, S. *Birth Defects and Drugs in Pregnancy.* Boston: John Wright PSG, 1977. P. 287.

Ho, C. K., Kaufman, R. L., and McAllister, W. H. Congenital malformations: Cleft palate, congenital heart disease, absent tibiae, and polydactyly. *Am. J. Dis. Child.* 129:714, 1975.

Dipyridamole (Persantine®)

Indications and Recommendations

Dipyridamole is indicated during pregnancy for the prevention of arterial thrombosis in patients with prosthetic heart valves. It is not indicated for the prophylaxis or treatment of venous thromboembolic disease. Although a full anticoagulant dosage of heparin has been the standard therapy for pregnant women with prosthetic valves, a combination of dipyridamole and aspirin has been used increasingly for this purpose.

Dipyridamole plus aspirin has been used to treat women who have been shown to have a circulating "lupus anticoagulant." This combination may prove to be useful as an adjunct to prednisone if active lupus erythematosus is present.

Dipyridamole is also used as a coronary vasodilator in patients with chronic angina pectoris. Fortunately, this condition is rare during pregnancy.

Special Considerations in Pregnancy

Dipyridamole has been used in an attempt to prevent preeclampsia-toxemia in women at risk for that condition. Administration of the drug to prevent preeclampsia-toxemia is controversial, and therefore, such therapy should only be attempted as part of a research protocol.

Dipyridamole given as a single 30-mg intravenous dose to 10 gravidas in the third trimester was demonstrated to increase uterine perfusion. There are no data available on the ability of dipyridamole to cross the placenta. In the cases reported to date, no adverse fetal effects have been noted.

Dosage

The usual oral dose is between 75 and 300 mg/day in three divided doses. When dipyridamole is used in combination with aspirin in patients who have the lupus anticoagulant, the dose is 225–300 mg/day.

Adverse Effects

In standard dosages, dipyridamole is nontoxic. Occasionally encountered side effects include nausea, vomiting, and diarrhea as well as headache and vertigo. With suprapharmacologic dosages of dipyridamole, peripheral vasodilatation and hypotension may occur.

Mechanism of Action

The mechanism of action of dipyridamole is not known. Like papaverine, it nonspecifically relaxes smooth muscle. It has been suggested that vasodilatation is related to a papaverinelike ability to inhibit cyclic nucleotide phosphodiesterase. Dipyridamole inhibits the uptake of adenosine by erythrocytes and other cells. In therapeutic dosages, the drug produces only slight alteration of systemic blood pressure or peripheral blood flow. Dipyridamole acts predominantly on the small resistance vessels of the coronary bed and seems to augment transcapillary exchange.

Dipyridamole in combination with aspirin prolongs the survival of platelets in patients with thrombotic disease. In this regard, the drug *by itself* has little or no clinical effect. It may interfere with platelet function by potentiating the effect of prostacyclin (PGI_2) or by inhibiting cyclic nucleotide phosphodiesterase activity, thereby increasing the intracellular concentration of cyclic AMP.

Absorption and Biotransformation

The drug is metabolized in the liver and is excreted unchanged or as its glucuronide conjugate in feces.

Recommended Reading

Beaufils, M., et al. Prevention of pre-eclampsia by early antiplatelet therapy. *Lancet* 1:840, 1985.

Biale, Y., et al. The course of pregnancy in patients with artificial heart valves treated with dipyridamole. *Intl. J. Gynaecol. Obstet.* 18:128, 1980.

Gilman, A. G., Goodman, L. S., and Gilman, A. *The Pharmacological Basis of Therapeutics* (6th ed.). New York: Macmillan, 1980. P. 830.

Lauchkner, W., Schwarz, R., and Retzke, U. Cardiovascular action of dipyridamole in advanced pregnancy. *Zentralbl. Gynakol.* 103:220, 1981.

Lubbe, W. F., et al. Lupus anticoagulant in pregnancy. *Br. J. Obstet. Gynaecol.* 91:357, 1984.

Moncada, S., and Korbut, R. Dipyridamole and other phosphodiesterase inhibitors act as antithrombotic agent by potentiating endogenous prostacyclin. *Lancet* 1:1286, 1978.

Disopyramide (Norpace®)

Indications and Recommendations

Disopyramide is relatively contraindicated during pregnancy because other therapeutic agents are preferable. This drug is an oral antiarrhythmic agent with electrophysiologic actions similar to those of quinidine and procainamide. It is used in the treatment of premature ventricular contractions and episodes of ventricular or supraventricular tachycardia. Its use during pregnancy has been associated with the initiation of uterine contractions that subsided when the drug was discontinued. Therefore, if a class 1 antiarrhythmic is required during pregnancy, quinidine should be given.

Recommended Reading

Befeler, B., et al. Electrophysiologic effects of the antiarrhythmic agent disopyramide phosphate. *Am. J. Cardiol.* 35:282, 1975.

Leonard, R. F., Braun, T. E., and Levy, A. M. Initiation of uterine contractions by disopyramide during pregnancy. *N. Engl. J. Med.* 299:84, 1978.

Disulfiram (Antabuse®)

Indications and Recommendations

The use of disulfiram (tetraethylthiuram disulfide) is contraindicated in pregnancy. This substance, if taken in combination with alcohol, causes extremely high acetaldehyde concentrations, which lead to generalized vasodilatation, feelings of warmth, throbbing headache, nausea, vomiting, respiratory difficulties, chest pain, hypotension, thirst, and other adverse signs and symptoms. Collectively, these are called the *acetaldehyde syndrome.* As a consequence, the drug is useful in helping to motivate alcoholic individuals to avoid alcohol.

Disulfiram has not been shown to be teratogenic in laboratory animals. Among nine exposed human infants uncovered by a literature search, two had clubfoot anomalies, one had phocomelia, one had a constellation of anomalies of the extremities and vertebral column, one had microcephaly and mental retardation, one had Pierre Robin syndrome, and three were normal. The true number of exposures in the population is not known. Although alcohol is known to be a teratogen, the mothers of these infants were reported to be alcohol free during their pregnancies. It is currently not known if alcohol intake before conception may be teratogenic.

Since alternative psychosocial interventions may be successful in treating alcoholism, the use of disulfiram appears to be unjustified during pregnancy. When a pregnant individual who has been taking disulfiram is counseled, she should be made aware of the available data and supported in whatever decision she makes regarding continuation of the pregnancy.

Recommended Reading

Dehaene, P., Titran, M., and DuBois, D. Syndrome de Pierre Robin et malformations cardiaques chez un nouveau-ne-role du disulfirame pendant la grossesse? *La Presse Médicale* 13:1394, 1984.

Favre-Tissot, M., and DeLatour, P. Psychopharmacologie et teratogenese a propos du disulfirame: Essai experimental. *Ann. Med. Psychol.* 1:735, 1965.

Gilman, A. G., Goodman, L. S., and Gilman, A. *The Pharmacological Basis of Therapeutics* (6th ed.). New York: Macmillan, 1980. Pp. 387–388.

Nora, A. H., Nora, J. J., and Blu, J. Limb-reduction anomalies in infants born to disulfiram-treated alcoholic mothers. *Lancet* 2:664, 1977.

Robens, J. F. Teratologic studies of carbaryl, diazinon, norea, disulfiram, and thiram in small laboratory animals. *Toxicol. Appl. Pharmacol.* 15:152, 1969.

Diuretics, Mercurial (Mercuhydrin®, Thiomerin®)

Indications and Recommendations

Mercurial diuretics should not be used during pregnancy. In the rare instances when diuretics are needed to treat the pregnant woman (e.g., chronic hypertension, cardiogenic edema, chronic renal disease), other agents are preferable (the thiazide diuretics or furosemide). The diuretic effect of mercurial diuretics is caused by the intrarenal release of free mercury cations. These act on the tubular cell membranes to inhibit the reabsorption of sodium and chloride and the excretion of potassium. Classic symptoms of systemic mercury poisoning may follow the injudicious use of these agents, especially in patients with poor renal function.

Poisoning of the fetus by organic mercury has been well documented in the tragic "natural experiment" that took place in Japan in the early 1960s. Local fishermen who consumed methylmercury in shellfish caught in Minamata Bay developed a bizarre neurologic syndrome. The methylmercury was traced to contamination of the bay by factory effluents. Affected individuals gave birth to congenitally anomalous babies with high perinatal mortality. Infants born to apparently asymptomatic mothers also developed cerebral palsy–like symptoms that varied in severity from mild spasticity to severe mental retardation and death. The type of compound used as a mercurial diuretic, however, was not implicated in this mercury poisoning syndrome.

Recommended Reading

Gilman, A. G., Goodman, L. S., and Gilman, A. *The Pharmacological Basis of Therapeutics* (6th ed.). New York: Macmillan, 1980. Pp. 896–899.

Joselow, M. M., Louria, D. B., and Browder, A. A. Mercurialism: Environmental and occupational aspects. *Ann. Intern. Med.* 76:119, 1972.

Diuretics, Thiazide: Chlorothiazide (Diuril®), Hydrochlorothiazide (HydroDIURIL®)

Indications and Recommendations

The use of the thiazides during pregnancy is controversial, and if used at all, they should be restricted to very specific situations. These drugs are diuretics and have antihypertensive activity in some patients with essential hypertension. The administration of thiazides does not prevent the development of preeclampsia-toxemia (PET), and these drugs have no role in the therapy of that condition. They also should not be used for the treatment of peripheral edema in the pregnant woman.

Since thiazides may decrease placental perfusion, controversy exists over the use of these drugs during pregnancy in patients with chronic hypertension. If started before conception, there is no strong evidence to suggest that continued therapy will compromise fetal growth. Some authors therefore recommend leaving a patient on this medication if it has been successfully used to control documented hypertension prior to the pregnancy. If, on the other hand, it becomes necessary to initiate treatment after the patient has become pregnant, the combination of a thiazide and methyldopa may reduce the potential for decreased placental perfusion. Some authors have recommended that the initiation of therapy with the thiazides be limited to the first half of pregnancy.

Frequent determinations of serum electrolytes should be made in pregnant women taking thiazide diuretics. Such women will frequently need oral potassium supplementation. Fetal growth should also be monitored closely throughout the period of therapy.

Thiazide diuretics may be given to breast-feeding mothers.

Special Considerations in Pregnancy

It is known that in PET many patients have a decreased intravascular volume. The administration of thiazides will reduce this further. Gant and colleagues have demonstrated a reduced metabolic clearance rate of dehydroepiandrosterone sulfate (MCR_{DS}) in 9 in 10 pregnant women studied on the seventh day of thiazide therapy, which may represent decreased placental perfusion. These facts suggest that the administration of thiazides may compromise optimal fetal oxygenation and nutrition, especially in fetuses of patients with PET.

Sibai, Grossman, and colleagues performed a randomized prospective investigation on 20 women with mild chronic hypertension who were receiving diuretics when seen in the first trimester. Half of these women were allowed to continue their diuretic medication throughout the pregnancy while the other 10 patients had this medication discontinued at the time of their first visit. The initial plasma volumes were similar in both groups, but serial studies showed a marked reduction of plasma volume in the diuretic as compared to the control group. While those who stopped taking the diuretics had a mean increase of 52% in plasma volume, as pregnancy progressed the diuretic group had a mean increase of only

18%. The difference was most pronounced at 26–32 weeks. Two patients in the diuretic group and one of the control subjects required the addition of methyldopa for blood pressure control. Despite the relative reduction in plasma volume in the treated group, there was no significant difference in gestational age at birth, birth weight, placental weight, or superimposed PET when compared to the control group. Although the number of patients studied was small, this well-designed study suggests that in chronic hypertensive pregnancies, diuretics may prevent normal plasma expansion without influencing perinatal outcome.

An additional problem that may occur when thiazides are given to pregnant women is maternal hyperuricemia. This rarely requires therapy but may mask the increase in serum uric acid that is often seen in association with developing PET. The thiazides cross the placenta and may cause symptomatic neonatal hyponatremia, hypokalemia, and thrombocytopenia.

Placental transfer of hydrochlorothiazide was studied in 10 term pregnancies in which mothers being treated for edema or hypertension were given 50 mg/day at least 2 weeks before delivery. Maternal and umbilical venous blood and amniotic fluid were collected at delivery in each of these cases. Analysis of the samples revealed that hydrochlorothiazide concentrations in umbilical cord plasma approached those in maternal plasma, while amniotic fluid levels were higher than those in either maternal or fetal blood.

The drugs are excreted in breast milk, but the amount of chlorothiazide that appears in the milk is probably too small to cause an adverse effect in the nursing infant.

Dosage

These drugs are usually given orally, with the diuretic effect occurring within 1–2 hours of absorption. The peak effect occurs in 4 hours and lasts about 6–12 hours. The two most commonly used thiazide diuretics are administered as follows:

Diuretic	Minimal	Usual	Maximal
Chlorothiazide	500 mg qd	500 mg bid	750 mg bid
Hydrochlorothiazide	50 mg qd	50 mg bid	75 mg bid

Adverse Effects

Side effects include hyponatremia, hypokalemia, and metabolic alkalosis. Hyperglycemia and allergic dermatitis with photosensitivity may occur. Occasionally pancreatitis, leukopenia, thrombocytopenia, and vasculitis may occur.

Mechanism of Action

The primary mode of action of thiazide diuretics is inhibition of electrolyte reabsorption in the distal tubules of the nephron. This results in an increase in sodium, chloride, and potassium excretion along with accompanying water. Uric acid excretion is also inhibited.

The thiazides cause an initial reduction in extracellular and plasma volume and a concurrent decrease in cardiac output. In nonpregnant patients, the effect is transient, and in 1–2 weeks, the plasma volume and cardiac output return to normal levels, although a reduction in peripheral resistance is maintained. The persistent hypotensive effect may be secondary to either a direct action on the arteriolar smooth muscle or to changes of electrolyte concentration in the vessel wall. The latter could influence tone or pressor responsiveness. The autonomic reflexes essential for cardiovascular homeostasis are unimpaired. Plasma renin increases in response to sodium depletion and may remain increased throughout the time the drug is administered.

Absorption and Biotransformation

The thiazides are not metabolized in the body. They are rapidly absorbed from the gastrointestinal tract, distributed throughout the extracellular space, and then excreted unchanged in the urine.

Recommended Reading

Beermann, B., et al. Placental transfer of hydrochlorothiazide. *Gynecol. Obstet. Invest.* 11:45, 1980.

Gant, N. F., et al. The metabolic clearance rate of dehydroisoandrosterone sulfate: III. The effect of thiazide diuretics in normal and future pre-eclamptic pregnancy. *Am. J. Obstet. Gynecol.* 123:159, 1975.

Gifford, R. W., Jr. A guide to the practical use of diuretics. *J.A.M.A.* 235:1890, 1976.

Gilman, A. G., Goodman, L. S., and Gilman, A. *The Pharmacological Basis of Therapeutics* (6th ed.). New York: Macmillan, 1980. Pp. 899–903.

Krumlovsky, F. A., and delGreco, F. Diuretic agents: Mechanisms of action and clinical uses. *Postgrad. Med.* 59:105, 1976.

Pritchard, J. A. Standardized treatment of 154 consecutive cases of eclampsia. *Am. J. Obstet. Gynecol.* 123:543, 1975.

Pritchard, J. A., and MacDonald, P. *Williams Obstetrics* (15th ed.). New York: Appleton-Century-Crofts, 1976.

Sibai, B. M., Grossman, R. A., and Grossman, H. G. Effects of diuretics on plasma volume in pregnancies with long-term hypertension. *Am. J. Obstet. Gynecol.* 150:831, 1984.

Sibai, B. M., et al. Plasma volume findings in pregnant women with mild hypotension: Therapeutic considerations. *Am. J. Obstet. Gynecol.* 145:539, 1983.

Werthmann, M. W., Jr., and Krees, S. V. Excretion of chlorothiazide in human breast milk. *J. Pediatr.* 81:781, 1972.

Docusates (over-the-counter) (Colace®, Doxinate®, Surfak®)

Indications and Recommendations

Docusates are safe to use during pregnancy. These drugs are used as stool softeners in people with hemorrhoids, anorectal disorders, hernias, and cardiovascular disease. They are widely used for women recovering from third- and fourth-degree perineal lacerations after delivery of their infants.

Special Considerations in Pregnancy

There are no special considerations to be kept in mind during pregnancy.

Dosage

Docusates vary in dosage from 50–480 mg/day taken by mouth. An effect is seen within 24–48 hours. Rectal preparations of 50–100 mg are also available.

Adverse Effects

An overdose may cause anorexia, diarrhea, and vomiting.

Mechanism of Action

Docusates soften the fecal mass by lowering surface tension, thus facilitating penetration of water and fats.

Absorption and Biotransformation

Docusates manifest no systemic effects because of their limited absorption, although a small portion is absorbed from the gastrointestinal tract and excreted in the bile.

Recommended Reading

Gilman, A. G., Goodman, L. S., and Gilman, A. *The Pharmacological Basis of Therapeutics* (6th ed.). New York: Macmillan, 1980. Pp. 1008–1009.

Nelson, M. M., and Forfar, J. O. Associations between drugs administered during pregnancy and congenital abnormalities of the fetus. *Br. Med. J.* 1:523, 1971.

Schenkel, B., and Vorherr, H. Non-prescription drugs during pregnancy: Potential teratogenic and toxic effects upon embryo and fetus. *J. Reprod. Med.* 12:27, 1974.

Dopamine (Intropin®)

Indications and Recommendations

The use of dopamine in pregnancy should be limited to the treatment of cardiogenic, traumatic, or hypovolemic shock. It is a potent sympathomimetic drug that has been used safely during pregnancy, but only in a small number of patients to date.

Special Considerations in Pregnancy

When dopamine was administered in doses of 2–4 μg/kg/minute to chronically instrumented pregnant sheep near term, a statistically significant increase in uterine blood flow was noted. When doses of 8–16 μg/kg/minute were given, the responses were variable. In another study, instrumented near-term pregnant sheep were subjected to autonomic blockade with spinal anesthesia. These animals demonstrated decreased systemic arterial pressure, heart rate, and uterine blood flow as well as increased uterine vascular resistance. Dopamine administered intravenously during the spinal hypotension corrected these disturbed circulatory parameters.

Published experience with the use of this drug during human pregnancy is limited. In one study, dopamine was given to 26 patients and found to be as effective as ephedrine in correcting postspinal hypotension before repeat cesarean section. No differences in Apgar scores or neonatal blood gases were observed in the two groups.

A Viennese series describes the use of dopamine to prevent renal failure in nine eclamptic patients. The drug was administered by continuous infusion at a dose of 3 μg/kg/minute in conjunction with a diuretic to improve renal perfusion and promote diuresis. All of the patients showed initial improvement in renal function with this regimen, and seven went on to complete recovery, but the other two died. No adverse fetal or neonatal effects attributed to the drug were described. More data are obviously needed before dopamine can be recommended for this indication.

No information is available at present on dopamine's disposition in breast milk.

Dosage

Dopamine is administered parenterally at an initial rate of 2–5 μg/kg/minute, and this may be gradually increased to 20–50 μg/kg/minute as the clinical situation demands. All patients require monitoring of blood volume, myocardial function, and urine production during therapy. Reduced urinary output, tachycardia, or the development of an arrhythmia may be an indication for slowing or terminating the infusion. Since the duration of action of dopamine is brief, the rate of administration can be used to control the intensity of effect.

Adverse Effects

Nausea, vomiting, tachycardia, anginal pain, arrhythmias, headache, hypertension, and vasoconstriction may be encountered during infusion of dopamine. Before dopamine is administered to patients in shock, hypovolemia should be corrected by transfusion of whole blood, plasma, or appropriate fluids.

Mechanism of Action

Dopamine exerts a positive inotropic effect on the myocardium, acting as an agonist at beta-1-adrenergic receptors. In low dosages, it causes renal and splanchnic vasodilatation through activation of dopaminergic receptors. Slightly higher dosages cause beta stimulation of the heart to increase cardiac output. Further increases in dosage elicit an increase in heart rate, although tachycardia is less prominent during infusions of dopamine than of isoproterenol. Still higher dosages cause alpha stimulation and vasoconstriction, which may impair generalized peripheral as well as renal and mesenteric perfusion.

Absorption and Biotransformation

Dopamine is ineffective when given orally. When administered parenterally, absorbed drug is rapidly biotransformed, primarily to 3,4-dihydroxyphenylacetic acid (DOPAC) and 3-methoxy-4-hydroxyphenylacetic acid (HVA); small amounts are also converted to norepinephrine and other compounds. About 80% of the metabolites are excreted in the urine within 24 hours. Very little, if any, dopamine crosses the blood-brain barrier.

Recommended Reading

Cabalum, T., et al. Effect of dopamine on hypotension induced by spinal anesthesia. *Am. J. Obstet. Gynecol.* 133:630, 1979.

Clark, R. B., and Brunner, J. A. Dopamine for the treatment of spinal hypotension during cesarean section. *Anesthesiology* 35:514, 1980.

Gerstner, G., and Grunberger, W. Dopamine treatment for prevention of renal failure in patients with severe eclampsia. *Clin. Exp. Obstet. Gynecol.* 7:219, 1980.

Gilman, A. G., Goodman, L. S., and Gilman, A. *The Pharmacological Basis of Therapeutics* (6th ed.). New York: Macmillan, 1980. Pp. 154–155, 479.

Grunberger, W., and Szalay, S. Uterine and systemic vascular responses to dopamine in pregnant ewes. *Arch. Gynecol.* 233:259, 1983.

Doxylamine (Bendectin®, When Combined with Pyridoxine)

Indications and Recommendations

The combination of doxylamine and pyridoxine (Bendectin®) has been removed from the market in the United States—not by the FDA, but by the manufacturer. This drug has been used widely and studied intensively in the pregnant woman. The manufacturer estimates that it was used in 29 million pregnancies between 1956 and 1979. At least 10 large epidemiologic studies have failed to demonstrate an association between use of the drug and the occurrence of birth defects in the offspring. Although a few of the studies have shown an association between some subcategories of birth defects and Bendectin®, the specific defects implicated were generally not the same from one study to another. It should be noted that when one is evaluating statistical significance, the usual test applied is the "0.05 level of probability." When this standard is met, it means that the likelihood of an association being due to chance is 5% (i.e., the odds are 20 to 1 that the finding is not artifactual). On the other hand, this also means that if no real association exists, it is likely that every 20 times such an association is looked for, one will by chance appear to be found. Thus, it is not surprising that when a myriad of individual birth defects are investigated, some will appear to be significantly associated with the drug under investigation. If the associations were real, one would expect that the same type of birth defects would recur from study to study; this has not been the case with Bendectin® to date. Two recent studies have reported a positive association between maternal Bendectin® use and the occurrence of pyloric stenosis in the offspring. However, neither study was able to determine whether the finding could be attributed to the Bendectin® use or to severe nausea during pregnancy. Furthermore, a third study found no such association, and the question is still open.

The manufacturer removed this product from the market for economic reasons. Beginning in 1981, an increasing number of lawsuits were filed against the manufacturer. They alleged that Bendectin® was responsible for a multitude of birth defects in children whose mothers had taken it during pregnancy. It should be noted that approximately 3% of all children have an identifiable birth defect, and that estimates of the percentage of pregnant women taking Bendectin® when it was available range from 5–25%. Thus, even if the drug *reduced* the occurrence of birth defects by half (no one has suggested that it does), there would be, among the 3–4 million babies born in the United States each year, between 2,250 and 15,000 babies with birth defects who were exposed to Bendectin® in utero. If we make the more reasonable assumption that this drug has no effect on birth defects, the numbers of such babies would be between 4,500 and 30,000 *each year*. By the time the manufacturer removed Bendectin® from the market in 1983, there had been well over 300 suits instituted, with no end in sight. Only two cases had been decided, one in favor of the manufacturer and the other in favor of the plaintiff (although this case is under appeal). In view of these events, the manufacturer made the projection that, even if it won all the suits filed, the cost of defending them would make the continued marketing of this drug financially prohibitive, and so the production of Bendectin® was discontinued. In addition, the manufacturer set up a fund to settle all outstanding and potential claims.

We have undertaken such a long discussion of an unavailable drug to explain why it is no longer being made and to point out that its discontinuance leaves a therapeutic gap in the care of pregnant women. Most cases of nausea in pregnancy can be dealt with by simple measures, and it is unlikely that the withdrawal of Bendectin® will drastically increase the incidence of hospitalization for hyperemesis gravidarum. However, persistent nausea in the first trimester continues to be a real clinical problem, and the physician is now faced with the prospect of prescribing medications about which much less is known when the usual nonpharmacologic forms of therapy fail. It is by no means clear that the removal of this drug from the market represents a "victory" for the pregnant consumer, as some have claimed.

Recommended Reading

Aselton, P. A., and Jick, H. Additional follow-up of congenital limb disorders in relation to Bendectin use. *J.A.M.A.* 250:33, 1983.

Aselton, P. A., et al. Pyloric stenosis and maternal Bendectin exposure. *Am. J. Epidemiol.* 120:251, 1984.

Cordero, J. F., et al. Is Bendectin a teratogen? *J.A.M.A.* 245:2307, 1981.

Eskenazi, B., and Bracken, M. B. Bendectin (Debendox) as a risk factor for pyloric stenosis. *Am. J. Obstet. Gynecol.* 144:919, 1982.

Fleming, D. M. Letter to the editor. *Am. J. Obstet. Gynecol.* 147:980, 1983.

Heinonen, O. P., Slone, D., and Shapiro, S. *Birth Defects and Drugs in*

Pregnancy. Littleton, Mass.: Publishing Sciences Group, 1977. Pp. 323–334.

Henderson, I. Congenital deformities associated with Bendectin. *CMA Journal* 117:721, 1977.

Indications for Bendectin narrowed. *FDA Drug Bull.* 11:1, 1981.

Jacobson, A. S. The withdrawal of Bendectin (editorial). *Medical Tribune* August 31, 1983. P. 22.

Jick, H., et al. First trimester drug use and congenital disorders. *J.A.M.A.* 246:343, 1981.

Michaelis, J., et al. Prospective study of suspected associations between certain drugs administered during early pregnancy and congenital malformations. *Teratology* 27:57, 1983.

Milkovich, L., and Van den Berg, B. J. An evaluation of the teratogenicity of certain antinauseant drugs. *Am. J. Obstet. Gynecol.* 125:244, 1976.

Mitchell, A. A., et al. Birth defects related to Bendectin use in pregnancy. I. Oral clefts and cardiac defects. *J.A.M.A.* 245:2311, 1981.

Mitchell, A. A., et al. Birth defects in relation to Bendectin use in pregnancy. *Am. J. Obstet. Gynecol.* 147:737, 1983.

Morelock, S., et al. Bendectin and fetal development. *Am. J. Obstet. Gynecol.* 142:209, 1982.

Shapiro, S., et al. Antenatal exposure to doxylamine succinate and dicyclomine hydrochloride (Bendectin) in relation to congenital malformations, perinatal mortality rate, birth weight, and intelligence quotient score. *Am. J. Obstet. Gynecol.* 128:480, 1977.

Ephedrine

Indications and Recommendations

The use of ephedrine during pregnancy should be limited to the correction of maternal hypotension unresponsive to rapid fluid infusion and left lateral uterine displacement following the administration of a spinal or epidural anesthetic. This drug should not be used to treat asthma in pregnant women as other agents for that purpose are preferable.

Special Considerations in Pregnancy

There is no information available as to whether the drug crosses the placenta, is secreted in breast milk, or whether it has teratogenic effects. Administration to normal pregnant ewes does not decrease uterine blood flow, alter fetal acid-base status, or produce changes in fetal heart rate. When ephedrine is used in combination with oxytocics, severe hypertension may develop. It must be used with extreme caution in patients with chronic hypertension or toxemia.

In one study, the administration of ephedrine to women who had been given epidural anesthesia was associated with significant increases in fetal heart rate and beat-to-beat variability. These changes were dose related, but did not have an observed effect on scalp blood pH or Apgar scores when compared with those of control subjects.

The prophylactic administration of intramuscular ephedrine in doses of 25 or 50 mg given 15–30 minutes before epidural anesthesia to women undergoing cesarean section was no more successful than intramuscular placebo in preventing hypotension. Furthermore, persistent hypertension developed in 8 in 12 women given the 50-mg dose.

In another study, ephedrine was administered to 44 healthy women undergoing elective, repeat cesarean section under spinal anesthesia. Twenty of these patients were given an infusion, starting at a dose of 5 mg/minute, immediately after induction of the anesthesia to maintain the maternal systolic blood pressure between 90 and 100% of the baseline value. The mean dose administered was 31.6 mg. The remaining 24 patients received a 20-mg IV bolus and additional 10-mg boluses if needed when the systolic blood pressure fell to 80% of baseline levels. The mean dose administered to this group was 26.8 mg. The infusion group had significantly less deviation of the systolic blood pressure from the baseline, and reactive hypertension did not occur. Furthermore, the group receiving ephedrine by infusion had significantly less nausea and vomiting. No appreciable difference was noted in Apgar scores, fetal blood gas tensions, or time for onset of neonatal respirations.

Dosage

For the treatment of hypotension, ephedrine is usually administered intravenously in 10–20-mg doses every 60 seconds as needed to keep the systolic blood pressure above 100 mm Hg. It is rarely necessary to use more than 60 mg for this purpose. Ephedrine's duration of action is several hours.

Adverse Effects

Side effects associated with the use of ephedrine include hypertension, cardiac arrhythmias, palpitations, insomnia, tremor, and anxiety.

Mechanism of Action

Ephedrine has both alpha- and beta-adrenergic actions. It acts by stimulating the release of stored norepinephrine and by direct stimulation of adrenergic receptors.

The effects of ephedrine in the body are widespread. Because it produces mild bronchodilatation, it has been used as an adjunct to theophylline therapy in asthma. It increases both systolic and diastolic blood pressures and decreases pulse pressure; heart rate is generally unchanged; cardiac output is increased; renal and splanchnic blood flow are decreased; and coronary, cerebral, and muscle blood flow are increased. Ephedrine decreases uterine activity (beta-2 effect). It also produces mydriasis when applied topically.

Absorption and Biotransformation

Ephedrine is well absorbed when given orally. Most of the drug is metabolized by deamination and conjugation. Both metabolites and unchanged drug are excreted in the urine.

Recommended Reading

Chen, K. K., and Schmidt, C. F. Ephedrine and related substances. *Medicine* 9:1, 1930.

Eng, M., Berges, P. V., and Ueland, K. The effects of methoxamine and ephedrine in normotensive pregnant primates. *Anesthesia* 35:354, 1970.

Kang, Y. G., Abouleish, E., and Caritis, S. Prophylactic intravenous ephedrine infusion during spinal anesthesia for cesarean section. *Anesth. Analg.* 61:839, 1982.

Ralstow, D. H., Schnider, S. M., and deLorimier, A. A. Effect of equipotent doses of ephedrine, metaraminol, mephentermine, and methoxamine on uterine blood flow in the pregnant ewe. *Anesthesia* 40:354, 1974.

Rolbin, S. H., et al. Prophylactic intramuscular ephedrine before epidural anaesthesia for cesarean section: Efficacy and actions on the fetus and newborn. *Can. Anaesth. Soc. J.* 29:148, 1982.

Schnider, S. M., deLorimier, A. A., and Holl, J. W. Vasopressor in obstetrics: I. Correction of fetal acidosis with ephedrine during spinal hypotension. *Am. J. Obstet. Gynecol.* 102:911, 1968.

Weinberger, M. Use of ephedrine in bronchodilator therapy. *Pediatr. Clin. North Am.* 22:121, 1975.

Wright, R. G., et al. The effect of maternal administration of ephedrine on fetal heart rate and variability. *Obstet. Gynecol.* 57:734, 1981.

Ergonovine Maleate (Ergotrate®)

Indications and Recommendations

Ergonovine maleate is contraindicated during pregnancy prior to delivery of the infant. Its use is indicated for the prevention and treatment of postpartum and postabortal hemorrhage due to uterine atony. It may also be used during the puerperium to promote involution of the uterus. It is a direct stimulant of gravid and nongravid uterine muscle, although the gravid uterus is much more sensitive to its effects. Due to the high degree of uterine stimulation produced, ergonovine is not recommended for antepartum use, nor should it be administered prior to delivery of the placenta. It should not be used for the induction or augmentation of labor because of its tendency to produce tetanic contractions.

Several studies have shown ergonovine to interfere with normal secretion of prolactin in the immediate puerperium. Lactation thus may be delayed or inhibited in nursing mothers when it has been administered.

Recommended Reading

Canales, R., et al. Effect of ergonovine on prolactin secretion and milk letdown. *Obstet. Gynecol.* 48:228, 1976.

Chase, G., et al. (eds.). *Remington's Pharmaceutical Sciences* (14th ed.). Easton, Pa.: Mack, 1970. Pp. 951–952.

Floss, H., Cassidy, J., and Robbers, J. Influence of ergot alkaloids on pituitary prolactin and prolactin-dependent processes. *J. Pharm. Sci.* 62:699, 1973.

Gilman, A. G., Goodman, L. S., and Gilman, A. *The Pharmacological Basis of Therapeutics* (6th ed.). New York: Macmillan, 1980. Pp. 939–947.

Reis, R. A., Gerbie, A. B., and Gerbie, M. V. Reducing hazards of the newborn during cesarean section. *Obstet. Gynecol.* 46:676, 1975.

Ergotamine Tartrate (Cafergot®, with Caffeine; Ergomar®; Ergostat®; Gynergen®)

Indications and Recommendations

Ergotamine tartrate is contraindicated during pregnancy. This drug, which is used to abort migraine and cluster headaches, produces alpha-adrenergic blockade and more importantly acts on the central nervous system and directly stimulates smooth muscle.

It should not be used during pregnancy because it can create tetanic uterine contractions. It may also cause a significant increase in blood pressure at therapeutic dosages. Administration of this drug during organogenesis has produced an increased incidence of fetal wastage in rats and fetal growth retardation in rats, mice, and rabbits. A case has been reported of a woman who ingested ergotamine tartrate daily during six pregnancies. Four ended in spontaneous abortion, one in the premature delivery of a small-for-date infant, and one in the premature delivery of an infant with multiple areas of jejunal atresia. The authors speculate that the atresia may have been due to the vascular effects of the drug.

Recommended Reading

AMA Drug Evaluations (3rd ed.). Littleton, Mass.: Publishing Sciences Group, 1977, Pp. 358–359.

American Hospital Formulary Service. *Monograph for Ergotamine Tartrate.* Section 12:16. Washington, D.C.: American Society of Hospital Pharmacists, 1959.

Floss, H., Cassidy, J., and Robbers, J. Influence of ergot alkaloids on pituitary prolactin and prolactin-dependent processes. *J. Pharm. Sci.* 62:699, 1973.

Gilman, A. G., Goodman, L. S., and Gilman, A. *The Pharmacological Basis of Therapeutics* (6th ed.). New York: Macmillan, 1980. Pp. 939–947.

Graham, J. M., Jr., Marin-Padilla, M., and Hoefnagel, D. Jejunal atresia associated with Cafergot ingestion during pregnancy. *Clin. Pediatr.* 22:226, 1983.

Grauwiler, J., and Schön, H. Teratological experiments with ergotamine in mice, rats and rabbits. *Teratology* 7:227, 1973.

Parkes, J. Relief of pain—headache, facial neuralgia, migraine and phantom limbs. *Br. Med. J.* 4:282, 1975.

Erythromycin (E-Mycin®, Erythrocin®)

Indications and Recommendations

Erythromycin is safe to use during pregnancy; however, preparations of the estolate ester should be avoided. It is an antibiotic used to treat gram-positive bacterial infections and syphilis in penicillin-allergic patients. It is also effective against gonococci, *Haemophilus* species, *Legionella pneumophila,* and *Mycoplasma pneumoniae.*

Special Considerations in Pregnancy

In one study, a significant proportion of pregnant women (10–15%) who received erythromycin estolate for 3 weeks developed subclinical, reversible hepatic toxicity. It is, therefore, recommended that erythromycin estolate be avoided during pregnancy. Use of oral erythromycin has been associated with declining maternal urinary estriol levels, with an almost immediate rise after cessation of therapy. The decline has been attributed to an alteration in the normal intestinal flora, which results in interference with estriol hydrolysis and reabsorption.

Fetal plasma concentrations are 5–20% of those found in maternal plasma. This drug is safe for the fetus and is often recommended to treat syphilis in penicillin-allergic pregnant women. Its efficacy in fetal syphilis is questionable.

Dosage

The usual oral dose is 250–500 mg q6h. The usual intravenous or intramuscular dose is 1–4 g/day. Parenteral administration is rarely indicated because of the severe pain and frequent phlebitis associated with its use.

Adverse Effects

Gastrointestinal disturbances are frequent with oral erythromycin use, while severe pain at the injection site is common with parenteral administration. Allergic reactions and transient deafness are rare side effects. Cholestatic hepatitis has been associated with erythromycin estolate use in adults.

Mechanism of Action

Erythromycin is an orally effective macrolide antibiotic that inhibits protein synthesis by binding to the 50S ribosomal subunits of sensitive microorganisms.

Absorption and Biotransformation

Erythromycin is well absorbed orally, but absorption varies with the salt and dosage form administered. It is concentrated in the liver and excreted in the bile. Only 2–5% of the oral dose is excreted by the kidneys, while 12–15% appears in the urine after parenteral administration.

Recommended Reading

Gallagher, J. C., Ismail, M. A., and Aladjem, S. Reduced urinary estriol levels with erythromycin therapy. *Obstet. Gynecol.* 56:381, 1980.

Gilman, A. G., Goodman, L. S., and Gilman, A. *The Pharmacological Basis of Therapeutics* (6th ed.). New York: Macmillan, 1980. Pp. 1222–1225.

McCormack, W. M., et al. Hepatotoxicity of erythromycin estolate during pregnancy. *Antimicrob. Agents Chemother.* 12:630, 1977.

Philipson, A., Sabath, L. D., and Charles, D. Transplacental passage of erythromycin and clindamycin. *N. Engl. J. Med.* 288:1219, 1973.

Thompson, S. E., and Dretler, R. H. Epidemiology of chlamydial infections in pregnant women and infants. *Rev. Infect. Dis.* 4:S747, 1982.

Estrogens (Synthetic and Natural)

Indications and Recommendations

Both steroidal and nonsteroidal estrogens are contraindicated in pregnancy. In the past, nonsteroidal estrogens were often prescribed for maintenance of diabetic pregnancies and the prevention of spontaneous abortions. However, it is now known that they are not effective for these therapeutic objectives.

Maternal side effects may include nausea, vomiting, skin changes, thrombophlebitis, pulmonary embolism, and cholestatic jaundice. Important fetal effects have been noted when nonsteroidal estrogen (specifically diethylstilbestrol [DES]) was administered during the first trimester. These include an increased incidence of adenocarcinoma and adenosis of the vagina, as well as cervical, uterine, and tubal deformities in females. A recent, well-controlled prospective study found that the incidence of cervical and vaginal dysplasia among DES daughters was approximately twice that seen in a matched control group of unexposed women. There are a number of reports of increased reproductive loss among DES daughters who become pregnant, with the strong possibility that incompetent cervix syndrome may be common among such patients. However, most of these studies have been based on selected groups of DES daughters, generally those presenting for care at a DES program. Thus, there are no accurate data regarding the incidence of reproductive loss among unselected DES daughters compared to the general population. Testicular cysts and oligospermia have been noted when developing male gonadal tissue has been exposed to these compounds in utero. The estrogens are secreted in breast milk.

It is recommended that estrogens, both steroidal and nonsteroidal, natural and synthetic, not be utilized during pregnancy. There is no proof that they are beneficial, and there is good evidence that the nonsteroidal estrogens may produce fetal genital tract anomalies and disease.

Recommended Reading

Bibbo, N., et al. Followup study of male and female offspring of DES exposed mothers. *Obstet. Gynecol.* 49:1, 1977.

Herbst, A. L. Diethylstilbestrol exposure—1984. *N. Engl. J. Med.* 311:1433, 1984.

Herbst, A. L., and Bern, H. A. (eds.). *Developmental Effects of Diethylstilbestrol (DES) in Pregnancy.* New York: Thieme-Stratton, 1981.

Herbst, A. L., et al. Reproductive and gynecologic surgical experience in diethylstilbestrol-exposed daughters. *Am. J. Obstet. Gynecol.* 141: 1019, 1981.

Jefferies, J. A., et al. Structural anomalies of the cervix and vagina in women enrolled in the Diethylstilbestrol Adenosis (DESAD) Project. *Am. J. Obstet. Gynecol.* 148:59, 1984.

Kaufman, R. H., et al. Upper genital tract abnormalities and pregnancy outcome in diethylstilbestrol-exposed progeny. *Am. J. Obstet. Gynecol.* 148:973, 1984.

Robboy, S. J., et al. Increased incidence of cervical and vaginal dysplasia in 3,980 diethylstilbestrol-exposed young women. *J.A.M.A.* 252:2979, 1984.

Sandberg, E. C., et al. Pregnancy outcome in women exposed to diethylstilbestrol in utero. *Am. J. Obstet. Gynecol.* 140:194, 1981.

Stillman, R. J. In utero exposure to diethylstilbestrol: Adverse effects on the reproductive tract and reproductive performance in male and female offspring. *Am. J. Obstet. Gynecol.* 142:905, 1982.

Wilson, J. G., and Brent, R. L. Are female sex hormones teratogenic? *Am. J. Obstet. Gynecol.* 141:567, 1981.

Ethacrynic Acid (Edecrin®)

Indications and Recommendations

The use of ethacrynic acid is relatively contraindicated during pregnancy because other therapeutic agents are preferable. It is a loop diuretic with activity similar to that of furosemide. The major complications associated with the use of ethacrynic acid in pregnancy are ototoxicity and hypokalemic alkalosis. These sequelae have been observed both in pregnant women and their offspring. It should be noted, however, that reports describing the uneventful use of this drug during pregnancy have been published. If a loop diuretic is indicated for an obstetric patient, furosemide is the drug of choice.

Recommended Reading

Finnerty, F. A. Hypertension in pregnancy. *Clin. Obstet. Gynecol.* 18:145, 1975.

Fort, A. T., Morrison, J. C., and Fish, S. A. Iatrogenic hypokalemia of pregnancy by furosemide and ethacrynic acid. *J. Reprod. Med.* 6:207, 1971.

Gilman, A. G., Goodman, L. S., and Gilman, A. *The Pharmacological Basis of Therapeutics* (6th ed.). New York: Macmillan, 1980. Pp. 903–907.

Harrison, K. A. Ethacrynic acid in blood transfusion—its effects on plasma volume and urine flow in severe anaemia in pregnancy. *Br. Med. J.* 4:84, 1968.

Jones, H. C. Intrauterine ototoxicity—a case report and review of the literature. *J. Natl. Med. Assoc.* 65:201, 1973.

Schneider, W. J., and Becker, E. L. Acute transient hearing loss after ethacrynic acid. *Arch. Intern. Med.* 117:715, 1966.

Wilson, A. L., and Matzke, G. R. The treatment of hypertension in pregnancy. *Drug Intell. Clin. Pharm.* 15:21, 1981.

Young, B. K., and Haft, J. I. Treatment of pulmonary edema with ethacrynic acid during labor. *Am. J. Obstet. Gynecol.* 107:330, 1970.

Ethambutol (Myambutol®)

Indications and Recommendations

Ethambutol is recommended as an adjunct to isoniazid in the treatment of active tuberculosis in pregnancy. It is a synthetic tuberculostatic agent that is used in conjunction with other antitubercular drugs because of the rapid development of resistance when it is used alone.

Special Considerations in Pregnancy

Ethambutol appears to have no maternal effects unique to pregnancy. Large-scale studies of women who received combination isoniazid-ethambutol therapy during pregnancy indicate that in the usual antitubercular dosages, the treatment is not associated with an increase in fetal anomalies when compared to untreated mothers.

In a review of 650 women who received ethambutol during 655 pregnancies, 14 infants or fetuses with congenital anomalies were found, for an incidence of approximately 2%. This rate is similar to that observed in the general population. No pattern to the anomalies was noted, and the rates of stillbirths and prematurity were not increased.

Dosage

The usual adult dose is 15 mg/kg/day, given in combination with isoniazid, for a total of 18–24 months.

Adverse Effects

Ethambutol use is relatively free of side effects. The most important adverse reaction is optic neuritis, which occurs primarily in patients who receive more than 25 mg/kg/day or in those with renal impairment. It appears gradually, usually as blurred vision, color blindness, and restriction of visual fields, and is generally reversible with prompt discontinuation of therapy. Hyperuricemia due to impaired urinary excretion of uric acid may occur.

Mechanism of Action

The mechanism of action of ethambutol is unknown. It has no effect on bacteria other than mycobacteria. Primary resistance among mycobacteria is rare, but resistance develops rapidly when the drug is used alone.

Absorption and Biotransformation

About 80% of an oral dose is absorbed. The drug is concentrated in erythrocytes, which may serve as a depot from which ethambutol slowly enters the plasma. Of the absorbed dose, nearly 100% is recovered in the urine within 24 hours, 80% as unchanged ethambutol. The half-life is 3–4 hours and increases significantly with renal failure.

Recommended Reading

Bobrowitz, I. D. Ethambutol in pregnancy. *Chest* 66:20, 1974.
Gilman, A. G., Goodman, L. S., and Gilman, A. *The Pharmacological Basis of Therapeutics* (6th ed.). New York: Macmillan, 1980. Pp. 1206–1207.

Lewat, M. D., et al. Ethambutol in pregnancy: Observations on embryogenesis. *Chest* 66:25, 1974.

Scheinhorn, D. J., and Angelillo, V. A. Antituberculosis therapy in pregnancy: Risks to the fetus. *West. J. Med.* 127:195, 1977.

Snider, D. E., et al. Treatment of tuberculosis during pregnancy. *Am. Rev. Respir. Dis.* 122:65, 1980.

Ethchlorvynol (Placidyl®)

Indications and Recommendations

The use of ethchlorvynol is relatively contraindicated during pregnancy because other therapeutic agents are preferable. It is used primarily as a hypnotic agent in the treatment of insomnia. This drug offers no therapeutic advantage over barbiturate or nonbarbiturate sedatives. Little is known about its effects on the pregnant woman or fetus. In dogs, it has been shown to achieve significant fetal blood levels within 90 minutes of maternal ingestion. Symptoms resembling congenital narcotic withdrawal have been described in the human newborn after the mother has ingested ethchlorvynol.

No sedative has been found to be absolutely safe during pregnancy as most cross the placenta and produce sedation and withdrawal symptoms in the newborn. Should such therapy be required during pregnancy, phenobarbital may be used (see *Phenobarbital*).

Recommended Reading

Gilman, A. G., Goodman, L. S., and Gilman, A. *The Pharmacological Basis of Therapeutics* (6th ed.). New York: Macmillan, 1980. Pp. 363–364.

Hume, A. S., Williams, J. M., and Douglas, B. H. Disposition of ethchlorvynol in maternal blood, fetal blood, amniotic fluid and chorionic fluid. *J. Reprod. Med.* 6:229, 1971.

Rumack, B. H., and Walravens, P. A. Neonatal withdrawal following maternal ingestion of ethchlorvynol. *Pediatrics* 52:714, 1973.

Ethosuximide (Zarontin®)

Indications and Recommendations

Ethosuximide may be administered to pregnant women in the treatment of absence seizures. This condition is rare in women of childbearing age, and its effects on the fetus have not been studied in depth. If absence seizures persist during childbearing years and require treatment, therapy with ethosuximide may be continued through pregnancy.

Special Considerations in Pregnancy

The placental transfer of ethosuximide has been demonstrated in rats; fetal and maternal tissue levels appear to be similar. There is no information regarding adverse effects of this drug on human pregnancy, although in animal experiments it is considered to be one of the least teratogenic of the antiseizure medications.

Although ethosuximide is detectable in breast milk, the amount has never been quantified; pharmacologic effects on infants being breast-fed have not been described.

Dosage

The starting dose should be 500 mg/day, which may be slowly increased to 20–40 mg/kg/day. Dosage should be adjusted to maintain a therapeutic plasma level of 40–100 μg/ml.

Adverse Effects

Side effects include drowsiness, headache, hiccup, euphoria, and disequilibrium. Ethosuximide may cause local irritative effects on the stomach, with anorexia, gastric discomfort, nausea, and vomiting. These problems often occur at the onset of therapy, are transient, and are not clearly dose related. Other reported associations include urticarial rash, Stevens-Johnson syndrome, a lupuslike syndrome, and rarely, leukopenia, pancytopenia, and aplastic anemia.

Mechanism of Action

The site and mechanism of action of ethosuximide are unexplained. However, since its antiseizure activity is similar to that of valproic acid, it may work by augmenting gamma-aminobutyric acid (GABA) activity. The drug also affects brain metabolism and enzyme function. It inhibits membrane $(Na^+ - K^+)$-ATPase, depresses oxygen utilization, and depresses cerebellar cyclic GMP, but these effects may not be related to its antiseizure activity.

Absorption and Biotransformation

Absorption is fairly rapid and complete from the alimentary tract, with peak plasma levels occurring 1–4 hours after a single oral dose. It has been demonstrated that ethosuximide is absorbed faster from a syrup preparation than from capsules. It is fairly uniformly distributed throughout the body, except in adipose tissue, where levels are lower than elsewhere. The drug is minimally bound to plasma and spinal fluid proteins. Ten to twenty percent of ethosuximide is excreted unchanged in the urine. The remaining drug is metabolized in the liver.

Recommended Reading

Gilman, A. G., Goodman, L. S., and Gilman, A. *The Pharmacological Basis of Therapeutics* (6th ed.). New York: Macmillan, 1980. Pp. 460–471.

Sullivan, F. M., and McElnatton, P. R. A comparison of the teratogenic activity of the antiepileptic drugs carbamazepine, clonazepam, ethosuximide, phenobarbital, phenytoin, and primidone in mice. *Toxicol. Appl. Pharmacol.* 40:365, 1977.

Wilder, B. J., and Bruni, J. *Seizure Disorders: A Pharmacological Approach to Treatment.* New York: Raven, 1981.

Woodbury, D. M. Penry, J. K., and Pippenger, C. E. *Antiepileptic Drugs* (2nd ed.). New York: Raven, 1982.

Evans Blue Dye (T 1824)

Indications and Recommendations

Evans blue dye, an azo dye used in the determination of maternal plasma volume, may be used after the first trimester of pregnancy. Because one series of studies has suggested teratogenicity in rats, this dye should probably not be utilized during the first trimester. Although Evans blue dye has also been injected intraamniotically to diagnose rupture of membranes and as a marker when performing amniocentesis in multiple gestations, indigo carmine is more commonly used for this purpose.

Special Considerations in Pregnancy

In a series of experiments in which 1 ml of a 1% solution of various azo dyes was injected subcutaneously into female rats on days 1, 8, and 9 of gestation, Evans blue dye was associated with a 10% maternal death rate, a 25% fetal reabsorption rate, and a 14% malformation rate among surviving fetuses. These rates were higher than those observed with any of the 14 other dyes utilized, with the exception of trypan blue. The malformations seen were primarily in the central nervous system. No information is available as to the mechanism of these problems, nor are dose-response curves described. Nevertheless, it would appear prudent to avoid the use of this agent during the time of organogenesis.

An association between reduced intravascular volume and both hypertensive disorders of pregnancy and intrauterine growth disorders has led to the widespread use of plasma volume determination as an investigative tool in patients at risk for these complications. Evans blue dye is the standard agent used in such measurements. There is evidence that this dye may disappear more rapidly from the circulation of women with preeclampsia than from that of normal pregnant women. Adverse pregnancy effects of the intravenous use of Evans blue dye have not been reported.

Dosage

With the patient lying on her side, Evans blue dye is injected intravenously in a known quantity (usually 2 ml of 0.5% solution). Preinjection and timed postinjection blood samples are obtained. These are then centrifuged, and the optical density of the plasma is measured at 620 nm. Optical density values are compared with those obtained when samples of the same lot of dye are diluted with pooled plasma, so that the concentration of the dye can be calculated from this formula:

Plasma volume (ml) = dye injected (mg)
$\div$ concentration obtained (mg/ml)

Investigators have generally either extrapolated back to time zero or used the dye concentration at 10 minutes after injection to calculate plasma volume.

Adverse Effects

No information is available.

Mechanism of Action

See Dosage.

Absorption and Biotransformation

Little information is available concerning the half-life of Evans blue dye in the circulation. It is known to be strongly protein bound. In one study, 5% of the dye had disappeared from the circulation by 1 hour after injection and 41% by 24 hours.

Recommended Reading

Atlay, R. D., and Sutherst, J. R. Premature rupture of the fetal membranes confirmed by intraamniotic injection of dye (Evans blue T-1824). *Am. J. Obstet. Gynecol.* 108:993, 1970.

Campbell, D. M., and Campbell, A. J. Evans blue disappearance rate in normal and pre-eclamptic pregnancy. *Clin. Exp. Hypertens.* B2:163, 1983.

Chesley, L. C., and Duffus, G. M. Posture and apparent plasma volume in late pregnancy. *J. Obstet. Gynaecol. Br. Commw.* 78:406, 1971.

Durocher, J., and Moutquin, J. Standardisation de la méthode de mesure du volume serique par le bleu Evans, chez la femme enceinte. *Clin. Biochem.* 16:234, 1983.

Goodlin, R. C., et al. Clinical signs of normal plasma volume expansion during pregnancy. *Am. J. Obstet. Gynecol.* 145:1001, 1983.

Hays, P. M., Cruikshank, D. P., and Dunn, L. J. Plasma volume determination in normal and preeclamptic pregnancies. *Am. J. Obstet. Gynecol.* 151:958, 1985.

Sibai, B. M., et al. Plasma volume determination in pregnancies complicated by chronic hypertension and intrauterine fetal demise. *Obstet. Gynecol.* 60:174, 1982.

Soffronoff, E. C., Kauffmann, B. M., and Connaughton, J. F. Intravascular volume determinations in hypertensive diseases of pregnancy. *Am. J. Obstet. Gynecol.* 127:4, 1977.

Wilson, J. G. Teratogenic activity of several azo dyes chemically related to trypan blue. *Anat. Rec.* 123:313, 1955.

Furosemide (Lasix®)

Indications and Recommendations

Furosemide may be administered to pregnant women for the treatment of congestive heart failure and some cases of chronic renal disease. It is an extremely powerful saluretic that may rapidly decrease maternal intravascular volume and, consequently, diminish uteroplacental perfusion. For this reason, it must be used with extreme care in the obstetric patient. It is not indicated for the routine treatment of hypertension or peripheral edema during pregnancy.

Special Considerations in Pregnancy

Furosemide must be administered with great caution in the pregnant patient. As indicated above, hypovolemia may lead to decreased uterine blood flow, which can affect the fetus adversely. If the drug is used, the fetus should be carefully monitored for evidence of intrauterine compromise.

Animal studies have shown that furosemide causes unexplained maternal deaths and abortions in rabbits as well as an increased incidence of fetal hydronephrosis in rats.

Using ultrasonic measurements of human fetal bladder volume, Wladimiroff reported that the maternal administration of furosemide resulted in an increase of 80–150% in the hourly fetal urine production rate. As a result of this observation, the "furosemide challenge test" was advocated as a diagnostic tool for evaluating renal function in utero. Recent studies in chronically catheterized fetal sheep, however, have shown that maternally administered furosemide actually causes a reduction in mean hourly fetal urine production in that species. From these findings, the authors have suggested that failure to visualize the human fetal bladder ultrasonically after maternal furosemide administration should not be interpreted as an absolute indication of absent fetal renal function.

In a placental transfer study, furosemide was administered orally to 18 pregnant women on the day of delivery. The ratio between drug concentrations in maternal plasma and umbilical cord plasma decreased with time and was equal 8–10 hours after administration. The plasma half-life appeared to be longer in the mothers than in healthy nonpregnant volunteers.

The pharmacokinetics of furosemide have been studied in 12 newborns who had been exposed to the drug transplacentally and 21 neonates who received it therapeutically after birth. In the transplacental group, plasma half-lives ranged from 6.8–96.0 hours, and there was a significant inverse relationship between the gestational age and elimination rate. In neonates who received intravenous furosemide postnatally for therapeutic indications, premature neonates had prolonged plasma half-lives (26.8 ± 12.2 h) as compared to the full-term group (13.4 ± 8.6 h).

It has recently been reported that furosemide may increase the incidence of patent ductus arteriosus in premature infants with the respiratory distress syndrome (RDS). This presumably is due to stimulation of the renal synthesis of prostaglandin E_2. Furosemide readily crosses the placenta, and amniotic fluid may act as a reservoir for this drug. Its half-life in neonates is eightfold longer than that in adults and, as mentioned previously, this is increased further in premature infants. Since in normal infants the ductus arteriosus may not close until several days after birth, exposure to furosemide in utero may be detrimental, especially in the case of premature neonates who go on to develop RDS.

Dosage

Furosemide may be given intravenously or orally in the following range:

Route	Minimum	Usual	Maximum
Oral	20 mg qd	40 mg qd–qid	600 mg daily
Intravenous	10 mg/dose	20–40 mg/dose	600 mg daily

Adverse Effects

The most serious side effect of furosemide is severe hypovolemia. Hyponatremia, hypokalemia, hypochloremia, hyperuricemia, and metabolic alkalosis may also occur. Glucose intolerance, hearing loss, and interstitial nephritis have been reported. Occasionally, skin rash, paresthesias, gastrointestinal disturbances, thrombocytopenia, and neutropenia are seen.

Mechanism of Action

Furosemide acts directly on the ascending limb of the loop of Henle. It works primarily by inhibiting sodium and chloride reabsorption in the loop. In the normally functioning kidney, furosemide causes excretion of 30–40% of the filtered sodium load and produces a prompt diuresis where maximal sodium and water reabsorption has not already taken place in the proximal tubule. The drug's effectiveness decreases as the glomerular filtration rate approaches 20 ml/minute.

Absorption and Biotransformation

Furosemide is readily absorbed from the gastrointestinal tract and is strongly bound to plasma proteins. Two-thirds of an oral dose is excreted in the urine, the remainder being eliminated via the feces. Urinary excretion is accomplished by both glomerular filtration and proximal tubular secretion. Only a small fraction of the drug is metabolized.

Recommended Reading

Aranda, J. V., et al. Pharmacokinetic disposition and protein-binding of furosemide in newborn infants. *J. Pediatr.* 93:507, 1978.

Beerman, B., et al. Placental transfer of furosemide. *Clin. Pharmacol. Ther.* 24:560, 1978.

Chamberlain, P. F., et al. Ovine fetal urine production following maternal intravenous furosemide administration. *Am. J. Obstet. Gynecol.* 151:815, 1985.

Cohen, J. I. Promotion of patent ductus arteriosus by furosemide (letter). *N. Engl. J. Med.* 309:432, 1983.

Gant, N. F. The metabolic clearance rate of dehydroisoandrosterone sulfate: III. The effect of thiazide diuretics in normal and future preeclamptic pregnancies. *Am. J. Obstet. Gynecol.* 123:159, 1975.

Gifford, R. W., Jr. A guide to the practical use of diuretics. *J.A.M.A.* 235:1890, 1976.

Gilman, A. G., Goodman, L. S., and Gilman, A. *The Pharmacological Basis of Therapeutics* (6th ed.). New York: Macmillan, 1980. Pp. 903–907.

Green, T. P., et al. Furosemide promotes patent ductus arteriosus in premature infants with the respiratory distress syndrome. *N. Engl. J. Med.* 308:743, 1983.

Krunlovsky, F. A., and del Grew, C. Diuretic agents: Mechanism of action and clinical uses. *Postgrad. Med.* 59:105, 1976.

Peiker, G., et al. Pharmacokinetics and electrolyte balance following administration of furosemide in pregnant women with E gestosis. *Pharmazie* 39:336, 1984.

Pritchard, J. A. Standardized treatment of 154 consecutive cases of eclampsia. *Am. J. Obstet. Gynecol.* 123:543, 1975.

Pritchard, J. A., MacDonald, P., Gant, N. *Williams Obstetrics* (17th ed.). New York: Appleton-Century-Crofts, 1984. Pp. 549–550.

Riva, E., et al. Pharmacokinetics of furosemide in gestosis of pregnancy. *Eur. J. Clin. Pharmacol.* 14:361, 1978.

Vert, P., et al. Pharmacokinetics of furosemide in neonates. *Eur. J. Clin. Pharmacol.* 22:39, 1982.

Wladimiroff, J. W. Effect of furosemide on fetal urine production. *Br. J. Obstet. Gynaecol.* 82:221, 1975.

Gamma Benzene Hexachloride, Lindane (Kwell®)

Indications and Recommendations

Gamma benzene hexachloride may be administered to pregnant women for the treatment of scabies and lice. Head lice (*Pediculus humanus capitis*) and crab lice (*Phthirius pubis*) are treated with the cream, lotion, or shampoo form of the drug. Scabies (*Sarcoptes scabiei*) is treated with the cream or lotion form. Treatment should be such that only a minimal amount of drug is absorbed percutaneously.

Special Considerations in Pregnancy

There have thus far been no reports of adverse fetal effects associated with the topical use of gamma benzene hexachloride during pregnancy. Since it can be absorbed through the skin and is known to cause severe neurologic reactions in cases of overdosage, attempts should be made to minimize the amount of drug absorbed. For the treatment of scabies, the lotion or cream should be applied to dry, cool skin and washed off after 8 hours. Pediculosis should be treated with the shampoo, which must be rinsed thoroughly after application. Simultaneous application of lotions, ointments, or oils may enhance percutaneous absorption and should be avoided. Reapplication and retreatment should not be undertaken routinely.

Dosage

In the treatment of scabies a thin layer of the cream or lotion should be applied to the entire skin surface. It should be allowed to remain on the skin for 8 hours and then the skin should be washed thoroughly. A second or third application may be made at weekly intervals if necessary.

In the treatment of pediculosis, the affected and surrounding hairy areas should be wet with 30 ml shampoo. Water should then be added and the shampoo worked into a lather for at least 4 minutes. The area should then be rinsed thoroughly and dried with a towel. A fine-tooth comb should be used to remove any remaining nit shells. If necessary, the treatment may be repeated in 24 hours but not more than twice in 1 week.

Adverse Effects

Side effects are rare but may be dangerous when they occur. Fatal cases of aplastic anemia have resulted from prolonged exposure to the vaporized drug. In addition, very high doses applied percutaneously or taken orally have produced convulsions in humans.

Mechanism of Action

The mechanism of action of gamma benzene hexachloride is similar to that of DDT. It is absorbed through the exoskeletons of many arthropods and acts directly on their nervous tissue to produce convulsions and death. It is an excellent miticide and pediculocide that produces relief of symptoms usually within 24 hours of application.

Absorption and Biotransformation

The exact pharmacokinetics of gamma benzene hexachloride are unknown. The drug is absorbed through the skin. After local application of an 0.3% lotion, it reaches levels of 2–6 ng/ml in patients with intact skin and 30–200 ng/ml in patients with excoriated skin. The preparations available in the United States are 1% concentrations and would be expected to produce correspondingly higher levels. The toxic level measured in a child who had ingested the drug and had severe neurologic sequelae was 86 μg/ml.

Recommended Reading

Gamma benzene hexachloride (Kwell and other products) alert. *FDA Drug Bull.* 6:28, 1976.

Lange, M., Nitzsche, K., and Zesch, A. Percutaneous absorption of lindane in healthy volunteers and scabies patients. *Arch. Dermatol. Res.* 271:387, 1981.

Lee, B., and Groth, P. Scabies: Transcutaneous poisoning during treatment. *Pediatrics* 59:643, 1977.

Rasmussen, J. E. The problem of lindane. *J. Am. Acad. Dermatol.* 5:507, 1981.

Schacter, B. Treatment of scabies and pediculosis with lindane preparations: An evaluation. *J. Am. Acad. Dermatol.* 5:517, 1981.

Zesch, A., Nitzsche, K., and Lange, M. Demonstration of the percutaneous resorption of a lipophilic pesticide and its possible storage in the human body. *Arch. Dermatol. Res.* 273:43, 1982.

Gentian Violet (Genapax®)

Indications and Recommendations

Gentian violet is relatively contraindicated in pregnancy because other therapeutic agents are preferable. When applied topically, this triphenylmethane (rosaniline) dye is bacteriostatic and bactericidal to gram-positive bacteria and many fungi. Gram-negative and acid-fast bacteria are very resistant. It is used for the treatment of vaginal candidiasis and has largely been replaced by other antifungal agents because of its propensity to stain skin and clothing. Its maternal and fetal effects are unknown as no studies of the use of gentian violent during pregnancy have been performed. Should treatment for *Candida* vaginitis become necessary during pregnancy, nystatin is the drug of choice.

Recommended Reading

Gilman, A. G., Goodman, L. S., and Gilman, A. *The Pharmacological Basis of Therapeutics* (6th ed.). New York: Macmillan, 1980. P. 979.

Glycopyrrolate (Robinul®)

Indications and Recommendations

Although experience with glycopyrrolate administration in obstetric patients is limited, this drug appears to be safe when used as indicated during pregnancy. Glycopyrrolate is a synthetic, anticholinergic, quaternary ammonium compound used parenterally to decrease gastrointestinal secretions before elective surgery. This drug appears to be as effective as atropine as a preanesthetic agent and, on a theoretic basis, offers greater safety to the fetus since its transfer across the placenta is minimal.

Special Considerations in Pregnancy

The effectiveness of glycopyrrolate in reducing the volume and acidity of gastric secretions, especially when combined with magnesium trisilicate, has been demonstrated in obstetric patients treated before elective cesarean sections. Several studies have shown that this drug causes an increase in maternal heart rate and decrease in beat-to-beat variability as a result of vagal inhibitory effects on the sinoatrial pacemaker. Unlike atropine, however, glycopyrrolate crosses the placenta poorly and has no demonstrable effect on either fetal heart rate or variability. No adverse effects on neonates born to women who were premedicated with this drug have thus far been reported.

Dosage

The drug is given parenterally in a single dose of 1–2 mg. Glycopyrrolate may be given orally in doses of 1–2 mg q4–6h.

Adverse Effects

As with other anticholinergic drugs, side effects include dryness of mucous membranes, thirst, and constipation. Larger dosages may produce slurred speech, blurred vision, occasional disorientation, hallucinations, delirium, loss of taste, urinary retention, headache, tachycardia, and palpitations. Glycopyrrolate is contraindicated for use in patients with glaucoma, bladder neck or gastrointestinal obstruction, paralytic ileus, and severe ulcerative colitis.

Mechanism of Action

Glycopyrrolate acts as a competitive antagonist of acetylcholine at postganglionic muscarinic sites. Because it is a quaternary ammonium compound, physicochemical laws of membrane transport suggest that glycopyrrolate should be transferred poorly across the blood-brain and placental barriers. This is probably why the drug causes fewer maternal central nervous system and fetal side effects than do other anticholinergic agents.

Absorption and Biotransformation

Glycopyrrolate undergoes biotransformation in the liver and renal excretion.

Recommended Reading

Abboud, T. K., et al. Use of glycopyrrolate in the parturient: Effect on the maternal and fetal heart and uterine activity. *Obstet. Gynecol.* 57:224, 1981.

Diaz, D. M., Diaz, S. F., and Mary, G. F. Cardiovascular effects of glycopyrrolate and belladonna derivatives in obstetric patients. *Bull. N.Y. Acad. Med.* 56:245, 1980.

Gilman, A. G., Goodman, L. S., and Gilman, A. *The Pharmacological Basis of Therapeutics* (6th ed.). New York: Macmillan, 1980. P. 130.

Roper, R. E., and Salem, M. G. Effects of glycopyrrolate and atropine combined with antacid on gastric acidity. *Br. J. Anaesthesiol.* 53:1277, 1981.

Gold Salts: Auranofin (Ridaura®), Aurothioglucose (Solganal®), Gold Sodium Thiomalate (Myochrysine®)

Indications and Recommendations

The administration of gold salts during pregnancy for the treatment of rheumatoid arthritis is controversial. Animal data suggest teratogenicity when high dosages are used. However, approximately 75 uneventful human pregnancies have been reported. Because gold salts are extremely toxic, their use should be reserved for patients with rheumatoid arthritis refractory to other forms of treatment, such as salicylates and physiotherapy, and they should be discontinued before conception if possible. Patients who conceive while receiving gold therapy or within months of discontinuing therapy should be informed of the theoretic risks to the fetus and of the generally favorable pregnancy outcomes reported in humans.

Special Considerations in Pregnancy

Gold salts have been shown to be teratogenic in rats and rabbits, with ventral wall defects being the predominant anomaly in the rabbits. Dosages were considerably higher than those generally used in humans.

Gold was detected in the liver, kidney, and placenta of a human fetus whose gold-treated mother chose termination when pregnancy was discovered at 20 weeks' gestation. When another woman, treated with gold throughout gestation, delivered a healthy baby at term, umbilical cord serum gold concentration was 225 μg/dl, while simultaneous maternal venous plasma gold concentration was 392 μg/dl. These cases demonstrate that gold salts cross the placenta. Anecdotal reports of human fetal exposure to gold salts in the first trimester include 79 cases. One baby died of severe malformations; two had congenital hip dislocation; a fourth was stillborn due to a true knot in the umbilical cord but was normally formed. Thus, the incidence of major anomalies was 1 in 79 (1.3%). These anecdotal data do not support the recommendation that pregnancies conceived inadvertently during the administration of gold salts be terminated.

Dosage

Aurothioglucose is given by intramuscular injection, and is available in vials containing 10 ml of a 50-mg/ml solution in oil. Gold sodium thiomalate is also given intramuscularly, and is marketed in ampules of 10, 25, 50, and 100 mg/ml, and in multiple-dose vials similar in content to aurothioglucose. Various dosing regimens have been proposed. Most commonly, 10 mg is given in the first week, 25 mg in the second and third weeks, and 50 mg/week thereafter, up to a total dose of 750 mg. If remission occurs, dosage is reduced to 50 mg every 2 weeks for 4 doses, then every 3 weeks for 4 doses, and then every 4 weeks for a year. Some physicians individualize dosage to signs of toxicity or to plasma or urine concentration.

If a relapse occurs during the year of low-dose therapy, the dosage is increased. If a relapse occurs after the course of treatment has ended, it is reinstituted.

Auranofin, a newly available oral form of gold, is manufactured in capsules containing 3 mg. The usual dose is 6 mg/day, with an increase to 9 mg/day if the response is inadequate after 6 months.

Adverse Effects

Gold salts are exceedingly toxic, with an estimated incidence of adverse effects between 25 and 50% of treated individuals. Serious toxicity occurs in about 10% of patients. The mortality related to this drug is estimated to be approximately 0.4%.

Toxicity most commonly involves the skin and oral mucous membranes. These reactions may range from erythema to severe exfoliative dermatitis. Stomatitis, pharyngitis, tracheitis, gastritis, colitis, glossitis, and vaginitis may occur. A characteristic gray-blue pigmentation may appear in skin and mucous membranes, especially with exposure to light. This is called *chrysiasis*.

Severe blood dyscrasias may also result. Thrombocytopenia may be fatal and may not develop until many months after the initiation of therapy. It is believed to be related to an immunologic mechanism, with accelerated platelet destruction. Leukopenia, agranulocytosis, and aplastic anemia have been reported. Eosinophilia is common and may be an indication for temporary discontinuance of therapy.

Renal damage, localized in the proximal tubules, results in heavy proteinuria and microhematuria in 1–3% of cases. The predominant lesion is membranous glomerulonephritis when nephrosis occurs.

Encephalitis, peripheral neuritis, hepatitis, pulmonary infiltrates, and nitritoid crisis (resembling anaphylaxis) have all been reported.

Chelating agents have been used in cases of severe toxicity or overdosage.

Mechanism of Action

The mechanism of action of gold salts in rheumatoid arthritis is poorly understood. These compounds can suppress symptoms but do not cure the disease. They can decrease concentrations of rheumatoid factor and immunoglobulins and impair mitogen-induced proliferation of lymphocytes. They probably suppress cell-mediated immunity. It has been hypothesized that gold is taken up by macrophages, with resultant inhibition of phagocytosis and the activities of lysosomal enzymes.

Absorption and Biotransformation

The gold salts are absorbed rapidly after intramuscular injection, reaching peak plasma concentrations in 2–6 hours unless the salt is suspended in oil, in which case the absorption is more gradual. Approximately 25% of the gold in an oral dose of auranofin is absorbed.

In the blood, gold is first bound to albumin (about 95%). Early in the course of treatment, much of the gold is transferred to erythrocytes. Synovial fluid concentrations are approximately half the plasma levels. As therapy continues, gold is preferentially deposited in the joints affected by rheumatoid arthritis, as opposed to skeletal muscle, bone, and fat. Gold deposits are found in macrophages, in renal tubular epithelium, and in many other tissues.

The plasma half-life is approximately 7 days for a single 50-mg dose, but lengthens with chronic therapy, and may be as long as weeks to months after prolonged therapy. Gold remains in tissues for many years after therapy is discontinued.

Excretion is approximately 75% renal and 25% fecal (via biliary secretion). After a cumulative dose of 1,000 mg, blood concentrations fall to normal in 40–80 days, but urinary excretion can be detected for at least 1 year. Sulfhydryl chelating agents increase the excretion of gold.

Recommended Reading

Chaffman, M., et al. Auranofin: A preliminary review of its pharmacological properties and therapeutic use in rheumatoid arthritis. *Drugs* 27:378, 1984.

Cohen, D. L., and Orzel, J. Infants of mothers receiving gold therapy. *Arthritis Rheum.* 24:104, 1981.

Gilman, A. G., Goodman, L. S., and Gilman, A. *The Pharmacological Basis of Therapeutics* (6th ed.). New York: Macmillan, 1980. Pp. 713–717.

Hollander, J. L. Gold Therapy for Rheumatoid Arthritis. In J. L. Hollander (ed.), *Arthritis and Allied Conditions.* Philadelphia: Lea & Febiger, 1972.

Kidston, M. E., Beck, F., and Lloyd, J. B. The teratogenic effect of Myochrysine injection in rats. *J. Anat.* 108:590, 1971.

Miyamoto, T., et al. Gold therapy in bronchial asthma—special emphasis upon blood levels in gold and its teratogenicity. *Nippon Naika Gakkai Zasshi* 63:1190, 1974.

Moller-Madsen, B., and Danscher, G. Transplacental transport of gold in rats exposed to sodium aurothiomalate. *Exp. Mol. Pathol.* 39:327, 1983.

Rocker, I., and Henderson, W. J. Transfer of gold from mother to fetus. *Lancet* 2:1246, 1976.

Rogers, J. G., et al. Possible teratogenic effects of gold. *Aust. Paediatr. J.* 16:194, 1980.

Szabo, K. T., DiFebbo, M. E., and Phelan, D. G. The effects of gold-containing compounds on pregnant rabbits and their fetuses. *Vet. Pathol.* 15(Suppl. 5):97, 1978.

Szabo, K. T., Guerriero, F. J., and Kang, Y. J. The effects of gold-containing compounds on pregnant rats and their fetuses. *Vet. Pathol.* 15(Suppl. 5):89, 1978.

Tarp, U., and Graudal, H. A followup study of children exposed to gold compounds in utero. *Arthritis Rheum.* 28:235, 1985.

Griseofulvin (Fulvicin-U/F®, Grifulvin V®, Grisactin®)

Indications and Recommendations

Griseofulvin use is contraindicated during pregnancy. It is a systemic agent used to treat fungal infections of the skin, hair, and nails. Such infections are not life-threatening, and since griseofulvin is a known teratogen in laboratory animals and has been demonstrated to cross the human placenta, its use is contraindicated during pregnancy. Its use should be postponed until after delivery.

Recommended Reading

Gilman, A. G., Goodman, L. S., and Gilman, A. *The Pharmacological Basis of Therapeutics* (6th ed.). New York: Macmillan, 1980. Pp. 1238–1239.

Klein, M. F., and Beall, J. R. Griseofulvin: A teratogenic study. *Science* 175:1483, 1972.

Kucers, A., and Bennett, N. *The Use of Antibiotics* (2nd ed.). London: William Heinemann, 1975.

Rubin, A., and Dvornik, D. Placental transfer of griseofulvin. *Am. J. Obstet. Gynecol.* 92:882, 1965.

Guanethidine (Ismelin®)

Indications and Recommendations

Guanethidine is contraindicated during pregnancy. This drug is a powerful postganglionic sympatholytic compound and may be used as an antihypertensive agent. It acts by blocking norepinephrine release from nerve endings, which exposes more of the neurotransmitter to metabolic inactivation within the neuron and results in a depletion of the storage pool.

Many of the observed side effects of guanethidine are due to the combination of adrenergic inhibition and unopposed parasympathetic function. Adverse effects include significant orthostatic and exercise hypotension, bradycardia, increased gastric secretion, and frequent bowel movements or diarrhea. The drug must be present within neuronal endings in order to have an effect. Any agents that inhibit the storage of guanethidine or its transport across the neuronal membrane will therefore block its action. These agents include the tricyclic antidepressants, phenothiazines, amphetamines, methylphenidate, and reserpine.

Experience with guanethidine in the pregnant woman is limited, and its effects on the fetus are unknown. Pronounced postural hypotension and other annoying sequelae of this drug make it a poor choice for the therapy of hypertension in pregnancy. Guanethidine appears in breast milk in very small quantities and can probably be given to nursing mothers.

Recommended Reading

Gilman, A. G., Goodman, L. S., and Gilman, A. *The Pharmacological Basis of Therapeutics* (6th ed.). New York: Macmillan, 1980. Pp. 198–201.
Kelly, J. V. Drugs used in the management of toxemia of pregnancy. *Clin. Obstet. Gynecol.* 20:395, 1977.
Med. Lett. Drugs Ther. 676:107, 1984.

Haloperidol (Haldol®)

Indications and Recommendations

Haloperidol may be administered to pregnant women for the treatment of psychosis. This agent is similar to the phenothiazines and is used to treat delusions, hallucinations, disordered thought processes, paranoid symptoms, and withdrawal psychoses. It has also been used successfully to treat chorea gravidarum during the second and third trimesters of pregnancy. It is reported to be effective in the treatment of Gilles de la Tourette disease. Because of isolated case reports of teratogenicity, haloperidol use in pregnancy should be avoided in the first trimester if possible.

Haloperidol will calm the excited patient and induce sleep. It will also block apomorphine-induced emesis.

Special Considerations in Pregnancy

Congenital anomalies including phocomelia have been noted in infants whose mothers have taken haloperidol during pregnancy. However, only isolated cases have been reported. In one series of 38 infants with severe limb reduction defects, none of the mothers could recall having taken haloperidol during the index pregnancies. As there have been no prospective studies to date, the data available are insufficient to implicate haloperidol as the cause of the reported malformations.

Due to the pharmacologic similarities of this drug to the phenothiazines, fetal and neonatal responses to maternal administration may be similar. Haloperidol is excreted in breast milk, with a calculated daily dose to the suckling infant in the range of 10–25 μg/day. This is equivalent to 6 μg/kg/day and should be compared with a daily dose of 14 μg/kg in an average 70-kg individual taking 1.0 mg haloperidol each day. To date there are no reports of adverse effects in human infants nursed by mothers taking this drug.

Dosage

The drug is available in tablets of 0.5, 1.0, 2.0, 5.0, 10.0, and 20.0 mg; as an oral concentrate of 2 mg/ml; and for intramuscular injection at 5 mg/ml. The usual dosage is between 0.5 and 2.0 mg 2–3 times a day. Some patients given long-term treatment are drug resistant and may require 3–5 mg 2–3 times a day. The reported cases of chorea gravidarum were treated initially with 1 mg 4 times a day, then reduced to 0.5 mg 4 times daily. In rare cases, haloperidol has been used in doses in excess of 100 mg daily.

Adverse Effects

Haloperidol can cause galactorrhea. Its autonomic effects are less prominent than other antipsychotic drugs. The most frequent side effects are extrapyramidal symptoms, akathisia, dystonia, dry mouth, and constipation. Occasional side effects include blood dyscrasias, hypotension, drowsiness, and menstrual changes. Rare side effects are cholestatic jaundice, photosensitivity, and convulsions.

Mechanism of Action

The mechanism of action of haloperidol is only partly known and is thought to be similar to that of the phenothiazines. Its effects may be due to blockage of dopamine receptors in the caudate nucleus and inhibition of the activation of adenyl cyclase by dopamine.

Absorption and Biotransformation

Haloperidol is readily absorbed from the gastrointestinal tract, with peak effect being achieved approximately 3 hours after oral dosing. The drug is extensively degraded in the liver, so that less than 1% is excreted unchanged in the urine.

Recommended Reading

AMA Drug Evaluations (5th ed.). Chicago: American Medical Association, 1983. Pp. 235–237.

Ayd, F. J., Jr. Excretion of psychotropic drugs in human breast milk. *Int. Drug Ther. Newslett.* 8:33, 1973.

Baldessarini, R. J. *Chemotherapy in Psychiatry.* Cambridge: Harvard University, 1977. Pp. 12–56.

Donaldson, J. O. Control of chorea gravidarum with haloperidol. *Obstet. Gynecol.* 59:381, 1982.

Gilman, A. G., Goodman, L. S., and Gilman, A. *The Pharmacological Basis of Therapeutics* (6th ed.). New York: Macmillan, 1980. P. 410.

Hanson, J. W., and Oakley, G. P., Jr. Haloperidol and limb deformity. *J.A.M.A.* 231:26, 1975.

Klopelman, A. E., McCullar, F. G. W., and Heggeness, L. Limb malformations following maternal use of haloperidol. *J.A.M.A.* 231:62, 1975.

Patterson, J. F. Treatment of chorea gravidarum with haloperidol. *South. Med. J.* 72:1220, 1979.

Stewart, R. B., Karas, B., and Springer, P. K. Haloperidol excretion in breast milk. *Am. J. Psychiatry* 137:849, 1980.

Van Waes, A., Van De Velde, E. Safety evaluation of haloperidol in the treatment of hyperemesis gravidarum. *J. Clin. Pharmacol.* 9:224, 1969.

Whalley, L. J., Blain, P. G., and Prime, J. K. Haloperidol secreted in breast milk. *Br. Med. J.* 282:1746, 1981.

Heparin

Indications and Recommendations

Heparin is the anticoagulant of choice during pregnancy. Some researchers have recommended the use of oral anticoagulants during the second trimester, but since these compounds may induce fetal abnormalities throughout pregnancy, it is preferable to administer heparin whenever anticoagulation is necessary in an undelivered patient.

Anticoagulants are indicated in the treatment and prophylaxis of pulmonary embolism, venous thromboembolic disease, and atrial fibrillation with embolization; prevention of clotting in arterial and cardiac surgery; and the prevention of clotting with implanted prosthetic devices such as heart valves. The use of heparin to treat disseminated intravascular coagulation (DIC) of obstetric origin remains controversial.

When initiated before elective surgery, a course of heparin given subcutaneously and in subtherapeutic dosages has been reported to be effective in preventing postoperative deep vein phlebitis. Minidose therapy has also been given as prophylaxis against phlebitis in obese patients confined to bed for prolonged periods and in women with a history of deep vein problems in prior pregnancies.

Patients who are being fully anticoagulated with heparin may require continuous hospitalization throughout the course of the therapy, although selected individuals can be instructed to give their own intravenous or subcutaneous injections with outpatient monitoring. Minidose heparin prophylaxis can be given entirely on an outpatient basis with periodic monitoring. Heparin can be administered to breast-feeding mothers.

Special Considerations in Pregnancy

Since heparin does not cross the placenta, it has no direct effect on the fetus. An increased risk of spontaneous abortion and premature labor has been reported by some authors. Prospective studies, however, have not confirmed these findings. Heparin given to breast-feeding women does not have any demonstrable ill effect on the nursing infant.

Effective treatment of DIC rests with the recognition and adequate eradication of the underlying illness. To date, no controlled double-blind prospective study has demonstrated a beneficial effect of the use of heparin in treating DIC of obstetric origin. Moreover, its use has been reported to be deleterious rather than helpful in some cases.

Dosage

The anticoagulant potency of a given weight of heparin may vary from one preparation to another. It should always be ordered in USP units as opposed to cubic centimeters of solution. The effect is variable among patients, and the dosage therefore must be monitored with either Lee-White whole-blood clotting time or activated partial thromboplastin times (APTT). The Lee-White time should be 2.5–3.0 times control values, and the APTT time should be 1.5–

Table 6. Heparin administration: method, frequency, and dose

Method of administration	Frequency	Dose (units)
Full heparinization		
Subcutaneous	Initial dose	10,000
	q8h	8,000–10,000
	q12h	12,000–20,000
Intermittent IV	Initial dose	10,000
	q4h	5,000–10,000
Continuous IV	Continuous	5,000 (loading)
		20,000–40,000/day
Prophylactic preoperative miniheparinization		
Subcutaneous	q8–12h (begin the night before surgery)	5,000

Note: Some authorities suggest giving 5,000 units of heparin subcutaneously every 12–24 hours for outpatient prophylaxis in patients with a history of deep vein phlebitis in a prior pregnancy. These patients should be monitored with APTTs every 3–4 weeks.

2.5 times control values. Requirements for heparin may dramatically decrease as the thrombophlebitic process is brought under control.

Table 6 gives the frequency and dose of heparin used with each method of administration. Continuous infusion is the preferred method of administration: There are fewer bleeding complications, and monitoring is simplified. With this type of infusion too, blood may be drawn at any time, while blood for clotting studies must be drawn immediately prior to the next dose when intermittent schedules are used.

In the case of overdose, heparin is immediately discontinued. If it is necessary to reverse the anticoagulant effect, protamine sulfate is administered as a 1% solution in a dose of 1 mg for each 100 units of heparin thought to be present at the time of neutralization. (Consider 30 min to be the half-life of intravenous heparin and 60 min the half-life of subcutaneous heparin.) If protamine is given in excess, it may itself act as an anticoagulant by interfering with the action of thrombin on fibrinogen. Some clinicians therefore will give half of the projected dose and observe the effect on the APTT.

Adverse Effects

The most important side effect associated with heparin administration is hemorrhage in the mother. The anticoagulant action of this substance can be rapidly reversed with protamine sulfate. The following conditions have been considered by some authors to be contraindications to the use of heparin:

1. Any condition in which an increased bleeding tendency exists
2. Subacute bacterial endocarditis
3. Acute pericarditis
4. Threatened abortion
5. Suspected intracranial bleeding

Prolonged use of heparin has been associated with maternal osteoporosis. The exact mechanism is unknown, although interference with the metabolism of vitamin D has been observed. The development of osteoporosis seems to be related to the dose of heparin administered and the duration of treatment. Spinal fractures are unusual and have not been reported in patients receiving less than 10,000 units/day regardless of the duration of therapy. Conversely, the shortest reported time from initiation of therapy to radiologic demonstration of spinal fractures is approximately 4 months.

A retrospective analysis of 20 women treated during and after pregnancy has been performed within 2 years of terminating therapy. These patients had received subcutaneous heparin at doses ranging from 16,000–20,000 units/day for 6–32 weeks, and none of them showed evidence of thoracolumbar spine osteoporosis. However, significant phalangeal demineralization was found in patients after long-term therapy (>25 weeks) as compared to short-term therapy (<7 weeks). Whether these changes are reversible remains to be determined, since prospective long-term follow-up studies are lacking.

Hypersensitivity reactions are usually manifested by chills, fever, and urticaria, but true anaphylactoid reactions have also occurred. Unusual side effects include transient alopecia, reversible thrombocytopenia, and rebound hyperlipemia when the drug is discontinued.

When given simultaneously with heparin, the following drugs may cause excessive bleeding: aspirin and aspirin derivatives, phenylbutazone, indomethacin, clofibrate, glyceryl guaiacolate (guaifenesin), and dipyridamole. Drugs that may decrease the anticoagulant effect when given with heparin include d-tubocurarine and the quinine derivatives.

Mechanism of Action

Heparin is a complex anionic mucopolysaccharide with a molecular weight of approximately 12,000. It is stored and probably formed in the mast cells of animal tissues. Heparin inhibits factors involved in the conversion of prothrombin to thrombin. Its anticoagulant effect requires the presence of an alpha globulin known as antithrombin III, the heparin cofactor. Heparin combines with antithrombin III and, in doing so, alters the configuration of that molecule. Antithrombin III is then able to combine with many coagulation proteins and inhibit their activity. Heparin also directly interferes with platelet aggregation.

Absorption and Biotransformation

Heparin is not well absorbed after oral administration. Subcutaneous, intravenous, and intramuscular routes of administration are effective. Intramuscular injections may cause local or dissecting retroperitoneal hematomas. The drug is metabolized in the liver. A partially degraded form of heparin called *uroheparin* is excreted in the urine. Heparin *does not* cross the placenta or pass into the mother's milk.

Recommended Reading

Bell, W. R. Hematologic abnormalities in pregnancy. *Med. Clin. North Am.* 61:165, 1977.

Courtney, L. D. Amniotic fluid embolism. *Obstet. Gynecol. Surv.* 29: 169, 1974.

de-Swiet, M., et al. Prolonged heparin therapy in pregnancy causes bone demineralization. *Br. J. Obstet. Gynaecol.* 90:1129, 1983.

Hall, J. G., Pauli, R. M., and Wilson, K. M. Maternal and fetal sequelae of anticoagulation during pregnancy. *Am. J. Med.* 68:122, 1980.

Howell, R., et al. The risks of antenatal subcutaneous heparin prophylaxis: A controlled trial. *Br. J. Gynaecol.* 90:1124, 1983.

Jaques, L. B. *Anticoagulant Therapy: Pharmacological Principles.* Springfield, Ill.: Charles C Thomas, 1965.

Kakkar, V. V. Deep vein thrombosis, detection and prevention. *Circulation* 51:8, 1975.

Kakkar, V. V. Efficacy of low doses of heparin in prevention of deep vein thrombosis after major surgery. A double blind, randomized trial. *Lancet* 2:101, 1972.

Pritchard, J. A. Haematological problems associated with delivery, placental abruption, retained dead fetus, and amniotic fluid embolism. *Clin. Haematol.* 2:563, 1973.

Heroin

Indications and Recommendations

Heroin, or diacetylmorphine, is contraindicated during pregnancy. It is a class I drug, meaning that there are no valid indications for its use in the United States. It is highly addictive and the pregnant woman addicted to heroin represents a significant economic, social, and medical problem to our society.

Heroin easily crosses the placenta, and fetal withdrawal may occur if the mother undergoes rapid withdrawal. Fetal death in utero has been reported under these circumstances. Infants of heroin-addicted mothers tend to be of low birth weight, and other obstetric complications occur with increased frequency. On the other hand, it appears that fetal hepatic and pulmonary maturation are accelerated. It is not clear whether congenital anomalies are more common among infants of heroin-addicted mothers, although some evidence suggests this to be the case. Overall perinatal mortality is increased. Neonatal withdrawal symptoms are common.

Effects of maternal heroin addiction may persist in the offspring up to at least 6 years of age, with poor growth and development described in one follow-up study. These problems are compounded by the tendency of mothers addicted to street drugs to seek prenatal care late if at all, and for their home environments to be less than optimal with respect to nutrition, comfort, and stress. Many treatment programs have been aimed at this group of individuals, and some success at improving outcome has been reported. See *Methadone* and *Narcotic Analgesics* for discussion of fetal and maternal effects.

Recommended Reading

Connaughton, J. F., et al. Perinatal addiction: Outcome and management. *Am. J. Obstet. Gynecol.* 129:679, 1977.

Gilman, A. G., Goodman, L. S., and Gilman, A. *The Pharmacological Basis of Therapeutics* (6th ed.). New York: Macmillan, 1980. Pp. 496–497, 544–549.

Glass, L., Rajegowda, B. K., and Evans, H. E. Absence of respiratory distress syndrome in premature infants of heroin-addicted mothers. *Lancet* 2:685, 1971.

Nathenson, G., et al. The effect of maternal heroin addiction on neonatal jaundice. *J. Pediatr.* 81:899, 1972.

Ostrea, E. M., and Chavez, C. J. Perinatal problems in maternal drug addiction: A study of 830 cases. *J. Pediatr.* 94:292, 1979.

Pelosi, M. A., et al. Pregnancy complicated by heroin addiction. *Obstet. Gynecol.* 45:512, 1975.

Perlmutter, J. F. Drug addiction in pregnant women. *Am. J. Obstet. Gynecol.* 99:569, 1967.

Rementeria, J. L., and Nunag, N. N. Narcotic withdrawal in pregnancy: Stillbirth incidence with a case report. *Am. J. Obstet. Gynecol.* 116:1152, 1973.

Stone, M. L., et al. Narcotic addiction in pregnancy. *Am. J. Obstet. Gynecol.* 109:716, 1971.

Wilson, G. S., et al. The development of preschool children of heroin-addicted mothers: A controlled study. *Pediatrics* 63:135, 1979.

Zelson, C., Rubio, E., and Wasserman, E. Neonatal narcotic addiction: 10 year observation. *Pediatrics* 48:178, 1971.

Hydralazine (Apresoline®)

Indications and Recommendations

Hydralazine is safe to use during pregnancy. It is the drug of choice for the control of moderate to severe hypertension in a patient with preeclampsia-toxemia (PET). This drug may also be used in combination with other agents to control chronic hypertension in obstetric patients.

Significant iatrogenic hypotension can develop when hydralazine is used to treat an acute hypertensive episode in an intravascularly depleted patient with preeclampsia. In order to minimize the chances of this occurring, a 5-mg test dose may be given intravenously 10–15 minutes prior to the administration of more aggressive therapy.

A patient with mild preeclampsia whose fetus still is pulmonically immature may be treated with oral hydralazine in doses of 200 mg/day or less, oral phenobarbital, and bed rest. Failure to maintain diastolic blood pressures below 110 mm Hg on this regimen should prompt the physician to stabilize the patient quickly with intravenous medication and then deliver her of her infant. The renal function of patients with preeclampsia being maintained on oral antihypertensive medication should be monitored daily. Any deterioration of that function should alert the physician to the need for rapid delivery.

Hydralazine alone is a poor choice for the management of patients with chronic hypertension. In order to maximize its long-term effectiveness, it may be necessary to add diuretics and possibly propranolol to the regimen. Since there are objections to the use of these agents during pregnancy, we do not recommend hydralazine as primary therapy for the obstetric patient with chronic hypertension.

Special Considerations in Pregnancy

Acute hypotensive episodes can occur in response to an intravenous bolus of hydralazine given to a preeclamptic patient who is intravascularly depleted. The effect on the fetus of lowering maternal blood pressure with intravenous hydralazine has been studied in 33 women with diastolic pressures of 110 mm Hg or greater. All of these pregnancies were beyond 30 weeks' gestation. Thirty of the women responded to a dose of 12.5 mg hydralazine with a decrease in diastolic pressure to values between 70 and 90 mm Hg. Nineteen fetuses demonstrated electronic fetal monitoring evidence of heart rate decelerations with or without bradycardia, while the other 14 fetuses did not show any evidence of fetal heart rate abnormalities. In the first group, there were three stillborns and 13 neonates born with weights below the 10th percentile for gestational age. In the second group, there was only one neonate below the 10th percentile and no perinatal deaths. Despite the fact that this study utilized an initial dose that is more than twice the recommended test dose, the majority of patients did not have a fall in diastolic values below 70 mm Hg. With drops in pressure into the range of 70–90 mm Hg, however, it appears that growth-retarded fetuses are far more likely to demonstrate heart rate changes than those who are appropriately grown. This undoubtedly reflects a greater compromise in fetal reserve and suggests that a reasonable therapeutic objective in these patients is a diastolic pressure between 90 and 100 mm Hg.

Tachycardia and increased cardiac work and oxygen consumption accompany the intravenous use of hydralazine. This may precipitate angina or myocardial ischemia in a patient with occlusive coronary artery disease. The treatment of symptoms related to increased cardiac work is intravenous propranolol.

Tolerance to the antihypertensive action of hydralazine can develop with chronic administration if a beta-adrenergic blocker (e.g., propranolol) or a diuretic, or both, is not administered. Since there are objections to the use of these agents in pregnancy, methyldopa is a better initial choice for treatment of the pregnant woman with chronic hypertension.

Specific fetal side effects related to hydralazine therapy for the mother have only rarely been described in humans. An isolated case of neonatal thrombocytopenia has been reported, but there is very little supportive evidence to implicate hydralazine as the cause of this problem. In animals, however, skeletal defects can be produced that resemble those observed in experimentally induced manganese deficiency states.

Animal experiments have indicated that hydralazine may increase uteroplacental blood flow in sheep with hypertension. There is no convincing evidence in humans that fetal compromise occurs after the administration of this drug in the absence of significant systemic hypotension in the mother.

Table 7. Doses of hydralazine and methods of administration

Method of administration	Dose (mg)	Onset (min)	Maximal effect (min)	Duration (h)	Interval (h)
IV*	5–20	10–20	20–40	3–8	3–6
IM	5–20	20–40	40–60	3–8	3–6
PO	20–50	30–60	90–120	6–8	6–8

*The initial intravenous dose should never exceed 20 mg and may be repeated as necessary. The onset of action usually occurs in about 15 minutes. The dose and frequency of administration required for satisfactory blood pressure control are highly variable. After stabilization is achieved, the drug can be administered by a continuous intravenous drip. The daily dose should not exceed 300 mg.

Dosage

Table 7 details how onset, maximal effect, and duration differ with different dosages and methods of administration.

Adverse Effects

Side effects include palpitations, flushing, nasal congestion, headache, dizziness, anginal attacks, and electrocardiographic changes of myocardial ischemia. Side effects related to chronic use in doses greater than 200 mg/day include drug fever, skin eruptions, peripheral neuropathy, blood dyscrasias, mild gastrointestinal symptoms, and an acute rheumatoid state that can progress to the hydralazine-lupus syndrome. Approximately 10–20% of patients who receive more than 400 mg/day will develop this last problem. Occasionally, central nervous system toxicity may be manifested as an acute psychotic episode.

Mechanism of Action

Hydralazine reduces vascular resistance by directly relaxing arteriolar smooth muscle. Postcapillary capacitance vessels are much less affected than precapillary resistance vessels. It has been postulated that hydralazine may be able to chelate certain trace metals required for smooth muscle contraction.

Peripheral arterial vasodilatation is not uniform. Vascular resistance in the coronary, cerebral, splanchnic, and uterine circulations decreases more than in skin and muscle. Renovascular resistance decreases more than that in other vascular beds. Blood flow in the more dilated circulatory beds usually increases unless the hypotensive effect of the drug is profound. Both supine and standing blood pressures are decreased.

Hydralazine has no direct action on the heart; homeostatic circulatory reflexes mediated by the autonomic nervous system, however, remain fully functional. Decreased arterial pressure activates baroreceptors to mediate a sympathetic discharge. This results in increased heart rate, stroke volume, and cardiac output. Because this increase in cardiac output partially offsets the effect of arteriolar dilatation and limits the hypotensive effectiveness of the drug, hydralazine is usually combined with a drug that limits the increase in cardiac output when prescribed for long-term use.

Renal blood flow and glomerular filtration rates are either unaffected or increased. Hydralazine causes sodium and water retention, with expansion of plasma and extracellular volumes. This is a result of a direct renal mechanism as well as an increase in peripheral plasma renin activity. Increases in renin activity during hydralazine therapy are effectively minimized in the nonpregnant woman by the coadministration of propranolol.

Absorption and Biotransformation

Hydralazine is fairly completely absorbed after oral administration. Peak serum concentrations are reached 1–2 hours after an oral dose. Intravenous administration of a given dose results in higher serum levels than the same dose given orally. About 85% of the circulating drug is bound to albumin.

Acetylation in the liver is the major pathway of biotransformation. The rate of acetylation is dependent on the genetically determined activity of hepatic N-acetyltransferase. Therefore, when treated with the same dose of hydralazine, slow acetylators have higher serum concentrations than rapid acetylators. In addition, slow acetylators seem to be more prone to develop the hydralazine-lupus syndrome.

Very high serum levels may be found in patients with renal insufficiency. Renal excretion of the active drug is not usually an important route of elimination, so uremia probably interferes with biotransformation.

Recommended Reading

AMA Committee on Hypertension. The treatment of malignant hypertension and hypertensive emergencies. *J.A.M.A.* 228:1673, 1979.

Koch-Weser, J. Hypertensive emergencies. *N. Engl. J. Med.* 290:211, 1974.

Koch-Weser, J. Hydralazine. *N. Engl. J. Med.* 295:320, 1976.

Vink, G. J., Moodley, J., and Philpott, R. H. Effect of dihydralazine on the fetus in the treatment of maternal hypertension. *Obstet. Gynecol.* 55:519, 1980.

Widerlov, E., Karlman, I., and Storsater, J. Hydralazine-inducted neonatal thrombocytopenia (letter). *N. Engl. J. Med.* 303:1235, 1980.

Woods, J. R. and Brinkman, C. R., III. The treatment of gestational hypertension. *J. Reprod. Med.* 15:195, 1975.

Hydroxyzine (Atarax®, Vistaril®)

Indications and Recommendations

Hydroxyzine is safe to use after the first trimester of pregnancy and is commonly administered, alone or in combination with analgesic agents, for the relief of pain and anxiety during labor. In addition, it is often used as an antipruritic and antianxiety agent. Although human data are lacking, there is evidence that hydroxyzine in large dosages is teratogenic in laboratory animals, and therefore use of the drug is best avoided during the first trimester of pregnancy. Antihistamines are not recommended for lactating women.

Special Considerations in Pregnancy

In the Collaborative Perinatal Project, there were 3,248 infants with malformations among the more than 50,000 mother-infant pairs studied. Five in 50 mother-infant pairs exposed to hydroxyzine during the first 4 lunar months of pregnancy had congenital abnormalities, while three anomalies would have been expected. Thus, there appeared to be a relative risk of 1.55 for birth defects in neonates exposed to this drug during the first 4 months in utero. This is not a particularly strong association and has thus far not been confirmed by other investigations. Animal studies have demonstrated an increased incidence of facial clefts when hydroxyzine was administered in excessive dosages (200 mg/kg) during organogenesis.

Although one study has demonstrated a statistically significant decrease in fetal heart rate beat-to-beat variability when hydroxyzine was administered to laboring mothers, this effect was said to be clinically insignificant.

There is a single case report of an apparent neonatal withdrawal syndrome in a newborn whose mother required 600 mg/day of hydroxyzine throughout the pregnancy. The cord blood hydroxyzine level was 180 μg/dl (usual adult therapeutic level, 50 μg/dl).

Due to its anticholinergic properties, hydroxyzine might be expected to inhibit lactation. Such an effect has not yet been demonstrated.

Dosage

Hydroxyzine is available in capsules containing 25, 50, and 100 mg, and in 25-, 50-, 75-, and 100-mg vials for intramuscular injection. When used as an antipruritic, the usual dose is 25 mg tid or qid. When used orally as an antianxiety drug, the starting dose is usually 50–100 mg qid. When used intramuscularly as an antianxiety agent or in combination with an analgesic, doses of 25–100 mg are employed and may be repeated at 4–6-hour intervals.

Adverse Effects

Although hydroxyzine is often used intentionally to potentiate the effects of narcotic analgesics, it should be remembered that this drug also potentiates other central nervous system depressants, such as barbiturates and alcohol. Other adverse effects include drowsiness and dry mouth. Rarely, excessively high doses have been associated with involuntary motor activity, tremor, and convulsions. Tissue damage has been reported with inadvertent subcutaneous injection.

Mechanism of Action

Hydroxyzine is a piperazine antihistamine that is a competitive blocker of the H_1 receptor in effector cells. It inhibits the smooth muscle response to histamine in the gastrointestinal and respiratory tracts, antagonizes the increased capillary permeability induced by histamine (the wheal and flare), and suppresses the stimulant effect of histamine on the autonomic nervous system. It does not inhibit histamine release. The central nervous system and anti-motion sickness effects are poorly understood, as is the potentiation of narcotics, depressants, and alcohol. Anticholinergic side effects appear to be due to blockage of muscarinic receptors.

Absorption and Biotransformation

Hydroxyzine is rapidly absorbed after oral dosing, and clinical effects are noted within 15–30 minutes after ingestion. Effects are maximal within 1–2 hours and last for 3–6 hours. The drug is metabolized in the liver, with degradation products excreted in the urine within 24 hours.

Recommended Reading

Gilman, A. G., Goodman, L. S., and Gilman, A. *The Pharmacological Basis of Therapeutics* (6th ed.). New York: Macmillan, 1980. Pp. 622–629.

Heinonen, O. P., Slone, D., and Shapiro, S. *Birth Defects and Drugs in Pregnancy.* Boston: John Wright PSG, 1977. Pp. 335–337.

Petrie, R. H., et al. The effect of drugs on fetal heart rate variability. *Am. J. Obstet. Gynecol.* 130:294, 1978.

Prenner, B. M. Neonatal withdrawal syndrome associated with hydroxyzine hydrochloride. *Am. J. Dis. Child.* 131:529, 1977.

Walker, B. E., and Patterson, A. Induction of cleft palate in mice by tranquilizers and barbiturates. *Teratology* 10:159, 1974.

Idoxuridine (Stoxil®)

Indications and Recommendations

Idoxuridine (IDUR) is relatively contraindicated in pregnancy because other therapeutic modalities are preferable. It is used in the treatment of herpes simplex keratitis. These infections are usually not associated with grave prognoses; they are most often limited to the eye and resolve completely. Idoxuridine will often control the infection but will have no effect on accumulated scarring, vascularization, or resultant progressive loss of vision. It acts to block herpes simplex virus reproduction by alteration of DNA synthesis.

Experience with IDUR in pregnant women is lacking, and its effects on the fetus are unknown. In rabbits, however, dosages similar to those used clinically are associated with fetal malformation, including exophthalmos and clubbing of the forelegs.

Should treatment be required, mechanical debridement is preferred over IDUR therapy.

Recommended Reading

Garner, A., and Klintworth, G. K. *Pathobiology of Ocular Disease.* New York: Marcel Dekker, 1982. Pp. 258–262.

Gittinger, J. W. *Ophthalmology. A Clinical Introduction.* Boston: Little, Brown, 1984. Pp. 75–76.

Itoi, M., et al. Teratogenicities of ophthalmic drugs. I. Antiviral ophthalmic drugs. *Arch. Ophthalmol.* 93:46, 1975.

Indigo Carmine

Indications and Recommendations

Indigo carmine may be introduced into the amniotic fluid for documentation of ruptured membranes and for identification of individual amniotic sacs in multiple gestations. Inadequate data are available to evaluate its safety when administered intravenously during urologic procedures in pregnant women.

Special Considerations in Pregnancy

Indigo carmine has replaced methylene blue as a marker dye for amniotic fluid because of the risks of fetal methemoglobinemia with the latter. There are no data available to suggest fetal risk from this substance when it is injected intraamniotically.

When indigo carmine is used to identify the fluid from multiple sacs during amniocentesis for diagnosis of fetal hemolytic disease, its presence may obfuscate measurement of the delta optical density at 450 nm. The dye should therefore not be injected until a sample of fluid has been aspirated. If, however, the amniotic fluid is contaminated with dye, a chloroform extraction procedure can be performed to permit more accurate measurements.

Dosage

When indigo carmine is used for amniocentesis, 0.5–1.0 ml of 0.8% solution is diluted to a 10-ml volume.

Adverse Effects

Intravenously injected indigo carmine has been associated with increased peripheral resistance, increased blood pressure, increased central venous pressure, and lowered cardiac output with reflex-diminished stroke volume and pulse rate. These results resemble those associated with alpha-adrenergic stimulation. There is also a single case report of hypertension and tachycardia with ectopic ventricular beats in a patient given 5 ml of 0.8% indigo carmine while under halothane anesthesia. Thus, care should be exercised in administering this dye intravenously to patients with cardiovascular disease.

Mechanism of Action

When indigo carmine is instilled at amniocentesis, it colors the amniotic fluid blue. In the case of a multiple gestation, subsequent taps may be performed, with the absence of blue discoloration in the aspirated samples indicating success at puncturing the remaining sac(s). In the case of ruptured membranes, the appearance of blue fluid in the vagina confirms the diagnosis. However, since the dye can be absorbed into the maternal circulation and enter the urine, a sterile sponge or tampon placed in the vagina will help to differentiate between true amniotic fluid and maternal urine contamination.

Absorption and Biotransformation

Indigo carmine is injected into the amniotic fluid directly. It is absorbed into the maternal bloodstream and is excreted in the urine. Thus, the urine may be stained.

Recommended Reading

Elias, S., et al. Genetic amniocentesis in twin gestations. *Am. J. Obstet. Gynecol.* 138:169, 1980.

Erickson, J. C., and Widmer, B. A. The vasopressor effect of indigo carmine. *Anesthesiology* 29:188, 1968.

Fribourg, S. Safety of intra-amniotic injection of indigo carmine. *Am. J. Obstet. Gynecol.* 140:350, 1981.

Horger, E. O., and Moody, L. O. Use of indigo carmine for twin amniocentesis and its effect on bilirubin analysis. *Am. J. Obstet. Gynecol.* 150:858, 1984.

Kennedy, W. F., Jr., et al. Cardiovascular and respiratory effects of indigo carmine. *J. Urol.* 100:775, 1968.

Knuppel, R. A., et al. Rhesus isoimmunization in twin gestation. *Am. J. Obstet. Gynecol.* 150:136, 1984.

Ng, T. Y., Datta, T. D., and Kirimli, B. I. Reaction to indigo carmine. *J. Urol.* 116:132, 1976.

Schwerin, G. S. Severe reaction to indigo-carmine. *Ill. Med. J.* 101:48, 1952.

Indomethacin (Indocin®)

Indications and Recommendations

Indomethacin is relatively contraindicated in pregnancy because other therapeutic agents are preferable. It is used in the treatment of rheumatic and nonrheumatic inflammatory disease. It has been shown to be effective as an antipyretic in Hodgkin's disease when the fever is refractory to other therapy. Indomethacin inhibits prostaglandin synthetase, and its use in pregnancy may theoretically produce premature closure of the ductus arteriosus. When used late in pregnancy to delay labor, indomethacin has been associated with persistent fetal circulation and persistent pulmonary hypertension of the newborn.

Recommended Reading

Csaba, I. F., Sueyok, E., and Ertl, T. Relationship of maternal treatment with indomethacin to persistence of fetal circulation. *J. Pediatr.* 92:484, 1978.

Kumor, K. M., et al. Indomethacin as a treatment for premature labor: Neonatal outcome. *Pediatr. Res.* 13:370, 1979.

Manchester, D., Margolis, H. S., and Sheldon, R. E. Possible association between maternal indomethacin therapy and primary pulmonary hypertension of the newborn. *Am. J. Obstet. Gynecol.* 126:467, 1976.

Rubaltelli, F. F., et al. Effect on neonate of maternal treatment with indomethacin. *J. Pediatr.* 94:161, 1979.

Rudolph, A. M. The effects of nonsteroidal antiinflammatory compounds on fetal circulation and pulmonary function. *Obstet. Gynecol.* 58:63S, 1981.

Insulin

Indications and Recommendations

Insulin is safe to use during pregnancy. It is a naturally occurring polypeptide hormone given parenterally to diabetic patients to lower the blood glucose and correct some of the other metabolic abnormalities related to diabetes. It is the treatment of choice for management of pregnancy in the diabetic. Careful attention to diet is equally important. Frequent blood glucose monitoring is mandatory for any patient taking insulin.

Special Considerations in Pregnancy

Insulin administered exogenously to the mother does not cross the placenta in any appreciable amount. Fetal endogenous insulin, presumably increased due to the effect of maternal hyperglycemia on the fetus, may be responsible for macrosomia and hypoglycemia in the newborn. Fetal hypoglycemia accompanies maternal hypoglycemia. As yet, there is no convincing evidence that insulin-induced maternal-fetal hypoglycemia has a detrimental effect on the developing fetus.

Dosage

The dosage of insulin given to a pregnant diabetic must be individually tailored to that patient's needs. In general, insulin requirements may decrease slightly during the first one-third to one-half of pregnancy, and rapid swings of blood sugar with episodes of hypoglycemia are frequently observed. During the second half of pregnancy, insulin requirements often increase to 2–3 times the prepregnancy dose. There is a tendency toward diabetic ketoacidosis, and hypoglycemia is less common.

Most authorities agree that strict control of circulating glucose is extremely important in managing the pregnancy of a diabetic woman. It is well documented that diabetic ketoacidosis is associated with an extremely high perinatal mortality (in some studies as high as 50%). There is some controversy over how low the circulating glucose level should be allowed to fall. At most centers caring for large numbers of diabetic pregnancies, the aim is to render the patient euglycemic; that is, glucose should be maintained at levels comparable to those in normal nondiabetic pregnant women. Fasting blood glucose is kept in the range of 50–100 mg/dl, and postprandial values are kept below 120 mg/dl. Although transient hypoglycemia occurs in some patients, it is believed safer to have to treat this complication occasionally (with a high-protein snack) than to allow continuous hyperglycemia.

There are numerous schemata for the administration of insulin during pregnancy. Some involve split doses of mixed short- and intermediate-acting insulin, some involve multiple doses of short-acting insulin throughout the day, while still others utilize the insulin pump. None has been proved superior to the others. The detailed description of these protocols is beyond the scope of this book.

The use of low doses of insulin (10 units neutral protamine

Hagedorn [NPH] or 20 units NPH wth 10 units regular) has been investigated and found to be effective in reducing the incidence of macrosomia in the infants of mild gestational diabetics. These patients would not generally require insulin to maintain euglycemia, but it may be used prophylactically to prevent macrosomia.

Adverse Effects

An overdose of insulin can obviously create the side effect of hypoglycemia. Another side effect, not necessarily related to overdosing, is hypertrophy or atrophy of subcutaneous fat at injection sites. Allergic reactions to the impurities contained in insulin derived from animals are commonly reported. These symptoms often disappear when the patient is switched to highly purified animal species insulin or to human insulin. Circulating antibodies to exogenous insulin are consistently found in patients treated with animal species insulins, but their clinical significance is controversial. Theoretically, patients taking insulin intermittently are most likely to be placed at a disadvantage by the presence of these antibodies. Women who require insulin for the first time during pregnancy, either because their hyperglycemia has intensified or because they have gestational diabetes, are likely to discontinue this therapy after delivery. We therefore recommend that such patients be treated with human rather than pork or beef insulin.

Mechanism of Action

Insulin consists of 51 amino acids in the form of a 21–amino-acid A chain and a 30–amino-acid B chain connected by disulfide linkages. It is produced as a single 84–amino-acid proinsulin chain, but the C chain of 33 amino acids (known as *connecting peptide*) must be cleaved from between the A and B chains in order for the insulin to become metabolically active.

Insulin is necessary for the efficient transport of glucose from blood to tissues other than those of the central nervous system, renal medulla, pancreatic beta cells, and gut epithelium. It also favors hepatic glycogen synthesis and storage of glucose in adipose tissue as triglyceride. Insulin facilitates the transport of ingested amino acids into cells, thus increasing protein synthesis. It inhibits lipolysis and is therefore antiketogenic.

Exogenous insulin can reverse the symptoms of diabetes, that is, polyuria and polydipsia, by lowering the blood glucose level. It can also reverse diabetic ketoacidosis. It is controversial whether exogenous insulin reverses or slows the vascular complications of diabetes.

Diabetes is characterized as a disease state in which there is a deficiency of insulin that can be either relative or absolute. Many long-standing overt diabetics have virtually undetectable endogenous insulin secretion as measured by C-peptide assay. On the other hand, mild gestational diabetics can have elevated levels of endogenous insulin. In these cases, the metabolic abnormality is presumably caused by peripheral resistance to insulin and its increased degradation. This is probably related to the effects of insulinase activity as well as placental steroid and polypeptide hormone production.

Absorption and Biotransformation

Controversy exists as to the fate of different forms of insulin in humans. A detailed exploration of this subject is beyond the scope of this book. It is known that insulin is degraded in the liver, kidneys, lungs, and placenta and that some insulin is excreted in the urine. Although some dispute exists, most investigators agree that insulin administered to the mother does not cross the placenta into the fetal circulation to a clinically relevant extent.

In the past, insulin was generally derived from pigs (pork insulin), cattle (beef insulin), or a mixture of the two. Of the 51 amino acids in chains comprising the insulin protein structure, pork insulin and human insulin differ by a single amino acid, while beef insulin contains three amino acid differences. Recently, human insulin (produced by recombinant DNA technology or by a chemical substitution in the pork insulin B chain) has become widely available.

The duration of action of exogenously administered insulin varies according to the preparation. The action of purified crystalline zinc insulin (CZI), "regular" insulin, peaks at 1–2 hours and has a duration of 5–6 hours when administered subcutaneously. Semilente insulin, another rapid-acting form, has a peak similar to CZI, but a longer duration (12–16 hours). An intermediate-acting insulin, NPH, is a combination of regular insulin and protamine zinc insulin, and has a peak of action at 2–8 hours and a duration of approximately 24 hours. Lente insulin has a similar time course. These peaks and durations of action are related more to absorption than to metabolic rate.

Recommended Reading

Coustan, D. R., and Imarah, J. Prophylactic insulin treatment of gestational diabetes reduces the incidence of macrosomia, operative delivery and birth trauma. *Am. J. Obstet. Gynecol.* 150:836, 1984.

Felig, P., and Coustan, D. R. Diabetes Mellitus. In G. N. Burrow and T. F. Ferris (eds.), *Medical Complications During Pregnancy*. Philadelphia: Saunders, 1982. Pp. 36–61.

Galloway, J. D., and Kimberlin, P. *Diabetes Mellitus*. Indianapolis: Eli Lilly, 1980.

Pedersen, J. *The Pregnant Diabetic and Her Newborn* (2nd ed.). Baltimore: Williams & Wilkins, 1977.

Isoniazid (INH®)

Indications and Recommendations

Isoniazid is recommended for the treatment of tuberculosis during pregnancy. It is generally considered to be the primary drug used for chemotherapy of tuberculosis and appears to be the safest antitubercular agent available for use during pregnancy. Although the need for treatment of patients whose skin tests are first reactive during pregnancy is controversial, fear of exposing the fetus to isoniazid, particularly after the first trimester, should not be a determining factor.

Special Considerations in Pregnancy

There appear to be no unusual maternal effects of isoniazid use during pregnancy. Isoniazid is known to cross the placenta. Several large-scale studies of women who received isoniazid therapy during all trimesters of pregnancy have shown no significant increase in congenital malformations and no detectable patterns in the malformations that did occur. The authors of a review of 1,480 pregnancies in which isoniazid was used report that 95% of the patients delivered normal infants at term. Approximately 1% of the infants or fetuses were found to be abnormal.

Isoniazid is excreted in breast milk and should be used with caution in women who are breast-feeding, as the infant is at risk for hepatic toxicity. If INH is also being given to the neonate, its dosage may have to be reduced.

Dosage

The usual dose for treatment of active tuberculosis is 300 mg/day (5 mg/kg). This dose is usually given in combination with other antitubercular medications for 18–24 months. When isoniazid is administered to skin-test reactors without active disease, it is given without other antitubercular drugs at the dose specified above for 12 months. Pyridoxine, 50 mg/day, is usually given prophylactically whenever isoniazid is prescribed.

Adverse Effects

The most common, treatable side effect is a pyridoxine-responsive peripheral neuropathy, which occurs most commonly in malnourished patients receiving more than 5 mg/kg/day. Other common side effects include rash, fever, and jaundice. Subclinical hepatitis characterized by reversible, usually asymptomatic elevation of serum glutamic oxaloacetic transaminase (SGOT) and serum glutamic pyruvic transaminase (SGPT) is frequent. Clinical hepatitis is age dependent and is rare in patients who are under 35 years old.

Mechanism of Action

The exact mechanism of action of isoniazid is unknown. It inhibits the synthesis of mycolic acid, a component of mycobacterial cell walls, and probably has other actions. It is both tuberculostatic and tuberculocidal in vitro. Its bactericidal effects are seen only in actively growing bacilli, and "resting" organisms resume normal growth when removed from contact with the drug.

Absorption and Biotransformation

Isoniazid is rapidly and completely absorbed after oral administration. It is widely distributed into all body fluids and cells. Elimination is primarily by hepatic acetylation. The specific pattern of elimination depends on the acetylator phenotype of the individual. In rapid acetylators, the half-life is 0.5–1.5 hours; in slow acetylators, it is 2–4 hours. The half-life is significantly increased in patients with liver disease.

Recommended Reading

Gilman, A. G., Goodman, L. S., and Gilman, A. *The Pharmacological Basis of Therapeutics* (6th ed.). New York: Macmillan, 1980. Pp. 1200–1203.

Good, J. T., et al. Tuberculosis in association with pregnancy. *Am. J. Obstet. Gynecol.* 140:492, 1981.

Scheinhorn, D. J., and Angelillo, V. A. Antituberculosis therapy in pregnancy: Risks to the fetus. *West. J. Med.* 127:195, 1977.

Snider, D. E., et al. Treatment of tuberculosis during pregnancy. *Am. Rev. Respir. Dis.* 122:65, 1980.

Isoproterenol (Isuprel®)

Indications and Recommendations

Isoproterenol is used as a cardiac stimulant to raise systemic blood pressure and as a bronchodilator in the treatment of bronchospasm. It is relatively contraindicated during pregnancy because other therapeutic agents are preferable. A recent study has demonstrated marked hepatotoxicity caused by isoproterenol in chick embryos, but to date, this has not been reported in humans.

Isoproterenol is a pure beta-adrenergic stimulator that increases myocardial strength while relaxing arteriolar and bronchiolar smooth muscle tone. It therefore has positive cardiac inotropic and chronotropic effects in addition to causing peripheral vascular relaxation and bronchodilatation.

Sympathomimetics seem to influence the fetus indirectly by altering uterine blood flow. Uterine vessels only have alpha-adrenergic receptors, and under baseline conditions during pregnancy, they are thought to be maximally dilated. Peripheral vasodilation will therefore only shunt blood away from the uterus. This decrease in uterine blood flow may adversely affect the fetus.

Recommended Reading

Dusek, J., and Ostadal, B. Isoproterenol-induced damage to the liver of chick embryos. *Physiol. Bohemoslov.* 33:67, 1984.

Gilman, A. G., Goodman, L. S., and Gilman, A. *The Pharmacological Basis of Therapeutics* (6th ed.). New York: Macmillan, 1980, Pp. 153–154.

Smith, N. T., and Corbasciao, A. N. The use and misuse of pressor agents. *Anesthesiology* 33:58, 1970.

Isotretinoin (Accutane®)

Indications and Recommendations

Isotretinoin, a synthetic vitamin A derivative used in the treatment of severe cystic acne, is contraindicated during pregnancy. It is a known human teratogen. A pregnancy test should be documented as being negative before any woman begins therapy with isotretinoin, and effective contraception should be maintained throughout the treatment course.

When nonhuman primates were exposed to retinoic acid at appropriate stages of pregnancy, a high incidence of major structural abnormalities (craniofacial, limb reduction, ear) occurred. Among 21 abnormal children exposed to isotretinoin in utero and reported to the FDA over 2 years' time, all had small or absent ears, neurologic injuries, and cardiac defects. Some had facial dysmorphia as well. An additional 26 normal pregnancies and 12 spontaneous abortions were reported. Another 95 patients elected to terminate their pregnancies. Whether the women with normal pregnancies were exposed during the critical period in embryogenesis (28–70 days' menstrual age) is unknown. The true denominator (i.e., number of exposed pregnancies) is also unknown. A subgroup of 36 exposed pregnancies that were followed prospectively yielded 5 malformed infants, 23 normal infants, and 8 spontaneous abortions. Because these anomalies followed a similar pattern, and this pattern resembles the anomalies produced by the drug in laboratory animals, isotretinoin should be considered a human teratogen and avoided during pregnancy.

A single case report of limb reduction defects in a neonate exposed to isotretinoin from day 26 to day 40 of gestation has been published.

Recommended Reading

Benke, P. J. The isotretinoin teratogen syndrome. *J.A.M.A.* 251:3267, 1984.

De La Cruz, E., Vangvanichyakorn, K., and Desposito, F. Multiple congenital malformations associated with maternal isotretinoin therapy. *Pediatrics* 74:428, 1984.

Isotretinoin (Accutane) for acne. *Med. Lett. Drugs Ther.* 24:79, 1982.

Lammer, E. J., et al. Retinoic acid embryopathy. *N. Engl. J. Med.* 313:837, 1985.

McBride, W. G. Limb reduction deformities in child exposed to isotretinoin in utero on gestation days 26–40 only. *Lancet* 1:1276, 1985.

Roche Laboratories. Accutane (isotretinoin/Roche) package insert. 1982.

Tremblay, M., Voyer, P., and Aubin, G. Malformations congenitales dues a l'Accutane. *Can. Med. Assoc. J.* 133:208, 1983.

Update on isotretinoin (Accutane) for acne. *Med. Lett. Drugs Ther.* 25:105, 1983.

Isoxsuprine (Vasodilan®)

Indications and Recommendations

Isoxsuprine, which is a beta-2-adrenergic agonist and peripheral vasodilator, may be administered to pregnant women in order to stop premature labor. A number of such drugs are currently under investigation as tocolytic agents. Only ritodrine has thus far been approved by the FDA for this indication. Although isoxsuprine has been widely used as a tocolytic agent in the United States, the relatively higher incidence of cardiovascular side effects associated with this drug has made other beta agonists more popular choices for the treatment of premature labor.

Special Considerations in Pregnancy

Hypotension is the major threat to fetal well-being. This complication is usually mild, especially when the maternal intravascular volume is adequate. Some recent data suggest an acceleration of maturity of the fetus's pulmonary system when beta-2 agonists are administered to the mother.

A recent retrospective study of outcome for the neonate when the mother was treated with isoxsuprine before giving birth has caused some concern. In this series, 20 babies whose mothers were treated with isoxsuprine and who were delivered of their infants prior to 32 weeks' were compared with 20 nontreated controls. In the treated group, seven of the babies died in the neonatal period, as compared with two in the control group (not statistically significant). All of the isoxsuprine-exposed babies manifested some degree of hypotension during the first 6 hours of life, as compared to 75% of the babies in the control group ($p < 0.05$). Half of the treated babies developed clinically evident ileus, as opposed to 15% of the untreated babies ($p < 0.05$). These effects on the newborn were most likely to be seen if the interval between the administration of the loading dose of isoxsuprine and the delivery of the baby was short. Neonatal hypoglycemia has also been reported with exposure to beta-2 agonists in utero. Although reports of adverse outcomes in the newborn period are limited in scope and retrospective, they do point out the necessity of being as certain as possible that a woman is truly in premature labor before administering isoxsuprine or any other beta-2 agonist.

Dosage

A number of different dosage recommendations have been made. The usual dose is 0.25–0.5 mg/minute IV for 8–12 hours. This is followed by intramuscular or oral isoxsuprine at 5–20 mg every 3–6 hours. The intravenous infusion is stopped and considered a failure if laborlike activity persists beyond 1 hour. To prevent hypotension, the dose has to be carefully titrated, and the patient should be placed in the left lateral position.

An alternative method is as follows: An initial 20-mg loading dose is given intravenously over 20 minutes with a constant infusion pump. If contractions have not diminished markedly by 40 minutes after the conclusion of the infusion, another 20 mg is administered in the same manner. Once success has been achieved, isoxsuprine, 25 mg IM q4–6 h, is given for 48 hours. Then, oral administration is begun at a dose of 50 mg q6h.

Adverse Effects

Because beta-2 receptors are not confined to the uterine muscle but are also responsible for smooth muscle relaxation in arterioles and bronchi as well as being involved in glycogenolysis, the side effects of isoxsuprine may involve any of these systems. Thus, overdosage or rapid infusion may cause hypotension and tachycardia in the mother. Hyperglycemia has also been reported with this drug. The most common side effects are tremor, palpitations, and restlessness. Allergic dermatitis has also been reported.

Case reports of pulmonary edema occurring in women receiving the combination of a beta-2 agonist and glucocorticoid therapy (in an attempt to enhance the maturity of the pulmonary system in the fetus) suggest that caution be exercised when these classes of agents are combined.

Mechanism of Action

Isoxsuprine interacts with beta-2 receptors on the myometrial cell membrane to release adenyl cyclase within the cell. This catalyzes the intracellular formation of cAMP, which subsequently leads to relaxation of the uterine musculature, presumably through changes in calcium availability. In addition, isoxsuprine may act directly on smooth muscle, since the vasodilatation caused by this drug is not blocked by propranolol.

Absorption and Biotransformation

Isoxsuprine is largely metabolized by monoamine oxidase. Some is excreted by the kidneys, the rate of excretion being higher in acidic urine.

Recommended Reading

Barden, T. P. Premature Labor. In *Yearbook of Obstetrics and Gynecology*. Chicago: Year Book, 1977. P. 109.

Brazy, J. E., and Pupkin, M. J. Effects of maternal isoxsuprine administration on preterm infants. *J. Pediatr.* 94:444, 1979.

Casten, O., Gummerus, M., and Saarikoski, S. Treatment of imminent premature labour. *Acta Obstet. Gynecol. Scand.* 54:95, 1975.

Horowitz, J. J., and Creasy, R. K. Allergic dermatitis associated with administration of isoxsuprine during premature labor. *Am. J. Obstet. Gynecol.* 131:225, 1978.

Manley, E. S., and Lawson, J. W. Effect of beta adrenergic receptor blockade on skeletal muscle vasodilation produced by isoxsuprine and nyliorin. *Arch. Int. Pharmacodyn. Ther.* 175:239, 1968.

Stubblefield, P. G. Pulmonary edema occurring after therapy with dexamethasone and terbutaline for premature labor: A case report. *Am. J. Obstet. Gynecol.* 132:341, 1978.

Ketanserin

Indications and Recommendations

Ketanserin is relatively contraindicated in pregnancy because it has not been studied enough to verify its effectiveness or safety as an antihypertensive agent. This investigational drug is a competitive selective blocker of type 2 serotonin (5-hydroxytryptamine) receptors.

Serotonin produces vasospasm, oliguria, hypotension, and a lesion histologically similar to glomeruloendotheliosis in the kidneys of some pregnant animals. Furthermore, elevated plasma and placental serotonin levels as well as abnormal platelet function associated with decreased platelet serotinin concentrations have been reported in women with preeclampsia. These data provided the rationale for an investigation of ketanserin for the control of postpartum hypertension. In that study, 20 women with preeclamptic hypertension received intravenous ketanserin after delivery in a randomized double-blind crossover study with placebo. Each patient served as her own control. Parenteral ketanserin significantly reduced blood pressures from 167/105 mm Hg to 126/70 mm Hg, while no appreciable change was noted in the placebo group. Systolic, diastolic, and mean arterial pressures were all significantly reduced compared to pressures recorded during placebo administration, regardless of the drug sequence. Each patient again became hypertensive after the ketanserin infusion was stopped. An interesting observation from this study was that ketanserin normalized the blood pressure post partum in purely preeclamptic patients but failed to reduce the blood pressure to a similar degree in patients with chronic hypertension and superimposed preeclampsia.

A case report has been published in which a centrally monitored multiparous woman with a dead fetus in utero was successfully treated with intravenous ketanserin during a hypertensive crisis at 23 weeks' gestation.

Ketanserin appears to exert its pharmacologic effects by blockade of type 2 serotonin receptors. This should decrease or inhibit platelet aggregation, inhibit serotonin's vasoconstrictive effect on peripheral vessels, and block any amplifying effect serotonin has on the vasoconstrictive properties of other neurohumoral mediators such as norepinephrine. Ketanserin neither inhibits serotonin-mediated vasodilatation in other vascular beds via type 1 receptors nor produces a significant decline in blood pressure in healthy volunteers. The drug may also possess some alpha-adrenergic blocking activity.

Continued study of both the role of serotonin in preeclampsia-toxemia and the therapeutic use of ketanserin appears to be in order. However, since little is known regarding the relative effectiveness of this drug compared to more conventional forms of antihypertensive therapy, and virtually nothing is known about its effects on the fetus and neonate, further investigations are mandatory before ketanserin can be recommended for the treatment of obstetric patients.

Recommended Reading

Van Houtte, P. M., et al. Antihypertensive properties of ketanserin. *Fed. Proc.* 42:182, 1983.

Van Nueten, J. M., Janssen, P. A. J., and Van Houtte, P. M. Pharmacological Properties of Serotonergic Responses in Vascular, Bronchial and Gastrointestinal Smooth Muscle. In *Proceedings of the Fourth Symposium on Neuroeffector Mechanisms.* Kyoto, Japan: Rowens, 1981.

Waugh, D., and Pearl, M. J. Serotonin induced acute nephrosis and renal cortical necrosis in rats—a morphologic study with pregnancy correlations. *Am. J. Pathol.* 36:43, 1960.

Weiner, C. P., Galfan, R., and Socol, M. L. Intrapartum treatment of preeclamptic hypertension by ketanserin—a serotonin receptor antagonist. *Am. J. Obstet. Gynecol.* 149:576, 1984.

Weiner, C. P., Socol, M. L., and Vaisrub, N. Control of preeclamptic hypertension by ketanserin, a new serotonin receptor antagonist. *Am. J. Obstet. Gynecol.* 149:496, 1984.

Whigham, K. A. E., et al. Abnormal platelet function in preeclampsia. *Br. J. Obstet. Gynaecol.* 85:28, 1978.

Levodopa (Bendopa®, Dopar®, Larodopa®)

Indications and Recommendations

Levodopa (L-3,4-dihydroxyphenylalanine) is a drug used in the treatment of Parkinson's disease. Although insufficient data exist to comment on its safety during human pregnancy, reports of animal teratogenicity support withholding this drug in all but the most serious clinical situations.

Special Considerations in Pregnancy

Only one report has been published to date describing the outcome of pregnancies in which levodopa was taken throughout gestation. In that small series, two women were treated during three pregnancies, all of which resulted in the birth of healthy neonates at term. Follow-up study at 1.5, 5.0, and 7.0 years, respectively, revealed the infants to be developing normally. In one of these cases, the patient was taking amantadine hydrochloride for her Parkinson's disease at the time of conception. The authors chose to discontinue that drug because of reports of animal teratogenicity, as well as a single case of an infant who was born with a complex congenital cardiovascular lesion after exposure to amantadine in utero.

One other case has been reported in which levodopa was given to improve the level of consciousness during an episode of acute hepatic failure occurring in the fifth month of pregnancy. That patient also delivered a healthy infant at term.

In rodents and some other laboratory animals, levodopa has been found to cause skeletal malformations, stunting, and increased numbers of stillborns. Although the data are very sparse, there are no reports of teratogenicity in humans.

Levodopa inhibits lactation by blocking the neurohumoral secretion of prolactin. This, as well as the major pharmacologic effects of levodopa, is due to the action of dopamine, which is the drug's principal decarboxylation product.

Dosage

The usual initial dose is 0.5–1.0 g/day in 3–4 divided doses. The total daily dosage must then be titrated for optimal therapeutic effectiveness. The usual daily maintenance dose ranges from 3–8 g, and this is reached by gradual incremental increases of 100–750 mg every 3–7 days. A good therapeutic effect may not be reached in some patients for as long as 1–6 months.

Adverse Effects

Eighty percent of patients experience anorexia, nausea, vomiting, or epigastric distress, and these symptoms often occur early in therapy. Mild and asymptomatic orthostatic hypotension is frequently present, and some patients may develop cardiac arrhythmias. Long-term effects include abnormal involuntary movements and psychiatric disturbances. All of these side effects are reversible and can usually be controlled by a reduction in dosage.

Mechanism of Action

Levodopa itself is practically inert pharmacologically. Its principal effects are produced by dopamine, which is the product of its decarboxylation. About 95% of orally administered levodopa is rapidly converted in the periphery to dopamine, which, unlike the parent compound, does not cross the blood-brain barrier. Therefore, large doses of levodopa must be taken in order to allow sufficient accumulation of this drug in the brain, where its decarboxylation raises the central dopamine concentration. Although levodopa's mechanism of action in patients with Parkinson's disease is not completely clear, it acts, at least in part, by replenishing depleted striatal dopamine stores in the central nervous system (CNS).

Absorption and Biotransformation

Levodopa is rapidly absorbed from the small intestine after oral administration. Peak plasma concentrations occur 0.5–2.0 hours after a single oral dose. The half-life is between 1 and 3 hours.

Ninety-five percent of levodopa is decarboxylated peripherally by widely distributed extracerebral aromatic L-amino decarboxylase. An extensive first-pass effect occurs in the liver so that little unchanged drug reaches the cerebral circulation, and less than 1% penetrates into the CNS.

Most levodopa is converted into dopamine, small amounts of which are in turn metabolized to norepinephrine and epinephrine. Biotransformation of dopamine results in the formation of its principal excretion products, 3,4-dihydroxyphenylacetic acid (DOPAC) and 3-methoxy-4-hydroxyphenylacetic acid (homovanillic acid [HVA]), but at least 30 metabolites of levodopa have been identified. The metabolites of dopamine are rapidly excreted through the kidneys, and 80% of a radioactively labeled dose can be recovered in the urine within 24 hours.

Recommended Reading

Chajek, T., et al. Treatment of acute hepatic encephalopathy with L-dopa. *Postgrad. Med. J.* 53:262, 1977.

Cook, D. G., and Klawans, H. L. Levodopa during pregnancy. *Clin. Neuropharmacol.* 8:93, 1985.

Gilman, A. G., Goodman, L. S., and Gilman, A. *The Pharmacological Basis of Therapeutics* (6th ed.). New York: Macmillan, 1980. Pp. 477–482.

Stone, S. C., and Dickey, R. P. Management of nursing and non-nursing mothers. *Clin. Obstet. Gynecol.* 18:139, 1975.

Lidocaine (Xylocaine®)

Indications and Recommendations

Lidocaine may be administered to pregnant women as an antiarrhythmic agent. It is used primarily in the emergency treatment of ventricular arrhythmias. Its use as an anesthetic agent will not be considered in this discussion.

Special Considerations in Pregnancy

Lidocaine crosses the placenta, and high blood levels in the mother may be associated with neonatal depression and neurobehavioral changes in the first few days of life. Fortunately, blood levels that are in the therapeutic range for treatment of arrhythmias (2–5 µg/ml) are somewhat lower than the levels found to be associated with these adverse neonatal effects. Very high blood levels in sheep, as well as in experimentally isolated uterine artery segments, may be associated with a transient decrease in uterine blood flow. This has not been reported in humans given lidocaine in therapeutic dosages.

Dosage

In the emergency management of ventricular arrhythmias, therapy is started with 50–100 mg given IV with continuous cardiac monitoring. The rate of administration should be 25–50 mg/min. If the initial dose is not successful, it may be repeated in 5 minutes. Following this, a continuous intravenous infusion may be used (at rates of 1–4 mg/min) to titrate the response.

Adverse Effects

Toxic effects of lidocaine occur in the cardiovascular and central nervous systems. Central nervous system effects include lightheadedness, drowsiness, tremors, convulsions, and respiratory depression and arrest. Cardiovascular effects include hypotension, cardiovascular collapse, and bradycardia, which may lead to cardiac arrest. These toxic effects are usually seen at serum levels above 5 µg/ml.

Mechanism of Action

Lidocaine's antiarrhythmic activity is related to a depression in the automaticity of Purkinje cells and a decrease in membrane responsiveness. There is little electrophysiologic effect on atrial muscle.

Lidocaine can eliminate premature ventricular contractions and convert a ventricular arrhythmia to normal sinus rhythm. It is not recommended for treatment of supraventricular arrhythmias.

Absorption and Biotransformation

Lidocaine is not effective when given orally and should be given by the intravenous route. It is primarily metabolized in the liver.

Recommended Reading

Finster, M., Morishima, H. O., Boyes, R. N., and Covino, B. G. The placental transfer of lidocaine and its uptake by fetal tissues. *Anesthesiology* 36:159, 1972.

Gilman, A. G., Goodman, L. S., and Gilman, A. *The Pharmacological Basis of Therapeutics* (6th ed.). New York: Macmillan, 1980. Pp. 779–781.

Heymann, M. A. Correlations of fetal circulation and the placental transfer of drugs. *Fed. Proc.* 31:44, 1972.

Mann, L. I., Bailey, C., Carmichael, A., and Duchin, S. Effect of lidocaine on fetal heart rate and fetal brain metabolism and function. *Am. J. Obstet. Gynecol.* 112:789, 1972.

Shnider, S. M., and Levinson, G. *Anesthesia for Obstetrics.* Baltimore: Williams & Wilkins, 1979. Pp. 28–29, 217, 382.

Teramo, K., et al. Effects of lidocaine on heart rate, blood pressure, and electrocortigram in fetal sheep. *Am. J. Obstet. Gynecol.* 118:935, 1974.

Lithium Carbonate (Eskalith®, Lithane®)

Indications and Recommendations

Lithium carbonate may be administered to pregnant women for treatment of the manic phase of manic-depressive illness. If it is being used for prophylaxis, this drug should be discontinued during the first trimester of pregnancy unless withdrawal would seriously jeopardize the woman or the pregnancy. During pregnancy, the smallest dosage possible for acceptable therapeutic effects should be used. This is best accomplished by monitoring plasma lithium levels at least weekly. Frequent, small dosages should be used to avoid larger fluctuations in maternal plasma concentrations. Individual doses should not exceed 300 mg and should be spaced evenly throughout the day. Major changes in maternal dietary intake or excretion of sodium, especially those causing hyponatremia, should be avoided.

Whenever possible, it is advisable to reduce the daily lithium dose by 50% in the last week of gestation and to discontinue it entirely at the onset of labor. Lithium should be reinstituted at prepregnancy dosage immediately after delivery. Since the drug is excreted in the mother's milk and has been associated with toxicity in infants, many experts advise that breast-feeding be avoided. However, drug intoxication does not always occur in the suckling infants of women taking lithium. Therefore, some authorities recommend that nursing be permitted but that these mothers be instructed to watch for signs of toxicity.

Special Considerations in Pregnancy

Lithium is not known to have any unusual maternal effects, and the drug is cleared more quickly than it is in the nonpregnant state. Lithium clearance normally ranges from 15–30 ml/minute and increases by 50–100% during the course of pregnancy. This value drops to prepregnancy levels at the time of delivery. Lithium is known to cross the placenta, with concentrations being equal on both sides. It can be teratogenic in rodents if even transiently high lithium concentrations are delivered. Given in divided daily doses and maintained at steady serum concentrations in the human therapeutic range, however, lithium has been found to be without any deleterious effects on either mother or fetus in rodents, rabbits, and monkeys.

Among 217 pregnant women with first-trimester lithium exposure reported to the International Register of Lithium Babies, 25 (11.5%) had malformed infants. Eighteen of the 25 malformed neonates had cardiovascular anomalies, including six with Ebstein's anomaly. Other cases of Ebstein's anomaly have subsequently been reported in lithium-exposed pregnancies, and it is now generally accepted that there is an association between lithium exposure in utero (particularly at high blood levels) and this type of cardiac defect. In addition to heart defects, malformations of the central nervous system, external ear, ureters, and endocrine system have been reported. Children exposed to lithium in utero and born without malformation appear to be at no greater risk than other children for developing abnormalities later in life.

Infants born to mothers whose lithium plasma concentrations are in the therapeutic range may exhibit neonatal intoxication. Symptoms include cyanosis, lethargy, hypotonia, jaundice, hypothermia, duskiness, poor sucking, poor respiratory effort, low Apgar scores, absent Moro reflex, altered thyroid, and altered cardiac function. There are case reports of neonatal goiters in babies born to mothers taking lithium who themselves had goiters. These babies were euthyroid, and their goiters were transient.

Lithium is secreted in breast milk and has been measured at levels up to half of those found in the mother's serum. Infants breast-fed by mothers taking lithium have been reported to be hypotonic, hypothermic, and cyanotic, and to have electrocardiographic changes.

Dosage

Dosage is determined by the severity of the illness and the patient's physical state, body weight, and age. In the treatment of acute mania, the usual dose range is 900–3,000 mg/day with therapeutic serum concentrations in the range of 0.9–1.4 mEq/liter. Plasma concentrations greater than 1.5 mEq/liter produce no clinical advantage and increase the incidence of side effects. As the manic episode subsides, the lithium requirement decreases; the dosage therefore should be decreased fairly rapidly to about 600–1,200 mg/day with plasma levels of 0.7–1.2 mEq/liter. This maintenance dosage must be individually adjusted according to symptoms and side effects.

There is a 4- to 10-day lag period in the onset of therapeutic effect due to the slow rate at which lithium crosses cell boundaries. Should more immediate treatment be required, an antipsychotic agent such as haloperidol or chlorpromazine is generally recommended.

Adverse Effects

Initial lithium therapy is associated with a transient increase in the excretion of 17-hydroxycorticosteroids, sodium, potassium, and water. Polydipsia and polyuria frequently occur, and the drug has been implicated in cases of nephrogenic diabetes insipidus. Circulating thyroid hormone levels fall, thyroid ^{131}I uptake is elevated, and plasma protein-bound iodine and free thyroxine levels are reduced. Patients usually remain euthyroid, although some may develop a goiter and become clinically hypothyroid. Reversible electrocardiographic changes can occur. Patients may also develop a fine tremor of the hands.

At toxic levels ($\geq$ 2.0 mEq/L), severe persistent nausea, vomiting and diarrhea, gross hand tremor, slurred speech, muscle twitching, lethargy, seizures, and stupor progressing to coma may appear.

Mechanism of Action

The precise mechanism of lithium's action is unknown, although it influences nerve excitation, synaptic transmission, and neuronal metabolism in the central nervous system. These effects may be due to altered ion transport or inhibition of adenyl cyclase.

Absorption and Biotransformation

Lithium is completely absorbed from the gastrointestinal tract within 8 hours, with peak plasma levels occurring in 2–3 hours. It is excreted unchanged, with 95% appearing in the urine, 4–5% in perspiration, and less than 1% in feces. Approximately 80% of filtered lithium is actively reabsorbed and is competitive with sodium. Sodium depletion will result in a greater reabsorption of lithium and possible toxicity. The plasma half-life in the average adult is 24 hours, with steady-state blood levels being reached in 5–6 days.

Recommended Reading

Ananth, J. Side effects in the neonate from psychotropic agents excreted through breast feeding. *Am. J. Psychiatry* 135:801, 1978.

Ayd, F. J. Hazards to women given lithium during pregnancy and delivery. *Int. Drug. Ther. Newsletter* 8:26, 1973.

Gilman, A. G., Goodman, L. S., and Gilman, A. *The Pharmacological Basis of Therapeutics* (6th ed.). New York: Macmillan, 1980. Pp. 430–434.

Kallen, B., and Tandberg, A. Lithium and pregnancy. A cohort study on manic-depressive women. *Acta Psychiatr. Scand.* 68:134, 1983.

Linden, S., and Rich, C. The use of lithium during pregnancy and lactation. *J. Clin. Psychiatry* 44:358, 1983.

Long, W. A., and Willis, P. W. IV. Maternal lithium and neonatal Ebstein's anomaly: Evaluation with cross-sectional echocardiography. *Am. J. Perinatol.* 1:182, 1984.

Schou, M., and Amdisen, A. Lithium and pregnancy—III. Lithium ingestion by children breast fed by women on lithium treatment. *Br. Med. J.* 2:138, 1973.

Singer, I., and Rotenberg, D. Mechanisms of lithium action. *N. Engl. J. Med.* 289:254, 1973.

Tunnessen, W. W., and Hertz, C. G. Toxic effects of lithium in newborn infants: A commentary. *J. Pediatr.* 81:804, 1972.

Weinstein, M. R., and Goldfield, M. D. Cardiovascular malformations with lithium use during pregnancy. *Am. J. Psychiatry* 132:529, 1975.

Local Anesthetics: Bupivacaine (Marcaine®), Chloroprocaine (Nesacaine®), Etidocaine (Duranest®), Lidocaine (Xylocaine®), Mepivacaine (Carbocaine®), Tetracaine (Pontocaine®)

Indications and Recommendations

Local anesthetics are generally safe to use for local infiltration and regional block for pain relief during labor and delivery as well as for cesarean section. Paracervical block is no longer recommended because of the high incidence of associated fetal bradycardias. Bupivacaine in a concentration of 0.75% has been found to have maternal cardiac toxicity when used as an epidural anesthetic, and therefore this concentration is no longer used in obstetric patients. In general, however, local anesthetics are highly selective with only minor systemic effects, making them ideal agents for use in pregnant women.

The use of lidocaine as an antiarrhythmic agent is discussed elsewhere in this book (see *Lidocaine*).

Special Considerations in Pregnancy

Although many local anesthetics are available, chloroprocaine, lidocaine, and bupivacaine have proved to be the most useful for epidural block during labor and delivery because they produce effective analgesia without excessive motor blockade. When used for epidural anesthesia, etidocaine and tetracaine produce profound motor block but suboptimal sensory blockade. Tetracaine, however, is one of the most effective drugs for subarachnoid block. Mepivacaine is not frequently used in obstetric anesthesia because of its greater propensity to reach the fetus as well as its long half-life in the neonate compared to other agents.

There are several reports of maternal deaths following ventricular arrhythmias and subsequent cardiac arrest after inadvertent intravascular injections of 0.75% bupivacaine during epidural anesthesia. Therefore, this concentration is no longer used in obstetric patients.

Paracervical blocks have been associated with a significant incidence of fetal bradycardias. In a prospective study of 92 patients who received 100 paracervical blocks with mepivacaine, it was found that 24 of the patients developed fetal bradycardias, the mean duration of which was 7.8 minutes. If the bradycardia lasted more than 10 minutes, there was a significant metabolic acidosis. All pH values returned to normal before delivery, but the one neonate born during the bradycardia had a 1-minute Apgar score of 3. All patients with bradycardias had 5-minute Apgars of 7 or above. Increased uterine tone was found in most patients with fetal bradycardia, presumably secondary to high local myometrial concentrations of the drug. In another study of 845 paracervical blocks administered to patients in labor, fetal heart rate changes were noted after 30% of the blocks. An increased incidence of these changes was observed in association with primiparity, prematurity, and preexisting fetal distress. Neonatal depression was significantly increased in those infants who had developed fetal heart rate changes following the paracervical block as compared to those infants whose heart rates had remained within the normal range.

Experiments in pregnant ewes and baboons have shown that local anesthetics administered intravenously or by paracervical block to produce clinically encountered blood levels stimulate myometrial contractility and vasoconstriction. This may result in a subsequent reduction in uteroplacental perfusion and decreased oxygen availability to the fetus. Other studies have shown that human uterine arteries constrict when exposed to lidocaine in vitro and that arteries from pregnant patients elicit significantly greater responses than those from nonpregnant women.

Based on their studies of uterine and fetal heart rate activity, along with continuous transcutaneous monitoring of oxygen tension (t_cPO_2) in the human fetus, Baxi and colleagues observed that post-paracervical block changes evolve in the following manner: After administration of the block, maternal and fetal blood levels of the drug rise rapidly. By 5 minutes, the t_cPO_2 has begun to decline. This is followed by increased fetal heart rate variability and then by visually appreciated fetal heart rate changes. Maximal changes in fetal and maternal blood levels of the anesthetic, fetal oxygenation, uterine activity, and fetal heart rate variability are noted at 9–12 minutes and last for only a short time. By 30–45 minutes, all values spontaneously return to preblock levels. These investigators believe that the changes they observed are primarily due to fetal hypoxia induced by uterine vasculature constriction after injection of the local anesthetic. In their study, mean uterine activity increased immediately following placement of the block, but there was sufficient patient variation to this response to make it appear that myometrial contractions only serve as a contributing factor in this sequence of events.

Local anesthetics may affect the fetus directly via transplacental transfer of the drug or indirectly via maternal effects such as hypotension. The latter is likely to occur when vasodilatation secondary to sensory blockade occurs in a relatively dehydrated patient. It is therefore recommended that prophylactic intravenous hydration with at least 1 liter of crystalloid solution be administered before an epidural or subarachnoid block is administered. Care should be taken, however, not to infuse an excessive glucose load. One study has shown that rapid infusions of 25 g or more of glucose into women prior to elective cesarean section was associated with fetal acidosis and neonatal hyperinsulinemia, hypoglycemia, and hyperbilirubinemia. These authors suggest that infusions be limited to 6 g dextrose per hour in preparation for elective cesarean section until a maximum safe level can be established. Additionally, when an epidural anesthetic is administered, a test dose should be delivered into the catheter before the full dose is injected in order to rule out the possibility that the drug is inadvertently being given intravenously.

All local anesthetics cross the placenta, but they do so at different rates. Transplacental diffusion is greater in those agents with the highest lipid solubility and the lowest maternal protein binding. The nonionized form of the drug is the most lipid soluble. Clinically, this could be significant during fetal acidosis, at which time the agent becomes ionized and therefore "trapped" in the fetal circulation, making fetal toxicity of the drug more likely.

In animal studies, fetal convulsions have been produced with high fetal blood levels of these agents. In dosages used in humans, no such effects have been reported.

Transient neonatal motor retardation during the first 8 hours of life has been reported by Scanlon et al. after epidural anesthesia using mepivacaine and lidocaine. However, no difference in Apgar scores was found between the epidural and control groups. Abboud and colleagues, in a later study, found no difference in neonatal neurobehavioral scores between epidural and control groups. The drugs used in this study were chloroprocaine, bupivacaine, and lidocaine.

Dosage

Local anesthetics are divided into two groups, depending on their molecular structure: those with ester-type linkage in the molecule and those with an amide linkage. The esters include chloroprocaine and tetracaine. The amide-linked agents include lidocaine, mepivacaine, bupivacaine, and etidocaine.

The total dosage of local anesthetic to be used depends on the route of administration, the specific agent used, and the level as well as duration of blockade desired (Table 8).

Adverse Effects

High maternal blood levels of local anesthetics may cause central nervous system (CNS) toxicity. They can initially stimulate the CNS, causing restlessness, nervousness, tremors, and convulsions. This stimulation is followed by depression and respiratory failure. The reported incidence of convulsions during obstetric regional anesthesia is low, varying from 0.03–0.50%.

Local anesthetics may affect the cardiovascular system by acting directly on the heart and peripheral vasculature, as well as indirectly by sympathetic blockade. In the myocardium, local anesthetics decrease electrical excitability, rate of conduction, and force of contractility. Arterial hypotension is the most common complication of spinal or epidural anesthesia. This is secondary to the sympathetic blockade as well as a direct effect on the arterioles when the drug is absorbed into the bloodstream.

Allergic reactions to local anesthetics are rare and more likely to be associated with the ester derivatives. These reactions include localized edema, urticaria, and pruritus, and are related to breakdown products of metabolized esters. Anaphylactic reactions are extremely uncommon.

Mechanism of Action

Local anesthetics reduce pain by inhibiting neural excitation via a direct effect on the nerve cell membrane. They are thought to obstruct the inward surge of sodium ions associated with depolarization. They do not affect either the resting membrane or threshold potentials of nerve cells. The predominant effect of these agents is to decrease the maximum rate of rise of the action potential. As a result, threshold cannot be achieved, and a propagated action potential fails to develop.

Table 8. Local anesthetics

Agent	Concentration	Protein binding (%)	Approximate lipid solubility	Maximum dose (mg)	Duration (min)
Low potency/short duration					
Chloroprocaine (Nesacaine®)	2.0–3.0	≈5	<1	1,000	45–69
Intermediate potency and duration					
Mepivacaine (Carbocaine®)	1.0–2.0	75	1	500	120–140
Lidocaine (Xylocaine®)	1.0–2.0	65	4	500	90–200
High potency/long duration					
Tetracaine (Pontocaine®)	0.15–0.25	85	80	200	180–600
Bupivacaine (Marcaine®)	0.25–0.75	95	30	300	180–600
Etidocaine (Duranest®)	0.5–1.5	94	140	300	180–600

Absorption and Biotransformation

The absorption of local anesthetics depends on the site of injection, the dosage, the addition of a vasoconstrictor agent, and the specific agent employed. Comparison of blood levels of local anesthetics after various types of obstetric regional anesthesia reveals that the most rapid rate of absorption occurs after paracervical blocks. This is followed, in order of diminishing blood levels, by administration of the agent into the caudal canal, lumbar epidural space, and subarachnoid space. The blood level of local anesthetic agents is related to the total dosage of drug given rather than the volume or concentration.

The rate of absorption of these drugs can be reduced considerably by the incorporation of a vasoconstrictor agent such as epinephrine. However, absorbed epinephrine may cause reduction of uterine blood flow and inhibition of uterine activity, making its use in obstetric anesthesia controversial.

The esters are broken down in the bloodstream by plasma pseudocholinesterase at different rates, with chloroprocaine having the fastest rate of hydrolysis. Since the amide-linked agents are metabolized in the liver, their half-lives are longer.

All local anesthetics employed for obstetric anesthesia diffuse across the placenta. The rate of placental diffusion is related to the degree of plasma-protein binding in maternal blood and the rate of fetal-tissue uptake. Fetal-tissue uptake in turn is higher with the more lipid-soluble agents. Fetal-plasma binding of local anesthetic agents is approximately 50% less than binding in maternal plasma, so that more unbound drug is present in the fetus. Those drugs that have the highest degree of protein binding also tend to be more lipid soluble (see Table 8), so that the rate of tissue uptake of the unbound drug is enhanced. Therefore, maternal-fetal anesthetic blood concentrations can differ markedly between agents, but the total amount of drug transferred across the placenta may be similar for agents of higher and lower protein-binding capacity. It was originally thought that agents such as bupivacaine, 95% of which is bound to maternal protein, did not cross the placenta in significant amounts. It is now believed, however, that this agent's high lipid solubility increases the fetal-tissue uptake of the drug that is transferred. The clinical significance of these findings is not certain, but it may be true that the potential for fetal toxicity is similar for all local anesthetic agents.

Recommended Reading

Abboud, T. K., et al. Maternal, fetal and neonatal responses after epidural anesthesia with bupivacaine, 2-chloroprocaine, or lidocaine. *Anesth. Analg.* 61:638, 1982.

Baxi, L. V., Petrie, R. H., and James, L. S. Human fetal oxygenation following paracervical block. *Am. J. Obstet. Gynecol.* 135:1109, 1979.

Covino, B. G., and Vasallo, H. G. *Local Anesthetics. Mechanisms of Action and Clinical Use.* New York: Grune & Stratton, 1976.

Freeman, R. K., et al. Fetal cardiac response to paracervical block anesthesia. *Am. J. Obstet. Gynecol.* 113:583, 1972.

Gibbs, C. P., and Noel, S. C. Human uterine artery responses to lidocaine. *Am. J. Obstet. Gynecol.* 126:313, 1976.

Gilman, A. G., Goodman, L. S., and Gilman, A. *The Pharmacological*

Basis of Therapeutics (6th ed.). New York: Macmillan, 1980. Pp. 300–320.

Greiss, F. C., Jr., Still, J. G., and Anderson, S. G. Effects of local anesthetic agents on the uterine vasculatures and myometrium. *Am. J. Obstet. Gynecol.* 124:889, 1976.

Kenepp, N. B., et al. Fetal and neonatal hazards of maternal hydration with 5% dextrose before cesarean section. *Lancet* 1:1150, 1982.

Morishima, H. O., et al. Bradycardia in the fetal baboon following paracervical block anesthesia. *Am. J. Obstet. Gynecol.* 140:775, 1981.

Ostheimer, G. W. *Manual of Obstetric Anesthesia.* New York: Churchill Livingstone, 1984. Pp. 99–125.

Scanlon, J. W., et al. Neurobehavioral responses of newborn infants after maternal epidural anesthesia. *Anesthesiology* 40:121, 1974.

Shnider, S. M., and Levinson, G. *Anesthesia for Obstetrics.* Baltimore: Williams & Wilkins, 1979.

Shnider, S. M., et al. Paracervical block anesthesia in obstetrics. I. Fetal complications and neonatal morbidity. *Am. J. Obstet. Gynecol.* 107:619, 1970.

Magnesium Sulfate

Indications and Recommendations

Magnesium sulfate is the drug of choice for the prevention of seizures in patients with preeclampsia-toxemia (PET). Women whose toxemia is severe enough to warrant administration of this drug should be delivered of their infants soon after stabilization has been accomplished.

When this drug is given, deep tendon reflexes should be elicited each hour, respirations should be 12/minute or more, and urinary output should exceed 30 ml/hour. The administration of magnesium sulfate should be discontinued if respiratory depression is noted. A serum magnesium level should be obtained if deep tendon reflexes are lost but the urinary output and respiratory rate are normal. Since diminished urinary output may result in dangerously high serum levels, the rate of infusion should be decreased and serum magnesium levels checked frequently when this occurs. Although magnesium sulfate can be given by either the intramuscular or intravenous route, the latter is recommended both in order to ensure adequate therapeutic levels and to allow maximal control over administration.

The drug should be continued for approximately 24 hours following delivery as prophylaxis against postpartum seizures. If hyperreflexia persists, longer periods of administration may be necessary.

Magnesium sulfate has also been used as a tocolytic agent in attempts to arrest premature labor. In this setting, it is currently the drug of choice for patients with insulin-dependent diabetes, heart disease, or other relative contraindications to more conventional beta-mimetic tocolytic therapy. Magnesium sulfate may also be given to patients who have failed a trial of beta-mimetic therapy. It is administered intravenously when given for tocolysis.

Special Considerations in Pregnancy

Magnesium sulfate may diminish the frequency and intensity of uterine contractions by direct action on the myometrium. In one study comparing the effectiveness of this drug with other agents, magnesium sulfate was successful in arresting premature labor in 77% of cases as opposed to 45% for intravenous ethanol and 44% for dextrose in water.

Magnesium crosses the placenta, and hypotonia, lethargy, weakness, and low Apgar scores have been attributed to fetal hypermagnesemia. Magnesium levels in the cord blood of neonates have been shown to reflect those of their mothers.

Dosage

When administered as seizure prophylaxis in PET, magnesium sulfate may be given intravenously or intramuscularly as is shown below:

Intravenous administration via infusion pump
Loading dose: 4 g in 250 ml 5% D/W over 20 minutes
Maintenance dose: 2–3 g/hour, titrated by deep tendon reflexes and serum levels

Intramuscular administration
Loading dose: 5 g in 50% solution in each buttock (total, 10 g) along with 4 g given intravenously as above
Maintenance dose: 5 g in 50% solution q4h after checking deep tendon reflexes, respiratory rates, and urinary output

The intravenous route is preferred in the treatment of PET and is always used when treating premature labor. The presence or absence of deep tendon reflexes is not always a reliable predictor of the serum magnesium level and should not, by itself, lead to an increase in dosage or a cessation of the infusion. The only reliable indicator of adequate dosage is a serum magnesium level of 4–7 mEq/dl or 5–8 mg/dl.

Magnesium sulfate toxicity in the mother can be treated by administering 1 g calcium gluconate intravenously into a peripheral vein over a 3-minute period.

Adverse Effects

Toxic signs and symptoms associated with magnesium sulfate administration do not appear until blood levels exceed 8–10 mEq/liter. At or near this level, knee jerks disappear. Between 10 and 12.5 mEq/liter, heart block and peaked T waves on electrocardiogram may be noted, the patient can become obtunded, and respirations may cease. Above this level, cardiac arrest can occur.

Fetal hypermagnesemia is known to be associated with hypotonia, lethargy, and respiratory depression of the neonate. Some authors believe that this neonatal symptom complex is more severe when maternal administration of the drug has been intravenous, but to date there have been no prospective studies that have conclusively demonstrated this.

Mechanism of Action

In pharmacologic dosages, magnesium sulfate is a central nervous system (CNS) depressant. It also blocks neuromuscular impulse transmission by diminishing the amplitude of the end plate potential and decreasing its sensitivity to the depolarizing action of acetylcholine. Furthermore, the excitability of muscle fibers to direct stimulation is diminished.

By its action on the CNS and peripheral neuromuscular functions, magnesium sulfate reduces the hyperreflexia associated with PET and is an effective prophylaxis against eclamptic seizures. By acting directly on blood vessel walls, this drug causes some vasodilatation. This may result in a modest decline in blood pressure and an increase in uterine blood flow in patients with PET.

Absorption and Biotransformation

When used for the treatment of PET, magnesium sulfate is administered either intravenously or intramuscularly. When given by the latter route, there is a lag of 90–120 minutes before plasma levels reach a plateau. Thirty-five percent of the drug is protein bound while the rest remains in the ionic form. Magnesium is excreted entirely in the urine, and elevated serum levels may accumulate when standard dosages of the drug are given to patients with diminished renal function.

Recommended Reading

Creasy, R. K. Preterm Labor and Delivery. In R. K. Creasy and R. Resnick (eds.), *Maternal Fetal Medicine*. Philadelphia: Saunders, 1984. Pp. 415–443.

Gilman, A. G., Goodman, L. S., and Gilman, A. *The Pharmacological Basis of Therapeutics* (6th ed.). New York: Macmillan, 1980. P. 879.

Green, K. W., Key, T. C., Coen, R., and Resnick, R. The effects of maternally administered magnesium sulfate on the neonate. *Am. J. Obstet. Gynecol.* 146:29, 1983.

Pritchard, J. A. Standardized treatment of 154 consecutive cases of eclampsia. *Am. J. Obstet. Gynecol.* 123:545, 1975.

Pritchard, J. A., MacDonald, P. C., and Gant, N. F. *Williams Obstetrics* (17th ed.). East Norwalk, Conn.: Appleton-Century-Crofts, 1985. Pp. 525–560.

Roberts, J. M. Pregnancy-related Hypertension. In R. K. Creasy and R. Resnick (eds.), *Maternal Fetal Medicine*. Philadelphia: Saunders, 1984. Pp. 703–752.

Steer, C. H., and Petrie, R. H. A comparison of magnesium sulfate and alcohol for the prevention of premature labor. *Am. J. Obstet. Gynecol.* 129:1, 1977.

Wacker, W., and Parisi, A. Magnesium metabolism. *N. Engl. J. Med.* 278:712, 1968.

Mannitol (Osmitrol®)

Indications and Recommendations

Mannitol may be administered to critically ill pregnant patients. It is used to promote diuresis and to reduce intracranial pressure. The effect that changes in fetal extracellular fluid volume and intravascular tonicity have on the fetus at various stages of gestation is unknown. For this reason, an osmotic diuretic such as mannitol should only be used for life-threatening conditions during pregnancy.

Special Considerations in Pregnancy

The administration of hypertonic solutions to a pregnant woman results in changes in the composition of the maternal extracellular fluid with similar effects on tonicity and blood volume in the fetus. Mannitol crosses the placenta and can result in fetal dehydration. Both of these factors may lead to oxygen and acid-base imbalances in the fetus. In addition, maternal cardiac decompensation could seriously hinder uterine blood flow and thus adversely affect the fetus.

In a study involving the intravenous administration of mannitol to nine normal pregnant women at term, the drug was detected in amniotic fluid within 5 minutes. The concentration of mannitol continued to increase in the amniotic fluid up to 240 minutes after administration of the drug and reached values that were higher than those simultaneously obtained in maternal plasma. In one woman with a dead fetus at 29 weeks', however, intravenously administered mannitol appeared in amniotic fluid but increased very little over time and never reached values higher than those of the maternal plasma. When intravenous mannitol was given to pregnant sheep, it was found that drug concentrations in fetal urine were 10–20 times higher than drug concentrations in the fetal plasma.

Dosage

Mannitol is available for intravenous administration as a 5%, 10%, 15%, 20%, or 25% solution. Specific dosages depend on the underlying disease as well as renal response and fluid balance in a particular patient. Usual adult doses range from 50–200 g/24 hours. A test dose of 0.2 g/kg should be given to a patient with marked oliguria or one believed to have inadequate renal function.

Adverse Effects

Adverse effects are related to the load of solute administered and the effect of mannitol on fluids and electrolytes. The most serious side effect is cardiac decompensation secondary to circulatory overload. The patient's cardiovascular status, therefore, must be carefully monitored during administration.

Mechanism of Action

Mannitol is a nonelectrolyte, osmotically active solute that, when excreted by the kidneys, is accompanied by an obligatory osmotic diuresis. The solute prevents reabsorption of water, and urine volume thus can be maintained even in the presence of decreased glomerular function. The concentration of sodium in the tubular fluid is decreased, and the amount of sodium that is reabsorbed is therefore decreased. The excretion of sodium and chloride is increased. In the treatment of elevated intracranial pressure, mannitol again acts osmotically to draw excess fluid across the blood-brain barrier into the intravascular space.

Absorption and Biotransformation

The drug is poorly absorbed from the gastrointestinal tract and must be administered intravenously. It is confined to the extracellular space, only slightly metabolized, and rapidly excreted in the urine. Approximately 80% of a 100-g dose appears unchanged in the urine in 3 hours.

Recommended Reading

Basso, A., et al. Passage of mannitol from mother to amniotic fluid and fetus. *Obstet. Gynecol.* 49:628, 1977.

Gilman, A. G., Goodman, L. S., and Gilman, A. *The Pharmacological Basis of Therapeutics* (6th ed.). New York: Macmillan, 1980. P. 894.

Pritchard, J. A. Standardized treatment of 154 consecutive cases of eclampsia. *Am. J. Obstet. Gynecol.* 123:543, 1975.

Pritchard, J. A., MacDonald, P., and Gant, N. *Williams Obstetrics* (17th ed.). East Norwalk, Conn.: Appleton-Century-Crofts, 1985. Pp. 549–551.

Ross, M. G., et al. Bulk flow of amniotic fluid water in response to maternal osmotic challenge. *Am. J. Obstet. Gynecol.* 147:697, 1983.

Marijuana

Indications and Recommendations

Marijuana is contraindicated during pregnancy. A number of factors are responsible for this recommendation. First, the hazards of cigarette smoking (see *Tobacco*) are, if anything, greater with marijuana, since the smoke is generally inhaled deeply into the lungs and kept there for as long as possible. Second, there is no approved indication for its use, although research into its efficacy as an antiglaucoma agent, an antiemetic, and a tranquilizer is ongoing. Third, delta-9-tetrahydrocannabinol (THC), the active ingredient of marijuana, is known to cross the placenta, depressing the fetal heart rate and changing fetal electroencephalographic patterns. Finally, indirect data suggest an increased incidence of fetal wastage, prematurity, meconium passage, congenital anomalies, and possibly a predisposition to the dysmorphic features of the fetal alcohol syndrome among offspring of marijuana users. Tetrahydrocannabinol has been demonstrated to accumulate in the breast milk of lactating women who use marijuana and to be absorbed by the nursing baby. For these reasons, it would seem judicious to abstain from marijuana use during pregnancy and lactation.

Recommended Reading

Blackard, C., and Tennes, K. Human placental transfer of cannabinoids. *N. Engl. J. Med.* 311:797, 1984.

Fried, P. A., Watkinson, B., and Willan, A. Marijuana use during pregnancy and decreased length of gestation. *Am. J. Obstet. Gynecol.* 150:23, 1984.

Gibson, G. T., Baghurst, P. A., and Colley, D. P. *Aust. N.Z. J. Obstet. Gynaecol.* 23:15, 1983.

Gilman, A. G., Goodman, L. S., and Gilman, A. *The Pharmacological Basis of Therapeutics* (6th ed.). New York: Macmillan, 1980. Pp. 560–563.

Greenland, S., Staisch, K. J., Brown, N., and Gross, S. J. The effects of marijuana use during pregnancy. I. A preliminary epidemiologic study. *Am. J. Obstet. Gynecol.* 143:408, 1982.

Hingson, R., et al. Effects of maternal drinking and marijuana use on fetal growth and development. *Pediatrics* 70:539, 1982.

Mantilla-Plata, B., Clewe, G. L., and Harbison, R. D. Teratogenic and mutagenic studies of delta-9-tetrahydrocannabinol in mice. *Fed. Proc.* 32:746, 1973.

Perez-Reyes, M. Presence of delta-9-tetrahydrocannabinol in human milk. *N. Engl. J. Med.* 307:819, 1982.

Mebendazole (Vermox®)

Indications and Recommendations

Mebendazole is contraindicated during pregnancy. It is a broad-spectrum antihelminthic agent effective in the treatment of ascariasis, enterobiasis, trichuriasis, and hookworm disease. It has been found to be embryotoxic and teratogenic at single doses of 10 mg/kg body weight in rats and is therefore not recommended for use during pregnancy.

Recommended Reading

Brugmans, J. P., et al. Mebendazole in enterobiasis. *J.A.M.A.* 217:313, 1971.

Drugs for parasitic infections. *Med. Lett. Drugs Ther.* 20:17, 1978.

Keystone, J. S., and Murdoch, J. K. Mebendazole. *Ann. Intern. Med.* 91:582, 1979.

Leah, S. K. K. Mebendazole in the treatment of helminthiasis. *Can. Med. Assoc. J.* 115:777, 1976.

Sargent, R. G., et al. A clinical evaluation of the efficacy of mebendazole in the treatment of trichuriasis. *South. Med. J.* 68:38, 1975.

Meclizine (Antivert®, Bonine®)

Indications and Recommendations

Meclizine is probably safe to use during pregnancy. It has been shown to be teratogenic in rodents, but large-scale studies in humans do not show any increase in the rate of severe congenital anomalies when it has been used. It is effective in the prevention of the nausea, vomiting, and dizziness associated with motion sickness, and it may be effective for the relief of vertigo associated with diseases affecting the vestibular system. It is listed in the *Physicians' Desk Reference* as being contraindicated in pregnancy because of the teratogenicity in rodents. Because of the controversy involved, patients should be made aware of this fact before the drug is given.

Special Considerations in Pregnancy

Meclizine crosses the placenta. Large-scale studies in humans show that the rate of severe congenital anomalies in children of mothers who took meclizine during pregnancy is not significantly different from that in the group of mothers who did not receive antinauseants during pregnancy.

Dosage

For prevention of motion sickness, meclizine is given in a dose of 25–50 mg 1 hour prior to departure. It may be repeated every 24 hours as needed for the duration of the journey.

For the control of vertigo it is given 25–100 mg/day in divided doses.

Adverse Effects

The most common side effects of meclizine include drowsiness, dry mouth, and rarely, blurred vision.

Mechanism of Action

Meclizine is a piperazine antihistamine that depresses labyrinth excitability and vestibular-cerebellar pathway conduction. It inhibits the effects of histamine on capillary permeability and on smooth muscle by competitive inhibition at H_1 receptors. Either stimulation or depression of the central nervous system may occur through an unknown mechanism. It has anticholinergic activity, although no significant effects on the cardiovascular system occur at normal therapeutic dosages.

Absorption and Biotransformation

Meclizine is readily absorbed from the gastrointestinal tract and is widely distributed to body tissues. The exact nature of elimination in humans is unknown, but it appears to be extensively metabolized in the liver and excreted in the urine.

Recommended Reading

Biggs, J. S. G. Vomiting in pregnancy: Causes and management. *Drugs* 9:299, 1975.

Gilman, A. G., Goodman, L. S., and Gilman, A. *The Pharmacological Basis of Therapeutics* (6th ed.). New York: Macmillan, 1980. P. 628.

Heinonen, O. P., Slone, D., and Shapiro, S. *Birth Defects and Drugs in Pregnancy*. Littleton, Mass.: Publishing Sciences Group, 1977. Pp. 322–327.

Long, J. W. *The Essential Guide to Prescription Drugs*. New York: Harper & Row, 1977. Pp. 368–370.

Milkovich, L., and VandenBerg, B. J. An evaluation of the teratogenicity of certain antinauseant drugs. *Am. J. Obstet. Gynecol.* 125:244, 1976.

Nishimura, H., and Tanimura, T. *Clinical Aspects of the Teratogenicity of Drugs*. Amsterdam: Excerpta Medica, 1976.

Meperidine (Demerol®)

Indications and Recommendations

Meperidine may be used as a short-term analgesic throughout pregnancy and may be used for the relief of pain during labor at term. A narcotic indicated for the relief of moderate to severe pain, it is commonly used in laboring patients, often in combination with a tranquilizer.

It is recommended that if this drug is used in pregnant women, the lowest effective dosage should be administered. Infants born to mothers who received meperidine as antepartum analgesia should be observed for respiratory depression. This can be reversed by naloxone. The degree of neonatal respiratory depression produced by any narcotic administered during labor depends on the gestational age and condition of the infant. The magnitude of this effect is inversely proportional to gestational age and may be made greater by birth asphyxia. Meperidine therefore should be used with extreme caution, if at all, during labor that could produce a premature infant.

Special Considerations in Pregnancy

Teratogenicity has not been associated with the use of meperidine during human pregnancies. When given before delivery, this drug does not appear to delay labor or to decrease uterine motility. It does not increase the incidence of postpartum hemorrhage, nor does it interfere with postpartum contractions or involution of the uterus.

Placental transfer of meperidine is very rapid, with fetal blood levels reaching approximately 80% of maternal levels. Administering meperidine to the mother before delivery has been associated with neonatal respiratory depression and lower psychophysiologic test scores. Both of these effects appear to be more marked when the dose is administered more than 1 hour and up to 4 hours before birth. These are relatively short-term effects, lasting several days, and seem to have no long-lasting impact on the infant. These effects may be related to the presence of normeperidine, an active metabolite with a long half-life, in the fetus. Recent data suggest that multiple dosages of both meperidine and normeperidine to the mother create a continued diffusion gradient resulting in maximum fetal exposure. If neonatal respiratory depression does occur in a meperidine-exposed newborn, naloxone should be administered to the baby.

As with all narcotic analgesics, infants born to meperidine-addicted mothers are addicted at birth and will experience withdrawal.

Meperidine is secreted into breast milk, but only in small amounts. It does not appear to have significant effects on the infant at dosages normally prescribed for analgesia.

Dosage

The usual analgesic dose is 50–100 mg IM every 3–4 hours. This dose must be increased if the oral route is used. Intravenous use increases the incidence and severity of untoward effects and subcutaneous administration causes local irritation and tissue induration.

Adverse Effects

The most frequently observed side effects seen with meperidine use include light-headedness, nausea, vomiting, dizziness, and sedation. Other less frequent side effects include euphoria, dysphoria, dry mouth, flushing, syncope, and palpitations. Meperidine produces less constipation and urinary retention than other narcotic analgesics. Excitation and convulsions may occur at higher dosages. Overdosage is characterized by respiratory depression; cold, clammy skin; and extreme somnolence progressing to coma. Death may result from respiratory arrest and cardiovascular failure.

Mechanism of Action

Meperidine exerts its analgesic effect on the central nervous system. Its exact nature remains unknown, but analgesia is thought to occur through effects on the sensory cortex of the frontal lobes and the diencephalon. In addition, meperidine may interfere with pain conduction or may affect the patients' emotional response to pain.

Meperidine's physiologic effects are similar to all of the narcotic analgesics. It produces prompt relief of moderate to severe pain, and the duration of its analgesia is between 2 and 4 hours. Meperidine has little or no antitussive activity in analgesic dosages.

Absorption and Biotransformation

Meperidine is poorly absorbed when given orally; an oral dose is less than half as effective as an identical parenteral dose. Following oral administration, peak analgesia occurs within 1 hour, and its duration is between 2 and 4 hours. After intramuscular injection, peak analgesia occurs within 40–60 minutes and subsides after 2–4 hours. Meperidine is primarily metabolized in the liver by hydrolysis and N-demethylation. One metabolite, normeperidine, is active, although less so than meperidine. Five percent of a dose is excreted unchanged.

Recommended Reading

Gilman, A. G., Goodman, L. S., and Gilman, A. *The Pharmacological Basis of Therapeutics* (6th ed.). New York: Macmillan, 1980. Pp. 513–517.

Hodgkinson, R., and Husain, F. J. The duration of effect of maternally administered meperidine on neonatal behavior. *Anesthesiology* 56:51, 1982.

Kuhnert, B. R., et al. Meperidine and normeperidine levels following meperidine administration during labor. I. Mother. *Am. J. Obstet. Gynecol.* 133:904, 1979.

Kuhnert, B. R., et al. Meperidine and normeperidine levels following meperidine administration during labor. II. Fetus and neonate. *Am. J. Obstet. Gynecol.* 133:909, 1979.

Kuhnert, B. R., et al. Meperidine disposition in mother, neonate and non-pregnant females. *Clin. Pharmacol. Ther.* 27:486, 1980.

Kuhnert, B. R., et al. Disposition of meperidine and normeperidine following multiple doses during labor. I. Mother. *Am. J. Obstet. Gynecol.* 151:406, 1985.

Kuhnert, B. R., et al. Disposition of meperidine and normeperidine following multiple doses during labor. II. Fetus and neonate. *Am. J. Obstet. Gynecol.* 151:410, 1985.

Morrison, J. C., et al. Meperidine metabolism in the parturient. *Obstet. Gynecol.* 59:359, 1982.

Szeto, H. H., et al. Amniotic fluid transfer of meperidine from maternal plasma in early pregnancy. *Obstet. Gynecol.* 52:59, 1978.

Tomson, G., et al. Maternal kinetics and transplacental passage of pethidine during labour. *Br. J. Clin. Pharmacol.* 13:653, 1982.

Mephobarbital (Mebaral®)

Indications and Recommendations

Mephobarbital is relatively contraindicated during pregnancy because other therapeutic agents are preferable. This drug is metabolized to phenobarbital. It has properties and uses similar to phenobarbital, but larger dosages must be given. Mephobarbital may be prescribed for routine sedation as well as therapy for various forms of epilepsy. If a long-acting barbiturate is necessary during pregnancy, however, phenobarbital is preferable to mephobarbital because it is as effective and much better studied.

Recommended Reading

AMA Drug Evaluations (3rd ed.). Littleton, Mass.: Publishing Sciences Group, 1977.

American Hospital Formulary Service. *Monograph for Mephobarbital.* Washington, D.C.: American Society of Hospital Pharmacists, 1984.

Gilman, A. G., Goodman, L. S., and Gilman, A. *The Pharmacological Basis of Therapeutics* (6th ed.). New York: Macmillan, 1980. Pp. 351–458.

Metaproterenol (Alupent®, Orciprenaline®)

Indications and Recommendations

Metaproterenol may be administered to pregnant patients in aerosol form in the treatment of infrequent, mild episodes of bronchospasm. If the patient remains symptomatic, an oral bronchodilator should be used. Oral metaproterenol may be used as an adjunctive bronchodilator in a pregnant asthmatic who remains symptomatic on maximal dosages of theophylline. It should be stated that although no reports of adverse effects have been published thus far, there have not been any large series that have studied the effect of this drug on the human fetus.

The drug must be administered with caution to patients with hyperthyroidism, hypertension, diabetes, congestive heart failure, and coronary artery disease. Furthermore, if it is administered along with another sympathomimetic drug, the potential for adverse side effects may be significantly increased.

Special Considerations in Pregnancy

Metaproterenol has been used to arrest premature labor, although it has not been approved for that use in this country. No unusual maternal effects are reported. No information is available regarding the passage of metaproterenol across the placenta or into breast milk.

In rabbits, fetal loss and teratogenic effects have been observed at and above oral doses of 50–100 mg/kg respectively. There are no published reports of teratogenesis in humans using the drug, although no controlled studies are available to establish its safety during pregnancy.

Dosage

For oral administration, the dose is 20 mg q6–8h. The onset of action is about 30 minutes. Peak effect occurs in 2 hours, and the duration of action is 4–6 hours.

For aerosol administration, the dose is 1–3 puffs (0.65 mg/puff) q3–4h. The onset of action is about 2–10 minutes. Peak effect occurs within 30–90 minutes, and the duration of action is 1–5 hours.

Adverse Effects

In addition to causing bronchodilatation, metaproterenol increases heart rate, stroke volume, and pulse pressure. It also may cause hyperglycemia and an increase in free fatty acids and glycerol. Metaproterenol may also reduce gastrointestinal tone and motility and cause mild general central nervous system stimulation.

Side effects include tachycardia, hypertension, palpitation, nervousness, tremor, nausea, and vomiting. The incidence of side effects is greater when the drug is given orally as opposed to the aerosol route.

Mechanism of Action

Metaproterenol is a beta-sympathomimetic agonist with predominantly beta-2 activity. It seems to work by stimulating adenyl cyclase, the enzyme that catalyzes the conversion of adenosine triphosphate (ATP) to cyclic AMP. Cyclic AMP acts locally as a bronchodilator.

Absorption and Biotransformation

An average of 40% of an oral dose of metaproterenol is absorbed. This is primarily excreted in the urine as glucuronic acid conjugates. Metaproterenol's prolonged duration of action when compared to catecholamine beta-sympathomimetic agonists is due to the fact that it is not metabolized by catechol-O-methyltransferase.

Recommended Reading

Drewitt, A. H. First clinical experience with Alupent—A new bronchodilator. *Br. J. Clin. Pract.* 16:549, 1962.

Freedman, B. J., and Hill, G. B. Comparative study of duration of action and cardiovascular effect of bronchodilator aerosols. *Thorax* 26:46, 1970.

Holmes, T. H. A comparative clinical trial of metaproterenol and isoproterenol as bronchodilator aerosols. *Clin. Pharmacol. Ther.* 9:615, 1968.

Hurst, A. Metaproterenol: A potent and safe bronchodilator. *Ann. Allergy* 31:460, 1973.

Rebuck, A. S., and Real, J. Oral Orciprenaline in the treatment of chronic asthma. *Med. J. Aust.* 1:445, 1965.

Zilianti, A. Action of Orciprenaline on uterine contractility during labor, maternal cardiovascular system, fetal heart rate and acid-base balance. *Am. J. Obstet. Gynecol.* 109:1073, 1971.

Metaraminol (Aramine®)

Indications and Recommendations

Metaraminol, an alpha-adrenergic agent used to increase systemic blood pressure, is relatively contraindicated during pregnancy because other therapeutic agents are preferable. Uterine vessels have only alpha-adrenergic receptors and react to adrenergic stimulus solely by contracting. Such decrease in uterine blood flow may adversely affect the fetus. Should a pressor be needed to treat hypotension associated with conduction anesthesia in a pregnant woman, ephedrine is the agent of choice.

Recommended Reading

Avery, G. S. *Drug Treatment: Principles and Practice of Clinical Pharmacology and Therapeutics.* Sydney, Aust.: Adis, 1976.

Gilman, A. G., Goodman, L. S., and Gilman, A. *The Pharmacological Basis of Therapeutics* (6th ed.). New York: Macmillan, 1980. P. 164.

Smith, N. T., and Corbascio, A. The use and misuse of pressor agents. *Anesthesiology* 33:58, 1970.

Methadone

Indications and Recommendations

Methadone may be used as a short-term analgesic during pregnancy. It is a long-acting narcotic analgesic that is effective when given orally. Its principal use in women of childbearing age is in the treatment of heroin addiction. Patients who are maintained on methadone for treatment of heroin addiction should not be detoxified during pregnancy.

Special Considerations in Pregnancy

Teratogenicity has not been associated with the use of methadone during pregnancy. The primary problems associated with the administration of methadone for treatment of pregnant heroin addicts are low birth weights and neonatal withdrawal. Methadone-specific effects are difficult to evaluate, however, because patients in maintenance programs often consume a wide variety of drugs.

The neonatal withdrawal syndrome is seen in the majority of infants born to methadone-maintained mothers. It usually begins within 48 hours of delivery, but its onset can be delayed for up to 2 weeks. The intensity of the symptoms increases in proportion to the maternal dosage and may last up to 6 months. In addition, infants born to addicted mothers are frequently premature and suffer from intrauterine growth retardation. The long-term effects on the infant are unknown.

Maternal narcotic withdrawal during pregnancy is not recommended. It causes a marked response of the fetal adrenal gland and sympathetic nervous system. It is also associated with increased stillborn rates and neonatal mortality.

Methadone enters the breast milk in concentrations approaching maternal plasma levels and may prevent or ameliorate withdrawal symptoms in addicted infants.

Dosage

The usual oral analgesic dose is 5–15 mg q6–8h. The usual parenteral analgesic dose is 5–10 mg. Doses for the treatment of heroin addiction are titrated according to individual patient need and usually range from 10–40 mg/day.

Adverse Effects

The side effects of methadone are similar to those of other narcotic analgesics and include euphoria, light-headedness, dizziness, sedation, dry mouth, constipation, and urinary retention. Overdosage is characterized by respiratory depression. With chronic administration, additional side effects including excessive sweating, lymphocytosis, and increased concentrations of prolactin, albumin, and globulins in plasma can occur.

Mechanism of Action

As with the other narcotic analgesics, the mechanism of action of methadone is not fully understood. It appears to act in the central nervous system to alter the response of several systems of neurotransmitters. Methadone is a potent antitussive in analgesic dosages.

Absorption and Biotransformation

Methadone is well absorbed from the gastrointestinal tract, reaching peak concentrations approximately 4 hours after an oral dose. Approximately 85% of circulating methadone is bound to plasma proteins. With repeated administration, it gradually accumulates in tissues and is slowly released into the bloodstream after the drug is discontinued. It is extensively metabolized in the liver, and the metabolites as well as small amounts of unchanged drug are excreted in the urine and bile. In nontolerant patients, the half-life is 15 hours, but this increases to 22 hours in tolerant patients.

Recommended Reading

Chasnoff, I. J., Hatcher, R., and Burns, W. J. Early growth patterns of methadone-addicted infants. *Am. J. Dis. Child.* 134:1049, 1980.

Finnegan, L. P. The effects of narcotics and alcohol on pregnancy and the newborn. *Ann. N.Y. Acad. Sci.* 362:136, 1981.

Gilman, A. G., Goodman, L. S., and Gilman, A. *The Pharmacological Basis of Therapeutics* (6th ed.). New York: Macmillan, 1980. Pp. 518–520.

Harris, V. J., and Srinivasan, G. Infants of drug-dependent mothers. *Semin. Roentgenol.* 18:179, 1983.

Rementeria, J. L., and Nunag, N. N. Narcotic withdrawal in pregnancy: Stillbirth incidence with a case report. *Am. J. Obstet. Gynecol.* 116:1152, 1973.

Rosen, T. S., and Johnson, H. L. Children of methadone-maintained mothers: Follow-up to 18 months of age. *J. Pediatr.* 101:192, 1982.

Strauss, M. E., Andresko, M., and Stryker, J. C. Methadone maintenance during pregnancy: Pregnancy, birth and neonate characteristics. *Am. J. Obstet. Gynecol.* 121:233, 1975.

Wilson, G. S., Desmond, M. M., and Wait, R. B. Follow-up of methadone-treated and untreated narcotic-dependent women and their infants: Health, developmental and societal implications. *J. Pediatr.* 98:716, 1981.

Methenamine Hippurate (Hiprex®, Urex®)

Indications and Recommendations

Methenamine hippurate is relatively contraindicated during pregnancy because other therapeutic agents are preferable. It is a urinary tract antiseptic used primarily in the treatment of chronic urinary tract infections. Because the safety of the hippurate salt during pregnancy has not been established, methenamine mandelate should be administered when therapy of chronic urinary tract infections is required and when methenamine is the agent of choice.

Recommended Reading

Gilman, A. G., Goodman, L. S., and Gilman, A. *The Pharmacological Basis of Therapeutics* (6th ed.). New York: Macmillan, 1980. P. 1120.

Gleckman, R., et al. Drug therapy reviews: Methenamine mandelate and methenamine hippurate. *Am. J. Hosp. Pharm.* 36:1509, 1979.

Methenamine Mandelate (Mandelamine®)

Indications and Recommendations

Methenamine mandelate is safe to use during pregnancy. The treatment of choice for urinary tract infections during pregnancy is either a sulfonamide (in the first or second trimester) or ampicillin. Should chronic prophylaxis be required, methenamine mandelate may be used in the pregnant woman. It is most useful in the prophylaxis of *Escherichia coli* cystitis, but it can also usually suppress the common gram-negative offenders, as well as *Staphylococcus aureus* and *Staphylococcus epidermidis.*

Special Considerations in Pregnancy

Methenamine mandelate has been reported to lower falsely the 24-hour urine estriol concentration because formaldehyde destroys estrogen in the urine. The assay is reliable 2 days following discontinuance of the drug.

A study was made of 51 women who received methenamine mandelate during pregnancy at a dose of 4 g/day in divided doses. No difference in fetal outcome was found in this group when compared to controls.

Dosage

The recommended dose of methenamine mandelate is 1 g qid. It is usually given with an acidifying agent, commonly ascorbic acid, 500 mg qid.

Adverse Effects

Side effects of methenamine mandelate include nausea and vomiting, and dermatologic reactions such as skin rashes, urticaria, and pruritus. Following large dosages, bladder irritation, urinary frequency, dysuria, albuminuria, and hematuria may occur.

Mechanism of Action

Methenamine mandelate is decomposed by acids with the liberation of formaldehyde. It is this formaldehyde that is responsible for methenamine's antibacterial effects in the urinary tract. Acidification of the urine is necessary to promote the formaldehyde-dependent antibacterial action. For maximal effectiveness, the urine should be maintained at a pH less than 5.5.

Urea-splitting strains of *Pseudomonas, Aerobacter,* and *Proteus* raise urinary pH and render methenamine inactive unless supplemental urinary acidification is provided. *Candida* infections are resistant to this drug.

Absorption and Biotransformation

Methenamine is absorbed orally, but 10–30% decomposes in the gastric juice unless the drug is protected by an enteric coat. The drug is then rapidly excreted in the urine.

Recommended Reading

Gilman, A. G., Goodman, L. S., and Gilman, A. *The Pharmacological Basis of Therapeutics* (6th ed.). New York: Macmillan, 1980. P. 1120.

Gleckman, R., et al. Drug therapy reviews: Methenamine mandelate and methenamine hippurate. *Am. J. Hosp. Pharm.* 36:1509, 1979.

Gordon, S. F. Asymptomatic bacteriuria of pregnancy. *Clin. Med.* 79:22, 1972.

Methoxamine (Vasoxyl®)

Indications and Recommendations

Methoxamine, an alpha-adrenergic agent used to increase systemic blood pressure in emergency situations, is no longer available commercially. Under baseline conditions during pregnancy, the uterine vessels are thought to be maximally dilated. Alpha-adrenergic stimulation causes vascular contraction and a decrease in uterine blood flow, which may adversely affect the fetus. Methoxamine has been known to produce uterine tetany. When a pressor is needed to treat hypotension associated with conduction anesthesia in pregnancy, ephedrine is the drug of first choice.

Recommended Reading

Avery, G. S. *Drug Treatment: Principles and Practice of Clinical Pharmacology and Therapeutics* (2nd ed.). Sydney, Aust.: Adis, 1980. P. 1251.

Gilman, A. G., Goodman, L. S., and Gilman, A. *The Pharmacological Basis of Therapeutics* (6th ed.). New York: Macmillan, 1980. P. 165.

Smith, N. T., and Corbascio, A. The use and misuse of pressor agents. *Anesthesiology* 33:58, 1970.

Methsuximide (Celontin®)

Indications and Recommendations

Methsuximide is contraindicated for use during pregnancy since other therapeutic agents are preferable. It is one of the succinimide group of anticonvulsants used in the treatment of absence seizures. Experience with this drug in pregnancy is limited. First-trimester exposure to methsuximide has been reported in five pregnancies, and no adverse fetal outcomes were reported. Nevertheless, because this drug is known to be less effective than ethosuximide, the latter is the anticonvulsant of choice when absence seizures must be treated in obstetric patients.

Recommended Reading

Annegers, J. F., Elveback, L. R., Hauser, W. A., and Kurland, L. T. Do anticonvulsants have a teratogenic effect? *Arch. Neurol.* 31:364, 1974.

Fabro, S., and Brown, N. A. Teratogenic potential of anticonvulsants. *N. Engl. J. Med.* 300:1280, 1979.

Fedrick, J. Epilepsy and pregnancy: A report from the Oxford record linkage study. *Br. Med. J.* 2:442, 1973.

Gilman, A. G., Goodman, L. S., and Gilman, A. *The Pharmacological Basis of Therapeutics* (6th ed.). New York: Macmillan, 1980. Pp. 460–465.

Heinonen, O. P., Slone, D., and Shapiro, S. *Birth Defects and Drugs in Pregnancy*. Littleton, Mass.: Publishing Sciences Group, 1977. Pp. 358–359.

McMullin, G. P. Teratogenic effects of anticonvulsants. *Br. Med. J.* 2:430, 1971.

National Institutes of Health: Anticonvulsants found to have teratogenic potential. *J.A.M.A.* 241:36, 1981.

Methyldopa (Aldomet®)

Indications and Recommendations

Methyldopa is currently the drug of choice for pregnant women with mild to moderate chronic hypertension. The action of this drug may be potentiated by adding hydralazine or a thiazide diuretic to the treatment regimen. It is recommended that therapy with a thiazide diuretic *not* be initiated during the second half of pregnancy because of its potential for transiently reducing uterine blood flow.

Methyldopa should not be used as primary therapy in a hypertensive crisis.

Special Considerations in Pregnancy

A study of 24 full-term neonates born to mothers treated with methyldopa compared with 50 full-term control neonates matched for birth weight and gestational age revealed mean systolic pressure in the treated infants to be 4.5 mm Hg lower on the first day and 4.3 mm Hg lower on the second. No differences were apparent thereafter. Furthermore, there were no episodes of bradycardia in the neonates of treated mothers. An investigation of 200 infants born to methyldopa-treated mothers revealed a reduction in neonatal head circumference when compared to matched controls. This difference, however, was confined to neonates whose mothers were initially treated between 16 and 20 weeks' gestation. By age 4, no significant differences were seen in height, weight, general health, or frequency of visual and hearing problems between the two groups, but male children of the treated women had smaller heads. Mean intelligence quotients and growth did not differ in follow-up study at 7.5 years.

Although methyldopa crosses the placental barrier, it is not known whether the Coombs' test can be made positive in neonates of mothers who take this drug during pregnancy. This neonatal complication seems unlikely because of the duration of therapy necessary before its occurrence in adults. In a series of 117 women given methyldopa during their pregnancies, one mother and none of the neonates developed a positive Coombs' test. The same series showed no effect on birth weight and maturity when offspring of patients given the drug were compared to offspring of untreated controls. The authors of this study believed that methyldopa had been demonstrated to be a safe drug for both mother and fetus.

Dosage

When given orally, the dose is 250–500 mg q6–8h. The onset of action is 2–4 hours, and the maximum effect is seen in 4–6 hours. The duration of action is 24 hours. At fixed dosage levels, 2–3 days of therapy are required before the full effect of the drug is achieved. After discontinuation of the drug, there is a return to pretreatment blood pressure levels in 24–48 hours.

When given intravenously, the dose is 250–500 mg q6–12h. The onset of action is 2–3 hours. Because of its relatively slow onset of action, this is not the drug of choice for a hypertensive emergency. Given intravenously, this drug may cause enough drowsiness to interfere with the patient's sensorium.

Adverse Effects

Methyldopa causes a decrease in peripheral vascular resistance, and postural hypotension may be observed. Cardiac output is reduced by this drug but rarely to a significant degree. Renal and uterine blood flows are maintained in the presence of its hypotensive action, and in fact, there may be selective renal vasodilatation.

Side effects include sedation and drowsiness, depression, sodium retention, and nasal stuffiness. A positive Coombs' test, which is infrequently associated with hemolytic anemia, may occur. Positive Coombs' tests are said to be present in 20% of patients who take this drug for more than 6 months but are rare before that time. Hypertensive crises have been reported when methyldopa has been given in conjunction with propranolol. This is presumably due to a potentiation of the pressor action of alpha-methylnorepinephrine by propranolol. Allergic reactions manifested as drug fever may also be seen.

Mechanism of Action

Methyldopa functions as an antihypertensive agent in a variety of ways. It stimulates alpha-adrenergic receptor sites in the central nervous system. It inhibits dopa decarboxylase, which results in a reduction in the production of norepinephrine in postganglionic nerve endings. It is metabolized to alpha-methylnorepinephrine, which functions as a "false neurohumoral transmitter" at smooth muscle receptor sites. It also suppresses the release of renal renin.

Absorption and Biotransformation

When methyldopa is administered orally, only 50% or less is absorbed. Methyldopa and its metabolites are weakly bound to plasma proteins. It is metabolized in the gastrointestinal tract and liver and is excreted in the urine largely by glomerular filtration. Unabsorbed drug is eliminated in the feces unchanged. It can be used in patients with impaired renal function but in smaller than usual dosages and given at longer than usual intervals.

In a study of nine neonates born to hypertensive mothers who received methyldopa for several weeks before delivery, blood levels present in the infants at birth were comparable to those in the mother, and these levels persisted for several days. Elimination of the drug in the neonate is primarily controlled by the rate of the renal excretion of its conjugated product. Methyldopa is eliminated slowly from the neonate and its half-life seems to be 3–4 times that reported for adults.

Recommended Reading

Cockburn, J., et al. Final report of study on hypertension during pregnancy: The effects of specific treatment on the growth and development of the children. *Lancet* 1:647, 1982.

Cummings, A. J., and Whitelaw, A. G. A study of conjugation and drug elimination in the human neonate. *Br. J. Clin. Pharmacol.* 12:511, 1981.

Frohlich, E. D. The sympathetic depressant antihypertensives. *Drug Ther.* 5:24, 1975.

Jones, H. M., and Cummings, A. J. A study of the transfer of alpha-methyldopa to the human foetus and newborn infant. *Br. J. Clin. Pharmacol.* 6:432, 1978.

Jones, H. M., et al. A study of the disposition of alpha-methyldopa in newborn infants following administration to the mother for the treatment of hypertension during pregnancy. *Br. J. Clin. Pharmacol.* 8:433, 1979.

Koch-Weser, J. Hypertensive emergencies. *N. Engl. J. Med.* 290:211, 1974.

Moar, V. A., et al. Neonatal head circumference and the treatment of maternal hypertension. *Br. J. Obstet. Gynaecol.* 85:933, 1978.

Redman, C. W. G., Beilin, L. J., and Bonnar, J. Treatment of hypertension in pregnancy with methyldopa: Blood pressure control and side effects. *Br. J. Obstet. Gynaecol.* 84:419, 1977.

Redman, C. W. G., et al. Fetal outcome in trial of antihypertensive treatment in pregnancy. *Lancet* 2:753, 756, 1976.

Whitelaw, A. Maternal methyldopa treatment and neonatal blood pressure. *Br. Med. J. Clin. Res.* 283:471, 1981.

Woods, J. R., and Brinkman, C. R., III. The treatment of gestational hypertension. *J. Reprod. Med.* 15:195, 1975.

Methylene Blue

Indications and Recommendations

Methylene blue is contraindicated in pregnancy, as safer agents are available. This dye, whose chemical name is tetramethylthionine chloride, has been utilized for intraamniotic injection to aid in the diagnosis of ruptured membranes. Evans blue dye was originally proposed for diagnosing ruptured membranes and as a "marker" when amniocentesis is performed on patients with multiple gestations and is apparently harmless, but methylene blue was frequently substituted, presumably because of its wide availability on gynecologic services.

Methylene blue and its colorless reduced derivative, leukomethylene blue, form a reversible oxidation-reduction system. In low concentrations, methylene blue hastens the reduction of methemoglobin to hemoglobin, acting as an electron acceptor from reduced pyridine nucleotides, then passing the electron along to methemoglobin. It is used in the treatment of both idiopathic and drug-induced methemoglobinemia. However, in higher concentrations, it acts as an oxidant, producing methemoglobin by oxidizing the iron of reduced hemoglobin from the ferrous to the ferric form.

In addition, methylene blue may produce Heinz body hemolytic anemia in the fetus and newborn. The mechanism of this effect appears to be the production of leukomethylene blue, which reduces oxygen to hydrogen peroxide. When normal detoxification mechanisms are overwhelmed, the excess hydrogen peroxide oxidizes hemoglobin to produce sulfhemoglobin and consequently Heinz bodies. The lipid membrane of the red cell is damaged, and hemolysis results.

There have been numerous case reports of hemolytic anemia and hyperbilirubinemia in neonates whose mothers had methylene blue instilled in the amniotic fluid. When looked for, Heinz bodies have been present and methemoglobin levels have been high. In one case, severe fetal tachycardia occurred immediately after the intraamniotic injection of 2 ml of 1% methylene blue, and it was believed that a fetal intravascular injection caused immediate methemoglobinemia with resultant tissue hypoxia.

Methylene blue has been inadvertently injected into the uterus during the first trimester without apparent untoward effect. However, because of the previously mentioned problems, it is recommended that this dye not be utilized for amniotic injection for the diagnosis of ruptured membranes or in diagnostic amniocentesis for the identification of amniotic sacs in multiple gestations.

Recommended Reading

Atlay, R. D., and Sutherst, J. R. Premature rupture of the fetal membranes confirmed by intraamniotic injection of dye (Evans blue T-1824). *Am. J. Obstet. Gynecol.* 108:993, 1970.

Cowett, R. M., et al. Untoward neonatal effect of intraamniotic administration of methylene blue. *Obstet. Gynecol.* 48:74s, 1976.

Crooks, J. Haemolytic jaundice in a neonate after intra-amniotic injection of methylene blue. *Arch. Dis. Child.* 57:872, 1982.

Gilman, A. G., Goodman, L. S., and Gilman, A. *The Pharmacological Basis of Therapeutics* (6th ed.). New York: Macmillan, 1980. P. 980.

Katz, Z., and Lancet, M. Inadvertent intrauterine injection of methylene blue in early pregnancy. *N. Engl. J. Med.* 304:1427, 1981.

Kirsch, I. R., and Cohen, H. J. Heinz body hemolytic anemia from the use of methylene blue in neonates. *J. Pediatr.* 96:276, 1980.

McEnerney, J. K., and McEnerney, L. N. Unfavorable neonatal outcome after intraamniotic injection of methylene blue. *Obstet. Gynecol.* 61:35, 1983.

Plunkett, G. D. Neonatal complications. *Obstet. Gynecol.* 41:476, 1973.

Spahr, R. C., Salsburey, D. J., Krissberg, A., and Prin, W. Intraamniotic injection of methylene blue leading to methemoglobinemia in one of twins. *Int. J. Gynaecol. Obstet.* 17:477, 1980.

Methylergonovine Maleate (Methergine®)

Indications and Recommendations

The use of methylergonovine maleate is absolutely contraindicated in the pregnant woman. It may be administered post partum in the management of postpartum uterine atony, hemorrhage, and subinvolution after delivery of the placenta. It should not be given prior to the delivery of the anterior shoulder. It is said to be safer than ergonovine when used in preeclamptic or eclamptic patients since it is associated with fewer pressor effects.

Special Considerations in Pregnancy

Because of its stimulatory effect on uterine muscle—causing tetanic uterine contractions—methylergonovine should not be used at any time during pregnancy, although it may be used post partum. There are reports that methylergonovine decreases plasma prolactin levels, and controversy exists as to whether or not it has any effect on lactation.

Dosage

Oral administration of 0.2 mg every 4 hours for 6 doses is recommended. Intramuscular administration of 0.2 mg after delivery of the anterior shoulder, after delivery of the placenta, or during the puerperium has an onset of action within 2–5 minutes. This dose may be repeated at intervals of 2–4 hours. If essential, methylergonovine may be administered intravenously at a rate not exceeding 0.2 mg/minute. Blood pressure must be monitored at all times.

Adverse Effects

When given orally, methylergonovine has minimal peripheral vasoconstrictive properties, although it may have a mild pressor effect and cause decreased peripheral blood flow. When given intravenously, however, there may be a significant increase in blood pressure with a subsequent acute hypertensive and cardiovascular crisis. More common adverse reactions include nausea, vomiting, dizziness, headache, tinnitus, diaphoresis, palpitations, and dyspnea.

Mechanism of Action

Methylergonovine directly stimulates uterine muscle. Peripheral vasoconstriction is also a direct effect. Other complex and sometimes conflicting physiologic effects are outside the scope of this discussion.

Absorption and Biotransformation

The oral tablet is rapidly and adequately absorbed with an onset of action of 5–10 minutes. Methylergonovine is metabolized by the liver and excreted in the feces.

Recommended Reading

Chase, G., et al. (eds.). *Remington's Pharmaceutical Sciences* (14th ed.). Easton, Pa.: Mack, 1970. Pp. 952–953.
delPozo, E., Brun de Re, R., and Hinselmann, M. Lack of effect of methylergonovine on postpartum lactation. *Am. J. Obstet. Gynecol.* 123:845, 1975.

Floss, H., Cassidy, J., and Robbers, J. Influence of ergot alkaloids on pituitary prolactin and prolactin-dependent processes. *J. Pharm. Sci.* 62:699, 1973.

Gilman, A. G., Goodman, L. S., and Gilman, A. *The Pharmacological Basis of Therapeutics* (6th ed.). New York: Macmillan, 1980. Pp. 939–947.

Methylphenidate Hydrochloride (Ritalin®)

Indications and Recommendations

Methylphenidate hydrochloride may be administered to pregnant women with severe narcolepsy when treatment is considered essential. Although this drug is also used for minimal brain dysfunction in children, as a mild sedative, or as treatment for apathetic or withdrawn senile behavior, narcolepsy, a rare phenomenon, seems to be the only likely indication for its use in pregnant women.

Special Considerations in Pregnancy

No information is currently available regarding the effects of this compound on the fetus.

Dosage

The usual adult dose is 10 mg 2 or 3 times a day. Because of the possibility of degradation in the acid medium of the postprandial gastric fluid, the drug is taken 30–45 minutes before meals. In the treatment of narcolepsy methylphenidate is usually administered before important activities.

Adverse Effects

Side effects include tachycardia, hypertension, palpitations, anorexia, insomnia, dizziness, headache, dry mouth, and anxiety.

Mechanism of Action

Methylphenidate is a sympathomimetic central nervous system stimulant. Effects on mental function are somewhat greater than on motor activity. Patients suffering from narcolepsy experience a reduced number of sleep attacks when methylphenidate is combined with changes in daily habits.

Absorption and Biotransformation

Methylphenidate is deesterified in plasma with less than 1% excreted in urine. The plasma half-life is less than 3 hours.

Recommended Reading

AMA Drug Evaluations (3rd ed.). Littleton, Mass.: Publishing Sciences Group, 1977. Pp. 498–499.

Bioavailability data on Ritalin. Ciba Pharmaceutical Company. Summit, N.J., 1976.

Gilman, A. G., Goodman, L. S., and Gilman, A. *The Pharmacological Basis of Therapeutics* (6th ed.). New York: Macmillan, 1980. Pp. 589–591.

Product information on Ritalin. Ciba Pharmaceutical Company. Summit, N.J., 1973.

Safer, D. Depression of growth in hyperactive children on stimulant drugs. *N. Engl. J. Med.* 287:217, 1972.

Methysergide Maleate (Sansert®)

Indications and Recommendations

Methysergide maleate is contraindicated during pregnancy. It is a semisynthetic derivative of the ergot alkaloids. A theoretic risk of abortion or premature labor exists, and effects of the drug on the fetus are unknown. Effects of methysergide on the mother may be severe.

This drug is effective in the prophylaxis of all types of migraine headaches. It is of no value in treatment of acute attacks or prevention or management of tension headaches. Methysergide has also been of some value in combatting intestinal hypermotility in patients with carcinoid and in the postgastrectomy dumping syndrome. Uninterrupted, long-term therapy with methysergide is contraindicated since it may induce fibrotic conditions, including retroperitoneal fibrosis, pleuropulmonary fibrosis, and endocardial fibrosis. Cardiovascular complications include cardiac murmurs; cold, numb, and painful extremities with or without paresthesias; and diminished or absent pulses.

Recommended Reading

AMA Drug Evaluations (3rd ed.). Littleton, Mass.: Publishing Sciences Group, 1977. Pp. 360–361.

Bedard, P., and Bouchard, R. Dramatic effect of methysergide on myoclonus. *Lancet* 1:738, 1974.

Gilman, A. G., Goodman, L. S., and Gilman, A. *The Pharmacological Basis of Therapeutics* (6th ed.). New York: Macmillan, 1980. Pp. 638–639, 939–947.

Long, J. W. *The Essential Guide to Prescription Drugs.* New York: Harper & Row, 1977. Pp. 409–412.

Melmon, K., and Morelli, H. *Clinical Pharmacology—Basic Principles in Therapeutics.* New York: Macmillan, 1972. Pp. 128–129, 628–629.

Product information on Sansert (methysergide maleate). Sandoz Pharmaceuticals. East Hanover, N.J., April 12, 1976.

Metoclopramide (Reglan®)

Indications and Recommendations

Metoclopramide, a blocker of dopaminergic receptors, is probably safe to use in pregnancy. It was recently approved for use in the United States. Approved indications include symptomatic gastroesophageal reflux, diabetic gastric stasis, the prevention of nausea and vomiting associated with cancer chemotherapy, and the facilitation of small bowel intubation and radiologic examination. Metoclopramide has been used as an antiemetic, as a preanesthetic medication to reduce gastric volume, and as a lactation-enhancing agent, although it has not been specifically approved for these indications. Because of the relatively brief experience with this drug in pregnancy to date, it would be best to use other agents in situations in which metoclopramide shows no distinct advantage.

Special Considerations in Pregnancy

Animal studies have not documented teratogenicity for this drug, and there have not been any reports suggesting human teratogenicity. Metoclopramide crosses the placenta in humans at term, with fetal plasma concentrations approximately half of maternal levels. Neonates exposed to this drug during labor did not exhibit differences in Apgar scores or cardiovascular or neurobehavioral effects when compared with placebo-treated control subjects. Studies in the first and third trimesters have demonstrated a rapid and significant increase in maternal serum prolactin, but not in growth hormone levels after intravenous administration of metoclopramide. During the first trimester, the administration of this drug did not change maternal levels of progesterone, estradiol, human chorionic gonadotropin (HCG), or human placental lactogen (HPL). Fetal prolactin levels were not increased when laboring mothers were given the drug. Physiologic studies in all three trimesters have demonstrated a significant reduction in maternal gastric volume when metoclopramide was administered.

Metoclopramide has been advocated for improvement of "defective lactation" in nursing mothers and has been shown to increase milk volume. However, one study has demonstrated milk-plasma ratios greater than 1 in 5 of 7 mothers tested during the first 2 weeks post partum, with detectable levels of the drug in the plasma of two infants. The estimated infants' doses derived from mothers' milk were as high as 24 μg/kg/day in some instances. The recommended therapeutic dose in children is 500 μg/kg/day. Of greatest concern was the finding that four in seven newborns had serum prolactin levels above the highest seen in untreated control infants. More information is needed before the safety of metoclopramide for this indication can be determined.

Dosage

Metoclopramide is available as a tablet containing 10 mg, a syrup containing 5 mg/5 ml, and an intravenous solution containing 5 mg/ml. The oral dose is 5–15 mg, up to 4 times daily, 15–30 minutes before meals. This may be continued up to 12 weeks. An intravenous dose of 10–20 mg given over 2 minutes is administered when prevention of nausea and vomiting during chemotherapy is desired. The dose usually employed for improving milk production is 10 mg PO, 2–3 times daily. In studies of gastric volume reduction, the usual dose is 10 mg IV.

Adverse Effects

The principal side effect has been sedation. However, dystonic-dyskinetic head and neck movements have been reported in two pregnant patients who took metoclopramide as an antiemetic. These extrapyramidal effects seem to be most common in young females, and the reactions resemble oculogyric crisis. Diazepam or diphenhydramine can be used to reverse these problems.

Other side effects include occasional agitation, excitability, seizures, constipation or diarrhea, rash, and dry mouth. Methemoglobinemia and edema of the mouth, tongue, or orbital areas have occurred.

Metoclopramide should not be used in patients with pheochromocytoma, as hypertensive crisis may be precipitated. It is also contraindicated in epileptics and in patients with gastrointestinal obstruction.

Mechanism of Action

Metoclopramide relieves nausea and vomiting by blocking stimuli at the chemoreceptor trigger zone. It also increases tone in the esophageal sphincter, increases the tone and amplitude of gastric contractions, relaxes the pyloric sphincter and duodenal bulb, and increases peristalsis in the duodenum and jejunum. Gastric emptying and intestinal transit time are diminished. As was previously mentioned, prolactin release is potentiated. Additionally, there is a transient rise in aldosterone levels, which may be associated with fluid retention.

Absorption and Biotransformation

The onset of action is 1–3 minutes after an intravenous dose and 30–60 minutes following an oral dose. Pharmacologic effects persist for 1–2 hours, with a plasma half-life of about 3 hours. The drug is metabolized by the liver. Approximately 85% of an orally administered dose (or its metabolites) appears in the urine within 72 hours.

Recommended Reading

AMA Drug Evaluations (5th ed.). Chicago: American Medical Association, 1983. Pp. 536–537, 1275–1278.

Anderson, A. N., et al. Ovarian and placental hormones during prolactin suppression in early human pregnancy. *Clin. Endocrinol.* 13:151, 1980.

Askenasy, J. J., Streifler, M., and Felner, S. The synaptic significance of metoclopramide induced dyskinetic-dystonic head and neck movements in pregnancy. *J. Neural Transm.* 42:73, 1978.

Bohnet, H. G., and Kato, A. K. Prolactin secretion during pregnancy and puerperium: Response to metoclopramide and interactions with placental hormones. *Obstet. Gynecol.* 65:789, 1985.

Brandes, J. M., et al. The acute effect of metoclopramide on plasma prolactin during pregnancy. *Acta Obstet. Gynecol. Scand.* 60:243, 1981.

Brock-Utne, J. G., et al. The effect of metoclopramide on the lower oesophageal sphincter in late pregnancy. *Anaesth. Intensive Care* 6:26, 1978.

Bylsma-Howell, M., et al. Placental transport of metoclopramide: Assessment of maternal and neonatal effects. *Can. Anaesth. Soc. J.* 30:487, 1983.

Cohen, S. E., et al. Does metoclopramide decrease the volume of gastric contents in patients undergoing cesarean section? *Anesthesiology* 61:604, 1984.

deGezelle, H., et al. Metoclopramide and breast milk. *Eur. J. Obstet. Gynecol. Reprod. Biol.* 15:31, 1983.

Guzman, V., et al. Improvement of defective lactation by using oral metoclopramide. *Acta Obstet. Gynecol. Scand.* 58:53, 1979.

Hey, V. M. F., and Ostick, D. G. Metoclopramide and the gastrooesophageal sphincter: A study in pregnant women with heartburn. *Anaesthesia* 33:462, 1978.

Kauppila, A., Kivinen, S., and Ylikorkala, O. A dose response relation between improved lactation and metoclopramide. *Lancet* 1:1175, 1981.

Kauppila, A., et al. Metoclopramide and breast feeding: Transfer into milk and the newborn. *Eur. J. Pharmacol.* 25:819, 1983.

Messinis, I. E., et al. Effect of metoclopramide on maternal and fetal prolactin secretion during labor. *Obstet. Gynecol.* 60:686, 1982.

Reglan®. *Physicians' Desk Reference* (39th ed.). Oradell, N.J.: Medical Economics, 1985. Pp. 1659–1661.

Robuschi, G., et al. Effect of metoclopramide on maternal and fetal hyperprolactinemia. *J. Endocrinol. Invest.* 6:107, 1983.

Robuschi, G., et al. Failure of metoclopramide to release GH in pregnant women. *Horm. Metab. Res.* 15:460, 1983.

Sousa, P. L. R. Metoclopramide and breast feeding. *Br. Med. J.* 1:512, 1975.

Wyner, J., and Cohen, S. E. Gastric volume in early pregnancy: Effect of metoclopramide. *Anesthesiology* 57:209, 1982.

Metronidazole (Flagyl®)

Indications and Recommendations

The use of metronidazole during pregnancy is controversial and, if used at all, should be restricted to very specific situations. Metronidazole is a broad-spectrum antiprotozoal, antibacterial agent that has been used in treating amebiasis, anaerobic infections (especially *Bacteroides* species), giardiasis, trichomoniasis, and vaginitis caused by *Haemophilus vaginalis* and as a radiosensitizer in the treatment of various tumors.

In pregnant women, metronidazole should not be used when other therapeutic options exist. It passes freely through the placental barrier and is found in amniotic fluid and cord blood in significant concentrations. There is abundant evidence that metronidazole is mutagenic in bacteria and carcinogenic in rodents. Several investigators report that metronidazole has been used in all stages of pregnancy without apparent fetal sequelae. However, it would be most prudent to avoid its use, especially during the first trimester.

Although metronidazole is probably the single most effective agent available for treating *Trichomonas* infections, use of clotrimazole vaginal tablets or vaginal cream may offer relief from *Trichomonas* infections and is preferable during pregnancy.

Since metronidazole is excreted in breast milk, the same precautions should be kept in mind for the nursing mother as for the pregnant woman. Should treatment be necessary, a single 2-g dose should be administered and breast-feeding deferred for 48 hours.

Recommended Reading

Erickson, S. H., Oppenheim, G. L., and Smith, G. H. Metronidazole in breast milk. *Obstet. Gynecol.* 57:48, 1981.

Gilman, A. G., Goodman, L. S., and Gilman, A. *The Pharmacological Basis of Therapeutics* (6th ed.). New York: Macmillan, 1980. Pp. 1075–1077.

Gyne-Lotrimin for vaginal infections. *Med. Lett. Drugs Ther.* 18:66, 1976.

Morgan, I. Metronidazole treatment in pregnancy. *Int. J. Gynaecol. Obstet.* 15:501, 1978.

Robbie, M. O., and Sweet, R. L. Metronidazole use in obstetrics and gynecology: A review. *Am. J. Obstet. Gynecol.* 145:865, 1983.

Miconazole (Micatin®, Monistat®, Monistat 7®)

Indications and Recommendations

Miconazole may be administered topically to pregnant women for the treatment of candidal vulvovaginitis and fungal infections of the skin and nails. It is a broad-spectrum antifungal agent. It should not be used vaginally if membranes are ruptured. Use of the intravenous preparation should be reserved for the treatment of life-threatening systemic fungal infections.

Special Considerations in Pregnancy

Topical use of miconazole for the treatment of vulvovaginal candidiasis has not been associated with fetal effects. No information is available regarding the effects of intravenous miconazole on the fetus. In rats, doses of 30 mg/kg/day resulted in an increased incidence of stillbirths and deaths of dams due to difficult labor; no dysmorphic effects were seen. In rabbits, doses of up to 100 mg/kg/day are associated with an increased percentage of fetal resorptions.

Dosage

For the treatment of candidal vulvovaginitis, one applicator dose of the vaginal cream should be inserted high into the vagina at bedtime for 7 days. Recommended doses for intravenous management of systemic fungal infections range from 200–3,600 mg/day for 1–20 weeks, depending on the pathogen.

Adverse Effects

Untoward effects of topical miconazole therapy are uncommon and include vaginal burning and itching, pruritus, and cramps. Reported adverse effects of intravenous therapy include phlebitis, thrombocytosis, pruritus, vomiting, and hyperlipidemia.

Mechanism of Action

Miconazole is effective against pathogenic yeastlike and filamental fungi. It appears to increase the permeability of the cell membrane and to interfere with membrane transport of nutrients and toxins.

Absorption and Biotransformation

Small amounts of miconazole are absorbed from the vaginal mucosa and can be detected in the serum and urine. After intravenous administration, it is rapidly metabolized in the liver, and the inactive metabolites are excreted in the urine.

Recommended Reading

Abrams, L. S., and Weintraub, H. S. Disposition of radioactivity following intravaginal administration of 3H-miconazole nitrate. *Am. J. Obstet. Gynecol.* 147:920, 1983.

Boelaert, J., et al. Pharmacokinetic profile of miconazole in man. *Eur. J. Pharmacol.* 10:49, 1976.

Gilman, A. G., Goodman, L. S., and Gilman, A. *The Pharmacological Basis of Therapeutics* (6th ed.). New York: Macmillan, 1980. Pp. 982–983.

Heil, R. C., et al. Miconazole: A preliminary review of its therapeutic efficacy in systemic fungal infections. *Drugs* 19:7, 1980.

Mineral Oil (over-the-counter)

Indications and Recommendations

Mineral oil is relatively contraindicated during pregnancy because other therapeutic agents are preferable. This stool softener retards the reabsorption of water from the fecal mass. Because mineral oil may decrease the absorption of vitamin K, leading to a prolonged prothrombin time, docusates are preferable as stool softeners in pregnancy.

Recommended Reading

Gilman, A. G., Goodman, L. S., and Gilman, A. *The Pharmacological Basis of Therapeutics* (6th ed.). New York: Macmillan, 1980. P. 1009.

Nelson, M. M., and Forfar, J. O. Associations between drugs administered during pregnancy and congenital abnormalities of the fetus. *Br. Med. J.* 1:523, 1971.

Schenkel, B., and Vorherr, H. Non-prescription drugs during pregnancy: Potential teratogenic and toxic effects upon embryo and fetus. *J. Reprod. Med.* 12:27, 1974.

Naloxone (Narcan®)

Indications and Recommendations

Naloxone is the drug of choice for the treatment of narcotic-induced respiratory depression in either the mother or neonate. It should be administered immediately after birth to any depressed neonate whose mother has been treated with narcotic analgesics. It should not, however, be used routinely in narcotic-exposed newborns, nor is it recommended for administration to a mother just before delivery to reverse fetal and neonatal effects of maternally administered narcotic analgesics. In addition, it should not be used to "normalize" fetal heart rates that exhibit low beat-to-beat variability.

Naloxone administration to an addicted mother or infant may precipitate withdrawal. It should, therefore, not be administered to a pregnant woman in order to diagnose narcotic addiction, as sudden withdrawal may be deleterious to the fetus. Similarly, it should not be administered to asymptomatic infants of narcotic-addicted mothers, who may themselves be addicted.

Special Considerations in Pregnancy

Naloxone crosses the placenta and, when given antenatally, can reverse neonatal depression secondary to narcotic administration to the mother. Antenatal use for the prevention of neonatal respiratory depression is, however, contraindicated. It is hypothesized that enkephalins and endorphins play important regulatory functions in fetal physiology. Naloxone reversal of such functions may be deleterious. It should, therefore, be used only in the face of obvious neonatal depression.

Naloxone has been used to treat loss of fetal heart rate beat-to-beat variability unassociated with maternal narcotic use. In one reported case, such use was associated with fetal asphyxia with ensuing neonatal death. The authors hypothesize that fetal endorphins produce fetal tolerance to pain as well as abnormally "flat" heart rate patterns intrapartum and protect the fetus from asphyxia. The unopposed antagonism of fetal opioids in times of distress were, therefore, believed to be detrimental in this situation.

Naloxone has been shown to suppress enkephalin-mediated secretion of prolactin. Studies in nursing mothers, however, indicate that endogenous opioids do not play a major role in prolactin secretion during the puerperium. Lactation should, therefore, not be affected by naloxone use.

Dosage

For adults, the dose is 0.4 mg given IV, IM, or SQ, repeated at 2- to 3-minute intervals 2 times if there is no immediate effect. The intravenous route of administration produces the most rapid effect. Repeat doses may be required at 12-hour intervals, depending on the specific agent that is causing the depression. Supplemental intramuscular doses have a longer-lasting effect.

The neonatal dose is 0.01 mg/kg. That dose may need to be repeated in 30–90 minutes depending on the narcotic agent and dose to which the mother and newborn were exposed. It should be administered intravenously, as intramuscular or subcutaneous absorption may be delayed in the stressed and vasoconstricted infant.

Adverse Effects

In opiate-dependent subjects, naloxone produces a moderate to severe withdrawal syndrome that appears within minutes and lasts approximately 2 hours. Naloxone itself is devoid of narcotic agonist properties, and doses of up to 12 mg produce no discernible effect in the absence of a narcotic.

Mechanism of Action

Naloxone displaces morphinelike drugs from their specific receptor sites. It reverses narcotic-induced respiratory depression, analgesia, sedation, hypotension, and pupillary constriction. It also reverses the depressant effects of narcotic antagonists and congeners including nalorphine, levallorphan, pentazocine, and diphenoxylate.

Absorption and Biotransformation

Naloxone is readily absorbed from the gastrointestinal tract but is so quickly cleared by the liver that oral doses are for the most part ineffective. It is metabolized in the liver primarily by glucuronidation.

Recommended Reading

Chang, A., et al. The effects of nalorphine and naloxone on maternal and fetal blood gas and pH. *Med. J. Aust.* 1:263, 1976.

Gilman, A. G., Goodman, L. S., and Gilman, A. *The Pharmacological Basis of Therapeutics* (6th ed.). New York: Macmillan, 1980. Pp. 522–525.

Goodlin, R. C. Naloxone and its possible relationship to fetal endorphin levels and fetal distress. *Am. J. Obstet. Gynecol.* 139:16, 1981.

Kauffman, R. E. Why not use naloxone? (in Reply). *Pediatrics* 67:444, 1981.

Lodico, G., et al. Effects of naloxone infusion on basal and breast stimulation induced prolactin secretion in puerperal women. *Fertil. Steril.* 40:600, 1983.

Segal, S., et al. Naloxone use in newborns. *Pediatrics* 65:667, 1980.

Narcotic Agonist-Antagonist Analgesics: Butorphanol (Stadol®), Nalbuphine (Nubain®), Pentazocine (Talwin®)

Indications and Recommendations

Narcotic agonist-antagonist analgesics may be used during pregnancy for short-term relief of severe pain. When used, however, they should be taken at the lowest effective dosage for the minimum required period. They should not be prescribed to mothers who are suspected of being addicted to narcotic agents, as use of these drugs may precipitate withdrawal and be detrimental to the fetus.

Special Considerations in Pregnancy

Each of these agents crosses the placenta and reaches significant levels in the fetus. The abuse of pentazocine during pregnancy (often in combination with tripelennamine) as a substitute for heroin is known to cause maternal and fetal dependence. Infants exposed chronically to pentazocine in utero experience withdrawal symptoms within 24 hours of birth. The use of pentazocine during pregnancy has not been associated with congenital malformation.

These agents have been used for analgesia during labor. Like the pure narcotic analgesics, the narcotic agonist-antagonist analgesics can produce severe neonatal respiratory depression and lower psychophysiologic test scores. If neonatal respiratory depression occurs in an exposed newborn, naloxone should be administered immediately to the infant.

Dosage

Drug	Route	Analgesic dosage
Butorphanol	IM	1–2 mg q3–4h
Nalbuphine	SQ/IM/IV	10 mg q3–6h
Pentazocine	IM/IV	30–60 mg q3–4h
	PO	50–100 mg q3–4h (available in combination with aspirin and acetaminophen)

Adverse Effects

The most frequent side effects are nausea, lightheadedness and dizziness, and sedation. In addition, narcotic agonist-antagonist analgesics can produce euphoria, headache, nervousness, gastrointestinal cramping, and vomiting. Intramuscular use of pentazocine, but not butorphanol or nalbuphine, may cause soft tissue induration, nodules, and ulceration at the injection site. High dosages may produce marked respiratory depression and cardiovascular effects that are usually less severe than those produced by pure narcotic overdose.

Mechanism of Action

The narcotic agonist-antagonist analgesics are synthetic agents formulated to provide potent analgesia with a lower abuse potential than pure narcotic agonists. Like the pure narcotic analgesics, they appear to produce analgesia by acting at opiate receptors in the central nervous system. They also, however, weakly antagonize narcotic effects at the receptor site and may precipitate withdrawal in patients who take narcotic agents regularly.

Absorption and Biotransformation

Pentazocine is well absorbed from the gastrointestinal tract, but undergoes extensive first-pass metabolism, which significantly lowers oral bioavailability. When given parenterally, all of these agents are well absorbed from injection sites. They are primarily metabolized by the liver; metabolites are excreted in the urine.

Recommended Reading

Goetz, R. L., and Bain, R. V. Neonatal withdrawal symptoms associated with maternal use of pentazocine. *J. Pediatr.* 84:887, 1974.

Levy, D. L. Obstetric analgesia. Pentazocine and meperidine in normal primiparous labor. *Obstet. Gynecol.* 38:907, 1971.

Pittman, K. A., et al. Human perinatal distribution of butorphanol. *Am. J. Obstet. Gynecol.* 138:797, 1980.

Refstad, S. O., and Lindbaik, E. Ventilatory depression of the newborn of women receiving pethidine or pentazocine. *Br. J. Anaesth.* 52:265, 1980.

Scanlon, J. W. Pentazocine and neonatal withdrawal symptoms. *J. Pediatr.* 85:735, 1974.

Narcotic Analgesics: Codeine, Dihydrocodeine (Synalgos®), Fentanyl (Sublimaze®), Hydrocodone, Hydromorphone (Dilaudid®), Levorphanol (Levo-Dromoran®), Morphine, Oxycodone (Percocet-5®, Percodan®)

Indications and Recommendations

These various narcotic analgesics may be used during pregnancy for short-term relief of severe pain. When used, however, they should be taken at the lowest effective dosage for the minimum required duration. Fixed combinations of narcotics and aspirin or acetaminophen are not recommended as they do not allow independent adjustment of dosages. For analgesia during labor, however, alphaprodine and meperidine are recommended, as they have been intensively studied in this setting. They are each discussed separately elsewhere in this handbook.

Special Considerations in Pregnancy

With the exception of codeine, use of these agents during pregnancy has not been associated with teratogenicity. There have been no large-scale prospective studies of their use during pregnancy, however. In several retrospective studies, the use of codeine during the first trimester has been associated with such diverse anomalies as respiratory tract malformation, pyloric stenosis, inguinal hernia, cardiac and circulatory system defects, and cleft lip and palate. While none of the studies clearly implicate codeine as a causative factor, they do suggest that codeine and the other narcotic analgesics should not be used indiscriminately during pregnancy, especially in the first trimester.

All of these drugs readily cross the placenta and reach significant fetal levels. The use of fentanyl during general anesthesia has been associated with loss of fetal heart rate variability without fetal hypoxia. In addition, these drugs readily cross the immature blood-brain barrier and can produce severe neonatal respiratory depression and lower psychophysiologic test scores. If neonatal respiratory depression occurs in a narcotic-exposed newborn, naloxone should be administered immediately to the infant.

Infants born to narcotic-addicted mothers are addicted at birth and will experience withdrawal symptoms. The severity and duration of symptoms vary with the specific agent, dosage, and duration of maternal exposure. Withdrawal symptoms have been reported in infants whose mothers had taken antitussive doses of codeine for as few as 10 days before delivery.

Analgesic doses of narcotics appear in breast milk in small amounts, which appear to be insignificant.

Dosage

Drug	Route	Analgesic dosage
Codeine	PO/IM/SQ	15–60 mg q4–6h
Dihydrocodeine	PO	Available in combination with aspirin and acetaminophen
Fentanyl	IM	0.05–0.10 mg given as a single dose pre- or intraoperatively
Hydrocodone	PO	Available in combination with aspirin and acetaminophen
Hydromorphone	PO/IM/SQ	2 mg q4–6h
Levorphanol	PO/SQ	2 mg given in a single dose as an adjunct to anesthesia
Morphine	PO	10–30 mg q4h
	IM	10 mg q4–6h
Oxycodone	PO	5 mg q6h

Adverse Effects

The major hazards of narcotic use occur primarily with overdose and include respiratory depression, apnea, and circulatory depression. The most frequent side effects are lightheadedness, sedation, nausea, vomiting, and sweating. In addition, narcotics can produce euphoria, dysphoria, dry mouth, constipation, and urinary retention.

Mechanism of Action

The narcotic analgesics act at opiate receptors in the central nervous system to mediate analgesic activity. Narcotic analgesia is potentiated by the analgesia of aspirin and acetaminophen. In addition to analgesia, these agents possess antitussive, antiemetic, and antidiarrheal properties.

Absorption and Biotransformation

The narcotic analgesics are absorbed from the gastrointestinal tract at differing rates; codeine, hydromorphone, and oxycodone are relatively better absorbed than the other agents of this category. Intravenous administration is most reliable and rapid. Intramuscular and subcutaneous administration may delay absorption and effect. All are metabolized by the liver and excreted primarily in the urine.

Recommended Reading

Bracken, M. B., and Holford, T. R. Exposure to prescribed drugs in pregnancy and association with congenital malformations. *Obstet. Gynecol.* 58:336, 1981.

Gilman, A. G., Goodman, L. S., and Gilman, A. *The Pharmacological Basis of Therapeutics* (6th ed.). New York: Macmillan, 1980. Pp. 494–530.

Heinonen, O. P., Slone, D., and Shapiro, S. *Birth Defects and Drugs in Pregnancy.* Littleton, Mass.: Publishing Sciences Group, 1977. Pp. 287–295.

Johnson, E. S., and Colley, P. S. Effects of nitrous oxide and fentanyl anesthesia on fetal heart-rate variability intra- and postoperatively. *Anesthesiology* 52:429, 1980.

Mangurten, H. H., and Benawra, R. Neonatal codeine withdrawal in infants of nonaddicted mothers. *Pediatrics* 65:159, 1980.

Ransom, S. Oxymorphone as an obstetric analgesic—a clinical trial. *Anesthesia* 21:464, 1966.

Saxen, I. Epidemiology of cleft lip and palate: An attempt to rule out chance correlations. *Br. J. Prev. Soc. Med.* 29:103, 1975.

Nitrites and Organic Nitrates: Amyl Nitrite, Erythrityl Tetranitrate (Cardilate®), Isosorbide Dinitrate (Isordil®, Sorbitrate®), Nitroglycerin (Nitro-Bid®, Nitrol®, Nitrostat®), Pentaerythritol Tetranitrate (Peritrate®)

Indications and Recommendations

Nitrites and organic nitrates may be administered to pregnant women with angina pectoris. In such patients, however, it is best to treat the condition with bed rest rather than with these drugs. If, however, nitrates must be used, they should be given in the lowest effective dosage and for treatment of acute attacks only. Fortunately, angina pectoris is not a disease frequently encountered in women of childbearing age.

Special Considerations in Pregnancy

Snyder et al. reported the use of nitroglycerin in six severely hypertensive women given general anesthesia for cesarean section. The drug was successful in rapidly providing control of the hypertension and blunting the response to endotracheal intubation. No adverse effects on the neonates were detected. Writer et al., however, demonstrated that nitroglycerin infusion diminishes autoregulation of cerebral blood flow in hypertensive dogs, with an increase in blood flow to the brain occurring despite a reduction in mean arterial pressure (MAP). They caution that any further increase in MAP, such as occurs during endotracheal intubation, could significantly increase intracranial pressure. Since the intracranial dynamics of women with severe preeclampsia-toxemia (PET) may already be disturbed, a sudden increase in MAP could potentially have drastic consequences if nitroglycerin were being used. This issue should be further investigated before the use of nitroglycerin can be recommended for the treatment of hypertensive crises in women with PET.

Nitroglycerin with a molecular weight of 227 is expected to read-

Table 9. Dose, onset, and duration of the nitrites and organic nitrates

Drug	Dose and method of administration	Onset	Duration
Amyl nitrite	Inhale 0.18–0.30 ml	30 sec	3–5 min
Nitroglycerin	0.15–0.60 mg sublingual	1–3 min	10–30 min
Nitroglycerin ointment	2% topical to skin, 1–2 inches	20–60 min	2–12 h
Erythrityl tetranitrate	5–10 mg sublingual 10–30 mg/dose PO	5 min 30 min	2 h Variable
Pentaerythritol tetranitrate	10–40 mg/dose PO	30 min	4–5 h
Isosorbide dinitrate	2.5–10.0 mg sublingual 5–30 mg/dose PO	2–5 min 15–40 min	1–2 h 4–6 h

ily cross the placenta. However, significant hypotensive effects were not observed in the first 10 minutes of life in neonates delivered by cesarean section to preeclamptic mothers who received nitroglycerin intravenously during induction of anesthesia. This may be due to the extremely rapid rate of maternal hepatic metabolism of the drug via glutathione reductase. There are no available reports on fetal effects associated with maternal ingestion of these drugs.

Dosage

Table 9 details dose and method of administration, onset, and duration of action of the nitrites and organic nitrates. These drugs are used as needed for angina pectoris and in the average patient would not be used daily.

Adverse Effects

The most common side effects of nitrites are headache, dizziness, weakness, postural hypotension, and a typical flush on the head, neck, and clavicular area. In very high dosages, the nitrite ion can significantly oxidize hemoglobin to methemoglobin.

Mechanism of Action

These drugs are thought to act through nitrite receptors to nonspecifically relax smooth muscle. They are functional antagonists of norepinephrine, acetylcholine, and histamine and do not prevent cells from responding to appropriate stimuli.

Their predominant therapeutic actions are on vascular smooth muscle. Generalized vasodilatation occurs, but venous dilatation is a prominent factor in the blood pressure response to nitroglycerin. Blood pressure is decreased secondarily to generalized vasodilatation, but, since the sympathetic nervous system is not blocked, tachycardia may occur. The extent of the hypotension depends on the patient's position. In people with angina, venous dilatation presumably causes peripheral pooling of blood, with a decrease in cardiac output and work load.

The nitrites are effective in the treatment of acute attacks of angina. They also can prevent these attacks when taken shortly before periods of stress. The studies on the long-acting nitrates used for chronic prophylaxis of angina are difficult to assess. The lack of correlation between some clinical findings and pharmacologic data is difficult to explain. Chronic administration of long-acting nitrates may lead to the development of tolerance, thus making nitroglycerin ineffective in acute situations.

Absorption and Biotransformation

Most organic nitrates (nitroglycerin and the long-acting compounds) are readily absorbed from the sublingual mucosa. When administered by this route, their effects are more intense and predictable than when they are administered orally. Degradation of these compounds takes place rapidly in the liver, so that even though they are well absorbed from the gastrointestinal tract, little drug reaches the systemic circulation in active form. Sustained-release oral preparations have been formulated and may deliver enough drug to provide a prolongation in action. Nitroglycerin and other organic nitrates are also absorbed through the skin. These compounds are rapidly dinitrated in the liver, and metabolites are excreted in the urine.

Recommended Reading

American Hospital Formulary Service. *Monograph for Nitrostat.* Washington, D.C.: American Society of Hospital Pharmacists, 1975.

Diaz, S. F., and Marx, G. F. Placental transfer of nitroglycerin. *Anesthesiology* 51:475, 1979.

Gilman, A. G., Goodman, L. S., and Gilman, A. *The Pharmacological Basis of Therapeutics* (6th ed.). New York: Macmillan, 1980. Pp. 819–828.

Poulton, T. J., and James, F. M., III. Reply to correspondence. *Anesthesiology* 51:475, 1979.

Snyder, S. W., Wheeler, A. S., and James, F. M. The use of nitroglycerin to control severe hypertension of pregnancy during cesarean section. *Anesthesiology* 51:563, 1979.

Writer, W. D. R., et al. Intracranial effects of nitroglycerin—an obstetrical hazard? *Anesthesiology* 53:S309, 1980.

Nitrofurantoin (Furadantin®, Macrodantin®)

Indications and Recommendations

Nitrofurantoin may be administered to pregnant patients to treat asymptomatic or symptomatic bacteriuria caused by sensitive organisms, but should be avoided near term. It is an antimicrobial agent used in the treatment of acute, uncomplicated, lower urinary tract infections as well as for long-term suppression in patients with chronic bacteriuria. It is contraindicated when there is a possibility of bacteremia, as oral nitrofurantoin does not achieve therapeutic serum levels. It is effective against *Escherichia coli,* enterococcus, and staphylococcus, but ineffective against *Pseudomonas, Proteus,* or *Klebsiella* species. Nitrofurantoin should not be used in patients with compromised renal function, including those with hypertensive, toxemic, or diabetic nephropathy, and it may cause hemolysis in patients that have glucose 6-phosphate dehydrogenase (G6PD) deficiency.

Special Considerations in Pregnancy

There are no unique maternal problems when nitrofurantoin is taken during pregnancy. Low levels of glutathione may predispose the fetus to hemolytic anemia if it is exposed to nitrofurantoin shortly before birth. It may be best, therefore, to prescribe another antibiotic during the third trimester of pregnancy.

Dosage

The dose of nitrofurantoin for treatment of acute urinary tract infections is 50–100 mg qid. The dose used for long-term suppressive therapy is 50–100 mg PO at bedtime.

Adverse Effects

Nausea and vomiting frequently occur but are less common with use of the macrocrystalline form. The most serious side effect is peripheral neuritis, which is often seen in patients receiving high-dose therapy, with or without renal impairment. This complication is potentially fatal, and its most common manifestation is an ascending motor and sensory polyneuropathy. The drug should be discontinued in women who complain of paresthesias and other early signs of neuritis. Pulmonary reactions have been observed in patients on long-term therapy, although acute reactions may occur within the first week of therapy. Hemolytic anemia may be seen in patients with G6PD deficiency. Hepatotoxicity has also been reported.

Mechanism of Action

The exact mechanism of action of nitrofurantoin is unknown. Reactive metabolites may bind covalently to DNA.

Absorption and Biotransformation

Nitrofurantoin absorption from the gastrointestinal tract varies with the form administered. The macrocrystalline form is absorbed more slowly than the crystalline form and is associated with less gastrointestinal intolerance. Because of rapid elimination, the serum half-life is 20–60 minutes; therapeutically effective serum levels are, therefore, not reached. One-third of an oral dose appears in an active form in the urine. Uremic patients excrete very little drug in the urine, making it useless in such patients.

Recommended Reading

Gilman, A. G., Goodman, L. S., and Gilman, A. *The Pharmacological Basis of Therapeutics* (6th ed.). New York: Macmillan, 1980. Pp. 1121–1122.

Gleckman, R., Alvarez, S., and Joubert, D. W. Drug therapy reviews: Nitrofurantoin. *Am. J. Hosp. Pharm.* 36:342, 1979.

Kalowski, S., Radford, N., and Kincaid-Smith, P. Crystalline and macrocrystalline nitrofurantoin in the treatment of urinary tract infection. *N. Engl. J. Med.* 290:385, 1974.

Lenke, R. R., Van Dorsten, J. P., and Schifrin, B. S. Pyelonephritis in pregnancy: A prospective randomized trial to prevent recurrent disease evaluating suppressive therapy with nitrofurantoin and dose surveillance. *Am. J. Obstet. Gynecol.* 146:953, 1983.

Nonsteroidal Antiinflammatory Agents: Fenoprofen (Nalfon®), Ibuprofen (Advil®, Motrin®, Nuprin®, Rufen®), Meclofenamate (Meclomen®), Naproxen (Anaprox®, Naprosyn®), Sulindac (Clinoril®), Tolmetin (Tolectin®)

Indications and Recommendations

The use of nonsteroidal antiinflammatory agents (NSAIAs) should be avoided during pregnancy, if possible, especially in the last trimester (see *Indomethacin, Phenylbutazone*). If the administration of one of these drugs becomes necessary, ibuprofen appears to be the safest agent. In nonpregnant patients, NSAIAs are used in the treatment of various inflammatory states including osteoarthritis, rheumatoid arthritis, and dysmenorrhea. Their mechanism of action is similar to aspirin's but they are reported to produce fewer side effects.

Special Considerations in Pregnancy

Both ibuprofen and naproxen are known to cross the placenta, and it must be assumed that the other propionic acid derivatives have similar potential. Because NSAIAs act to inhibit the synthesis of prostaglandins, they have the potential to constrict and possibly close the fetal ductus arteriosus. Chronic administration, therefore, could produce prolonged pulmonary arterial hypertension and stimulate overdevelopment of medial smooth muscle in fetal precapillary vessels, which in turn might lead to persistent pulmonary hypertension of the newborn. In addition, they potentiate vasoconstriction under conditions of hypoxia.

Thus far, only naproxen use has been associated with these types of fetal hemodynamic problems. Hypoxemia due to persistent pulmonary hypertension, low prostaglandin E (PgE) levels, premature closure of the ductus arteriosus, increased bilirubin levels, and abnormalities in blood clotting and renal function have been anecdotally reported to occur in infants born to mothers who use naproxen to delay delivery. It seems advisable to avoid the use of this drug throughout pregnancy, but especially during the third trimester.

Ibuprofen and naproxen appear to be minimally excreted in breast milk. The significance of the dose presented to the infant is unknown.

Dosage

Drug	Daily dosage range for rheumatoid arthritis
Fenoprofen	2.4–3.2 g in 4 divided doses
Ibuprofen	1.6–2.4 g in 3–4 divided doses
Meclofenamate	200–400 mg in 3–4 divided doses
Naproxen	500–750 mg in 2 divided doses
Sulindac	300–400 mg in 2 divided doses
Tolmetin	1.2–2.0 g in 3–4 divided doses

Adverse Effects

The most common adverse effect of NSAIAs is gastric or intestinal irritation manifested as nausea, vomiting, diarrhea, and ulceration. Such irritation may lead to secondary anemia as a result of blood loss. Platelet function is also disturbed by NSAIAs, but this effect is quantitatively less and of shorter duration than that which occurs with aspirin. With long-term use, these agents may cause renal papillary necrosis and affect renal function. Dermatologic reactions have been reported in between 3 and 9% of patients taking these drugs.

Mechanism of Action

The NSAIAs belong to various chemical groups including propionic acid derivatives (ibuprofen, naproxen, and fenoprofen). They seem to act by selectively inhibiting prostaglandin biosynthesis and they produce a similar array of adverse reactions. Their action is like that of the salicylates. However, unlike the salicylates, their effects are reversible.

Absorption and Biotransformation

Nonsteroidal antiinflammatory agents are rapidly and almost completely absorbed from the gastrointestinal tract. Their elimination depends largely on hepatic biotransformation; metabolites are excreted in the urine.

Recommended Reading

Gilman, A. G., Goodman, L. S., and Gilman, A. *The Pharmacological Basis of Therapeutics* (6th ed.). New York: Macmillan, 1980. Pp. 682–728.

Rudolph, A. M. The effects of non-steroidal antiinflammatory compounds on fetal circulation and pulmonary function. *Obstet. Gynecol.* 58:63S, 1981.

Townsend, R. J., et al. Excretion of ibuprofen into breast milk. *Am. J. Obstet. Gynecol.* 149:184, 1984.

Wilkinson, A. R., Aynsley-Green, A., and Mitchell, M. P. Persistent pulmonary hypertension and abnormal prostaglandin E levels in preterm infants after maternal treatment with naproxen. *Arch. Dis. Child.* 54:942, 1979.

Norepinephrine, Levarterenol (Levophed®)

Indications and Recommendations

The use of norepinephrine in pregnancy is controversial, and if used at all, it should be restricted to life-threatening situations. It is an adrenergic agent that has a preponderance of alpha activity and is used to treat hypotension. An increased frequency of uterine contractions has been noticed with its use. In addition, the uterine vasculature, thought to be maximally dilated during pregnancy, reacts to adrenergic stimulus solely by contracting. Such a decrease in uterine blood flow may adversely affect the fetus. Should an adrenergic agent be required to treat hypotension associated with conduction anesthesia during pregnancy, ephedrine is the drug of choice. In other situations in which a vasopressor is needed to treat life-threatening hypotension, a more effective agent such as dopamine is the drug of choice.

Recommended Reading

Gilman, A. G., Goodman, L. S., and Gilman, A. *The Pharmacological Basis of Therapeutics* (6th ed.). New York: Macmillan, 1980. Pp. 151–153.

Smith, N. T., and Corbascio, A. The use and misuse of pressor agents. *Anesthesiology* 33:58, 1970.

Nystatin (Mycostatin®, Nilstat®)

Indications and Recommendations

Nystatin is safe to use during pregnancy for the treatment of *Candida* infections of the skin, mucous membranes, and intestinal tract. It should not be applied vaginally when membranes have ruptured.

Special Considerations in Pregnancy

Since nystatin is effectively contained at the site of application, it is safe to use during pregnancy. Its use has not been associated with teratogenesis.

Dosage

Oral (for intestinal fungal infections)
0.5–1.0 million units tid; continue for 48 hours after clinical cure

Oral (for thrush)
400,000–600,000 units qid; retain in mouth as long as possible

Topical (for cutaneous or mucocutaneous candidiasis)
Apply liberally bid; continue applications for 1 week after clinical cure

Vaginal (for vulvovaginal candidiasis)
100,000–200,000 units via applicator placed daily high in the
vagina for 2 weeks

Adverse Effects

Untoward effects of nystatin are uncommon. Mild nausea and
vomiting may occur after oral administration.

Mechanism of Action

Nystatin is bound to fungal cell membranes, creating a change in
permeability of the membrane. This change allows leakage of essential small molecules out of the cell.

Absorption and Biotransformation

Nystatin is poorly absorbed from intact skin and mucous membranes. Absorption from the gastrointestinal tract is negligible and
results in no detectable blood levels at recommended dosages.

Recommended Reading

Burrow, G. N., and Ferris, T. F. *Medical Complications During Pregnancy.* Philadelphia: Saunders, 1975. Pp. 470–471.
Gilman, A. G., Goodman, L. S., and Gilman, A. *The Pharmacological
Basis of Therapeutics* (6th ed.). New York: Macmillan, 1980. Pp.
1232–1233.

Paraldehyde (Paral®)

Indications and Recommendations

Paraldehyde is relatively contraindicated during pregnancy because other therapeutic agents are preferable. It is a short-acting
sedative-hypnotic used in the treatment of abstinence (from alcohol)
phenomena and other psychiatric states characterized by excitement. It has also been used in the emergency treatment of various
types of seizures.
　Because of numerous reports of death from paraldehyde intoxication, and because of the tendency of the drug to become contaminated by corrosive decomposition products, it has been replaced by
other drugs in most situations. Paraldehyde readily crosses the placenta and depression of the fetus has been reported with its use. It is
recommended that agents such as magnesium sulfate, used for the
prevention of convulsions in preeclampsia, and phenothiazine
drugs, used as psychotherapeutic agents, be administered instead of
paraldehyde.

Recommended Reading

American Hospital Formulary Service. *Monograph on Paraldehyde.*
Section 28:24. Washington, D.C.: American Society of Hospital Pharmacists, July, 1975.

Gilman, A. G., Goodman, L. S., and Gilman, A. *The Pharmacological Basis of Therapeutics* (6th ed.). New York: Macmillan, 1980.

Kittel, J. Paraldehyde toxicity. *Hosp. Pharmacy* 8:8, 1973.

Paramethadione (Paradione®)

Indications and Recommendations

Paramethadione is contraindicated during pregnancy because other therapeutic agents are preferable. Like trimethadione, it is an oxazolidinedione derivative used in the treatment of petit mal epilepsy and has largely been replaced by less toxic agents. Paramethadione shares trimethadione's teratogenic effects and produces malformations characteristic of the fetal paramethadione-trimethadione syndrome. These may include mental retardation, cardiac anomalies, failure to thrive, and an increased incidence of fetal wastage. If treatment for petit mal epilepsy is required during pregnancy, ethosuximide is preferred.

Recommended Reading

Fabro, S., and Brown, N. A. Teratogenic potential of anticonvulsants. *N. Engl. J. Med.* 300:1280, 1979.

German, J., et al. Possible teratogenicity of trimethadione and paramethadione. *Lancet* 2:261, 1970.

Gilman, A. G., Goodman, L. S., and Gilman, A. *The Pharmacological Basis of Therapeutics* (6th ed.). New York: Macmillan, 1980. P. 465.

National Institutes of Health. Anticonvulsants found to have teratogenic potential. *J.A.M.A.* 245:36, 1981.

Rutman, J. T. Anticonvulsants and fetal damage. *N. Engl. J. Med.* 189:696, 1973.

Pargyline (Eutonyl®)

Indications and Recommendations

Pargyline is contraindicated during pregnancy. It is a monoamine oxidase inhibitor that has been used as an antihypertensive agent and also has antidepressive properties.

Inhibition of monoamine oxidase in postganglionic nerve endings results in the accumulation of dopamine and octopamine at these sites. These substances act either as false neurohumoral transmitters or permit a negative feedback inhibition of tyrosine hydroxylase. The latter is an integral part of norepinephrine biosynthesis.

This drug may precipitate a severe hypertensive crisis when a patient eats food that is rich in tyramine while the drug is being ingested. A hypertensive crisis can also occur when pargyline is prescribed concurrently with amphetamine, ephedrine, imipramine, phenylephrine, metaraminol, and phenylpropanolamine.

Because other agents are more effective and less dangerous, pargyline has no role in the management of hypertension or depression in the pregnant woman.

Recommended Reading

Frohlich, E. D. The sympathetic depressant anti-hypertensives. *Drug Ther.* 5:24, 1975.

Gilman, A. G., Goodman, L. S., and Gilman, A. *The Pharmacological Basis of Therapeutics* (6th ed.). New York: Macmillan, 1980. Pp. 204–205, 427–430.

Levin, N. W., et al. Anti-hypertensive therapy. *Hosp. Formu. Manag.* 6:9, 1971.

Penicillamine (Cuprimine®, Depen®)

Indications and Recommendations

Penicillamine (dimethylcysteine), a chelating agent, may be used during pregnancy in patients with Wilson's disease, although the dose should be kept at or below 1 g/day. Dosage should be further reduced to 250 mg/day during the last 6 weeks of pregnancy because of possible effects on wound healing. Since other forms of therapy are available, case reports of congenital cutis laxa and growth retardation make the use of this drug during pregnancy controversial in patients with cystinuria and rheumatoid arthritis.

Special Considerations in Pregnancy

Penicillamine crosses the placenta and is capable of inducing fetal resorptions and congenital anomalies in laboratory animals. The mechanism for this is believed to be through fetal deficiency of certain metals, including copper and zinc. However, these speculations have not been confirmed to date.

A literature review reveals reports on 61 viable pregnancies with Wilson's disease, 57 with cystinuria, and 20 with rheumatoid arthritis that were exposed to penicillamine during at least the first 16 weeks of gestation. Four neonates, two from mothers with Wilson's disease and one in each of the other maternal diagnostic categories, were noted to have generalized loose skin, cutis laxa. Three of the four had inguinal hernias. The neonates whose mothers had rheumatoid arthritis or cystinuria were growth retarded and died of various complications, while the two infants of mothers with Wilson's disease survived and the skin abnormality apparently regressed. Serum copper levels in the latter two offspring were elevated rather than depressed. Copper levels were not reported in the former two cases. There is some suggestion that the effect of penicillamine on the offspring might be dose related, since one mother took 900 mg/day and the other three took 1.5–2.0 g/day throughout pregnancy. This has led to recommendations to reduce the dosage if possible.

If cutis laxa is related to penicillamine therapy, the case reports suggest that it is no more common than 4 in 138, or approximately 3% of exposures. It is problematic to make such an estimate in view of a lack of appropriate denominator figures; however, since normal outcomes are less apt to be reported than are abnormal ones, it is unlikely that the true incidence is higher than 3%. Reports of elevated serum copper levels in the two affected offspring of mothers with Wilson's disease suggest that the cause may not be related to copper depletion; other heavy metals may be depleted by this therapy, and some investigators believe that zinc deficiency may be at fault. Whether zinc supplementation would be helpful has not been established.

Continued treatment with penicillamine is necessary to prevent recrudescence of Wilson's disease. The effects of this disorder can be life-threatening, and it is thus reasonable to continue treatment during pregnancy, although at reduced dosage if possible. In cystinuria, the major problem is urinary calculus formation. High fluid intake and alkalinization may help prevent stones from forming. In patients who form stones despite these therapeutic interventions, penicillamine may be continued. The physician and patient must decide together whether the fetal risk outweighs the maternal benefit of this drug in a particular case. When the patient has rheumatoid arthritis, numerous other agents may be used. Thus, the physician is faced with a choice between the risk of fetal hemorrhage (salicylates), possible teratogenicity (gold), maternal adverse effects (corticosteroids), and so forth.

No data have been found regarding breast milk excretion or the safety of breast-feeding for women taking penicillamine.

Dosage

Penicillamine is available as 250-mg tablets and capsules. For Wilson's disease, the patient is maintained on a low copper diet and the drug is begun at 250–1,000 mg/day (depending on the patient's tolerance of side effects). The dose is titrated against urinary copper excretion, the goal being to maintain negative copper balance. It is rarely necessary to prescribe more than 2 g/day. During pregnancy, the dosage should be as low as is compatible with maintenance of negative copper balance.

For cystinuria, the drug is initiated at 250 mg/day and increased to the point at which urinary cystine excretion is below 100 mg/day; 2 g/day is a common dose. Patients with cystinuria should also be instructed to drink enough water to maintain the urinary specific gravity below 1.010, take enough alkali to maintain the urinary pH at 7.5, and maintain a diet low in methionine.

When penicillamine is used to treat rheumatoid arthritis, it is usually initiated at a dose of 250 mg/day and increased in 250-mg/day increments every 2–3 months to achieve a therapeutic effect. Usual maintenance doses are 500–750 mg/day.

Penicillamine should be taken on an empty stomach (at least 1 hour after the last meal and before the next meal) to ensure appropriate absorption and to minimize gastrointestinal side effects.

Adverse Effects

Allergic reactions have been reported in 5% of patients who take penicillamine, and these most often appear early in the course of therapy. They include fever, rashes, leukopenia, eosinophilia, and thrombocytopenia. For this reason, complete blood counts (including platelets) should be performed every 2 weeks during the first 6 months of therapy, and monthly thereafter. If allergic manifestations develop in a patient with Wilson's disease or one with cystinuria who has formed stones despite a high fluid intake and alkalinization, it may be necessary to desensitize the patient and resume therapy, since alternative forms of treatment are not available.

Penicillamine interferes with collagen formation and may delay wound healing. It is for this reason that reduction in dosage is recommended during the last 6 weeks of pregnancy.

Other adverse effects include gastrointestinal disturbance (anorexia, nausea, vomiting, abdominal pain), seen in 17% of patients, decreased taste sensation, proteinuria, tinnitus, optic neuritis, myasthenia gravis, and a variety of other problems. The development of insulin antibodies accompanied by severe hypoglycemia has been reported in two patients with rheumatoid arthritis who were treated with penicillamine.

It should be emphasized that penicillamine has many side effects, and that these problems occur in a high proportion of individuals who take the drug. It is only for conditions that are serious and not amenable to other forms of treatment that penicillamine is appropriate.

Mechanism of Action

Penicillamine is prepared by hydrolysis of penicillin. It is an effective chelator of copper, mercury, zinc, and lead, leading to an increased urinary excretion of these metals. In Wilson's disease, in which ceruloplasmin, the copper-carrying plasma protein, is deficient, copper builds up in various tissues. Penicillamine increases copper excretion. In patients with cystinuria, large amounts of cystine appear in the urine. Cystine (a disulfide composed of two cysteine molecules) is relatively insoluble and forms renal stones, especially in acid urine. Penicillamine forms a disulfide with cysteine, which is considerably more soluble than cystine, thus lowering the potential for stone formation. The mechanism of penicillamine's action against rheumatoid arthritis is not understood at present.

Absorption and Biotransformation

Penicillamine is rapidly absorbed after oral dosing, with peak plasma levels being achieved at approximately 130 minutes. Plasma half-life is 60.7 ± 8.2 minutes. Approximately 20% of an oral dose is excreted in the urine within 24 hours, and 50% appears in the stool.

Recommended Reading

Albukerk, J. N. Wilson's disease and pregnancy. A case report. *Fertil. Steril.* 24:494, 1973.

AMA Drug Evaluations (5th ed.). Chicago: American Medical Association, 1983. Pp. 134–135, 1870–1871.

Arbisser, A. I., Scott, C. I., Jr., and Howell, R. R. Mannosidosis and maternal penicillamine therapy. *Lancet* 1:312, 1976.

Benson, E. A., Healey, L. A., and Barron, E. J. Insulin antibodies in patients receiving penicillamine. *Am. J. Med.* 78:857, 1985.

Endres, W. D-Penicillamine in pregnancy—to ban or not to ban? *Klin. Wochenschr.* 59:535, 1981.

Fukuda, K., et al. Pregnancy and delivery in penicillamine treated patients with Wilson's disease. *Tohoku J. Exp. Med.* 123:270, 1977.

Gilman, A. G., Goodman, L. S., and Gilman, A. *The Pharmacological*

Basis of Therapeutics (6th ed.). New York: Macmillan, 1980. Pp. 1627–1628.

Gregory, M. C., and Mansell, M. A. Pregnancy and cystinuria. *Lancet* 2:1158, 1983.

Harpey, J. P., et al. Cutis laxa and low serum zinc after antenatal exposure to penicillamine. *Lancet* 2:858, 1983.

Keen, C. L., Lonnerdal, B., and Hurley, L. S. Drug-induced copper deficiency: A model for copper deficiency teratogenicity. *Teratology* 28:155, 1983.

Laver, M., and Fairley, K. F. D-Penicillamine treatment in pregnancy. *Lancet* 1:1019, 1971.

Linares, A., et al. Reversible cutis laxa due to maternal D-penicillamine treatment. *Lancet* 2:43, 1979.

Lyle, W. H. Penicillamine in pregnancy. *Lancet* 1:606, 1978.

Marecek, Z., and Graf, M. Pregnancy in penicillamine-treated patients with Wilson's disease. *N. Engl. J. Med.* 295:841, 1976.

Mjolnerod, O. K., et al. Congenital connective-tissue defect probably due to D-penicillamine treatment in pregnancy. *Lancet* 1:673, 1971.

Scheinberg, I. H., and Sternlieb, I. Pregnancy in penicillamine-treated patients with Wilson's disease. *N. Engl. J. Med.* 293:1300, 1975.

Solomon, L., et al. Neonatal abnormalities associated with D-penicillamine treatment during pregnancy. *N. Engl. J. Med.* 296:54, 1977.

Toaff, R., et al. Hepatolenticular degeneration (Wilson's disease) and pregnancy. *Obstet. Gynecol. Surv.* 32:497, 1977.

Walshe, J. M. Pregnancy in Wilson's disease. *Q. J. Med.* (new series) 181:73, 1977.

Penicillins: Amoxicillin (Amoxil®, Larotid®), Ampicillin (Omnipen®, Polycillin®), Azlocillin (Azlin®), Carbenicillin (Geopen®), Cloxacillin (Tegopen®), Dicloxacillin (Dycill®, Dynapen®), Hetacillin (Versapen®), Methicillin (Celbenin®, Staphcillin®), Mezlocillin (Mezlin®), Nafcillin (Nafcil®, Unipen®), Oxacillin (Bactocill®, Prostaphlin®), Penicillin G, Penicillin V, Piperacillin (Pipracil®), Ticarcillin (Ticar®)

Indications and Recommendations

Penicillins are safe to use during pregnancy in nonallergic patients. These compounds are among the most effective and least toxic antimicrobials available. The family consists of natural and semisynthetic compounds that have individual spectra and pharmacologic properties. There is a paucity of clinical experience with the more recently released penicillins (e.g., piperacillin, mezlocillin, and azlocillin). These drugs should, therefore, be considered only when another, better studied antibiotic cannot be used.

Special Considerations in Pregnancy

Penicillin G and most of the other penicillins appear in the amniotic fluid and fetal blood and tissues. Highly protein-bound penicillins reach much lower levels in the fetus and amniotic fluid than do those that are less bound. They do not appear to be teratogenic.

Plasma levels of ampicillin have been shown to be lower in pregnant patients than in nonpregnant women receiving equivalent dosages. Its volume of distribution and plasma clearance is higher and the half-life is shorter during pregnancy. While similar trends have been reported with other penicillins, further studies must be undertaken to elucidate the pharmacokinetics of each agent.

The use of ampicillin can lower urine estriols, presumably by destroying gastrointestinal flora and interfering with enterohepatic recirculation of estrogens. Estriol values return to normal 2 days after the drug is discontinued.

Penicillin appears in breast milk and may cause diarrhea and candidiasis in the nursing infant.

Dosage

Table 10 details recommended dosages of the penicillins.

Adverse Effects

The penicillins are reported to be among the most common causes of drug allergy. The severity of allergic reactions ranges from a mild rash to anaphylaxis. Interstitial nephritis has been associated primarily with methicillin while oxacillin has been implicated as the cause of a reversible hepatotoxicity and neutropenia. The most frequent side effects of orally administered penicillins are nausea, vomiting, epigastric distress, diarrhea, and black hairy tongue. Penicillins are irritating to the central and peripheral nervous systems, especially at very high dosages and in patients with impaired renal function. As parenteral formulations may contain large quantities of sodium or potassium, electrolyte imbalances may occur with intravenous therapy. Candidal vaginitis is a common sequel to penicillin therapy, presumably because of suppression of normal vaginal flora.

Mechanism of Action

This group of antibiotics acts by interfering with cell wall synthesis. They are therefore more effective when organisms are actively dividing.

In general, the penicillins are active against gram-positive cocci and bacilli and some gram-negative bacilli; some have a broader spectrum and are active against many gram-negative bacilli. None of the penicillins are active against viruses, mycobacteria, plasmodia, fungi, or rickettsiae.

Absorption and Biotransformation

The penicillins are variably absorbed from the gastrointestinal tract and are widely distributed throughout the body. They diffuse into ascitic fluid and attain high concentrations in lungs, intestine,

Table 10. Dosage chart for penicillins

Drug	Route	Usual dose[a]	Interval
Penicillin G	PO	250–500 mg	q6h
	IM	600,000–1.2 million units	q12–24h
	IV	1–5 million units	q4–6h
Penicillin V	PO	250–500 mg	q6h
Methicillin	IM/IV	1 g	q4–6h
Nafcillin	PO	250–1,000 mg	q4–6h
	IM/IV	500 mg	q4–6h
Oxacillin	PO	500 mg	q4–6h
	IM/IV	250–1,000 mg	q4–6h
Cloxacillin	PO	250–500 mg	q6h
Dicloxacillin	PO	125–500 mg	q6h
Ampicillin	PO	250–1,000 mg	q6h
	IM/IV	500–2,000 mg	q4–6h
Hetacillin	PO	225–450 mg	q6h
Amoxicillin	PO	250–500 mg	q8h
Carbenicillin	PO[b]	382–764 mg	q6h
	IM/IV	1–2 g	q6h
Ticarcillin	IM/IV	Depends on indication	q4–6h
Mezlocillin	IM/IV	2–4 g	q6h
Piperacillin	IM/IV	2–4 g	q4–6h
Azlocillin	IV	2–4 g	q4–6h

[a] Dosage may require reduction in the face of renal impairment.
[b] For treatment of urinary tract infections only.

and liver. The penicillins are concentrated in bile; only small amounts diffuse into cerebrospinal fluid, with penetration being greater through inflamed meninges. Penicillins are bound to plasma proteins to varying degrees; the free drug appears to be the active form. Most penicillins are primarily excreted unchanged in the urine, with only small amounts being inactivated by the liver. The latter mode of elimination assumes more importance in the presence of renal failure. The half-lives of the penicillins are in general short, ranging from 30–90 minutes. In an anuric patient, half-lives may be as high as 10 hours. Concomitant administration of probenecid increases and prolongs serum penicillin levels by competitively inhibiting renal tubular secretion and thus slowing the rate of penicillin elimination.

Recommended Reading

Adamkin, D. H., Marshall, E., and Weiner, L. B. The placental transfer of ampicillin. *Am. J. Perinatology* 1:310, 1984.

Adlercreutz, H., et al. Effect of ampicillin administration on plasma, conjugated and unconjugated estrogen, and progesterone levels in pregnancy. *Am. J. Obstet. Gynecol.* 128:266, 1977.

Landers, D. V., Green, M. D., and Sweet, R. L. Antibiotic use during pregnancy and the postpartum period. *Clin. Obstet. Gynecol.* 26:391, 1983.

Philipson, A. Pharmacokinetics of ampicillin during pregnancy. *J. Infect. Dis.* 136:370, 1977.

Wright, A. J., and Wilkowski, C. J. The pencillins. *Mayo Clin. Proc.* 58:21, 1983.

Phenacetin

Indications and Recommendations

Phenacetin is generally not available as a single drug. It is always used in combination with acetylsalicylic acid, salicylamide, caffeine, or similar agents. Because of concern about the antiplatelet activity of aspirin and its effect on fetal circulation, phenacetin in combination with aspirin-like compounds is not recommended for use during pregnancy (see *Salicylates*).

Recommended Reading

Gilman, A. G., Goodman, L. S., and Gilman, A. *The Pharmacological Basis of Therapeutics* (6th ed.). New York: Macmillan, 1980. Pp. 701–705.

Phenazopyridine (Pyridium®)

Indications and Recommendations

Phenazopyridine is relatively contraindicated in pregnancy because other therapeutic agents are preferable. It is an azo dye that exhibits an analgesic action on the urinary tract. It is used only to alleviate the symptoms of lower urinary tract mucosal irritation, including burning, urgency, and frequency. It is not a urinary tract antiseptic. No studies examining the use of phenazopyridine during pregnancy have been conducted. It has, however, been used in some obstetric patients without reported adverse fetal effects. Because it is indicated only for symptomatic treatment, it is best to treat the underlying cause of the irritation rather than to administer a drug with unknown fetal effect.

Recommended Reading

Heinonen, O. P., Slone, D., and Shapiro, S. *Birth Defects and Drugs in Pregnancy.* Littleton, Mass.: Publishing Sciences Group, 1977. Pp. 299–308.

Phenazopyridine and phenazopyridine hydrochloride. *I.A.R.C. Monogr. Eval. Carcinog. Risk Chem. Hum.* 24:163, 1980.

Phencyclidine (Angel Dust)

Indications and Recommendations

Phencyclidine, originally developed as an anesthetic agent but now widely used as a street drug, is contraindicated in pregnancy. It is administered by snorting, swallowing, or injecting, and may also be absorbed through the skin. Acute effects of phencyclidine use include euphoria, dizziness, ataxia, dysarthria, nystagmus, and psychosis. Deaths have been reported and have been attributed to convulsions, cardiac and respiratory arrest, or hypertensive crisis. There are no known indications for phencyclidine use, and there is animal, as well as anecdotal human, evidence suggesting possible teratogenicity. Phencyclidine crosses the placenta, with fetal concentrations approximately twice maternal levels. The placenta is also capable of phencyclidine biotransformation. Neonatal jitteriness and hypertonicity have been reported after chronic maternal phencyclidine use; this presumed behavioral teratogenesis was long lasting. Animal studies suggest that phencyclidine is concentrated in breast milk at as much as 10 times maternal blood levels. One survey in an urban population reports a 0.8% incidence of phencyclidine use during pregnancy.

Recommended Reading

Golden, N. L., Sokol, R. J., and Rubin, I. L. Angel dust: Possible effects on the fetus. *Pediatrics* 65:18, 1980.

Golden, N. L., et al. Phencyclidine use during pregnancy. *Am. J. Obstet. Gynecol.* 148:254, 1984.

Nicholas, J. M., Lipshitz, J., and Schreiber, E. C. Phencyclidine: Its transfer across the placenta as well as into breast milk. *Am. J. Obstet. Gynecol.* 143:143, 1982.

Petrucha, R. A., Kaufman, K. R., and Pitts, F. N. Phencyclidine in pregnancy: A case report. *J. Reprod. Med.* 27:301, 1982.

Rayburn, W. F., Holsztynska, E. F., and Domino, E. F. Phencyclidine: Biotransformation by the human placenta. *Am. J. Obstet. Gynecol.* 148:111, 1984.

Strauss, A. A., Modanlou, H. D., and Bosu, S. K. Neonatal manifestations of maternal phencyclidine (PCP) abuse. *Pediatrics* 68:550, 1981.

Phenmetrazine (Preludin®)

Indications and Recommendations

Phenmetrazine is contraindicated during pregnancy. It is used as a short-term (4–6 weeks) adjunct to a weight reduction program for obese patients. The anorexic effect of phenmetrazine is temporary and believed to be mediated through direct stimulation of the hypothalamic satiety center. Maternal side effects may include palpitations, elevation of blood pressure, and tachycardia.

Cases of skeletal and visceral anomalies in infants whose mothers had taken phenmetrazine during pregnancy have been reported, but no causal relationship has been proved. In the Collaborative Perinatal Project, no increase was seen in birth defects in the children of 58 mothers who took phenmetrazine during the first 4 months of pregnancy. Similarly, in a study comparing 1,824 women receiving anorectic drugs during pregnancy with 8,989 who did not receive these drugs, there was no increase in congenital anomalies (diagnosed by 5 years of age) among the 55 infants exposed to phenmetrazine within 84 days of the last menstrual period. Studies performed in weaning pups whose mothers were given phenmetrazine in pregnancy demonstrated a decrease in survival and growth rate.

Since it is not appropriate for pregnant women to participate in weight reduction programs, phenmetrazine has no role during pregnancy.

Recommended Reading

Cahen, M. L. Evaluation of the teratogenicity of drugs. *Clin. Pharmacol. Ther.* 5:480, 1964.

Craddock, D. Anorectic drugs: Use in general practice. *Drugs* 11:378, 1976.

Heinonen, O. P., Slone, D., and Shapiro, S. *Birth Defects and Drugs in Pregnancy.* Boston: John Wright PSG, 1977. Pp. 346–347, 439.

Milkovich, L., and van den Berg, B. J. Effects of antenatal exposure to anorectic drugs. *Am. J. Obstet. Gynecol.* 129:637, 1977.

Product information on Preludin. Boehringer Ingelheim Ltd., Ridgefield, Conn., May 1976.

Phenobarbital

Indications and Recommendations

Phenobarbital can be administered to pregnant women in the treatment of generalized tonic-clonic and simple partial seizures and can be given as a sedative to patients with mild to moderate preeclampsia. It is not recommended for the stimulation of fetal hepatic enzymes. Phenobarbital can be given to breast-feeding mothers, but drowsiness should be looked for in the nursing infant.

The following recommendations have been made in a bulletin published in 1979 by the American Academy of Pediatrics Committee on Drugs in collaboration with the American College of Obstetricians and Gynecologists (ACOG) Committee on Obstetrics: Maternal and Fetal Medicine.

> No woman should receive anticonvulsant medication unnecessarily. When possible, a woman who has been seizure free for many years should be withdrawn from her medication prior to pregnancy. When a woman who has epilepsy and requires medication asks about pregnancy, she should be advised that she has a 90% chance of having a normal child, but that the risk of congenital malformations and mental retardation is two to three times greater than average because of her disease or its treatment. . . .
>
> There is no reason at present to advise a woman to switch from phenytoin or phenobarbital to other anticonvulsants about which even less is known. Discontinuation of medication in a woman whose epilepsy is controlled by medicine may cause seizures, and prolonged seizures could cause serious sequelae to her and the fetus.*

**Pediatrics 63:331, summary 333, February 1979. Copyright © 1979 by American Academy of Pediatrics.

Special Considerations in Pregnancy

Phenobarbital rapidly crosses the placenta. It has been implicated as a possible teratogen causing cleft lip, congenital heart disease, and microcephaly. Thus far, the data are not conclusive.

Phenobarbital induces the production of fetal liver enzymes, including the glucuronyltransferase needed for bilirubin conjugation and excretion, and consequently has been recommended for both the prevention and treatment of neonatal hyperbilirubinemia. Enzyme induction is also associated with an increased rate of steroid metabolism and altered vitamin D metabolism. Neonatal hypocalcemia has been reported. Coagulopathies resulting from a decrease in vitamin K–dependent clotting factors have been seen in neonates after ingestion of phenobarbital by the mother. Withdrawal symptoms are commonly seen in neonates whose mothers have taken 90–120 mg phenobarbital daily for at least 12 weeks before delivery.

Nursing mothers can usually take anticonvulsant dosages of barbiturates without its affecting the infant. Drowsiness should be looked for in the nursing infant.

Dosage

In the treatment of epilepsy, the usual adult maintenance dose of phenobarbital is 60–200 mg (orally or parenterally) once daily. The therapeutic plasma concentration is 15–30 μg/ml. Dosage requirements increase during pregnancy. When phenobarbital is used as a mild sedative in preeclampsia, a dose of 30–60 mg q6h is given.

Adverse Effects

Side effects include sedation, paradoxic irritability or hyperactivity in children, and confusion in the elderly. Nystagmus and ataxia are seen at excessive dosages. Megaloblastic anemia and osteomalacia have been associated with long-term phenobarbital therapy. Rare idiosyncratic reactions include scarlatiniform or morbilliform rashes, exfoliative dermatitis, agranulocytosis, and hepatitis.

Mechanism of Action

Phenobarbital increases the seizure threshold and limits the spread of seizure activity. These effects may be due to an augmented response to gamma-aminobutyric acid (GABA), an inhibitory synaptic transmitter, without an increased level of this compound in the brain.

Barbiturates depress the activity of all excitable tissue, with the central nervous system being the most sensitive. There is little effect on skeletal, cardiac, or smooth muscle at therapeutic dosages. By its combination with cytochrome P-450 and induction of hepatic microsomal enzymes, phenobarbital alters the metabolism of other drugs.

Phenobarbital is effective in the treatment of status epilepticus and generalized tonic-clonic and simple partial seizures. It is only minimally effective against complex partial seizures and not useful in the treatment of absence seizures.

Absorption and Biotransformation

Phenobarbital is well absorbed through the small intestine and from intramuscular injection sites. Approximately 40–60% of the drug is protein bound. From 10–25% is excreted unchanged in the urine; this process is enhanced by alkalization and diuresis. The liver microsomal oxidizing system metabolizes the remaining drug, after which metabolites are excreted by the kidney. The half-life in adults is 2–6 days; it is longer in neonates and shorter in children.

Recommended Reading

Anticonvulsants and pregnancy. Prepared by AAP Committee on Drugs in collaboration with the ACOG Committee on Obstetrics: Maternal and Fetal Medicine. January 1979.

Friis, B., and Sardemann, H. Neonatal hypocalcemia after intrauterine exposure to anticonvulsant drugs. *Arch. Dis. Child.* 52:239, 1977.

Gilman, A. G., Goodman, L. S., and Gilman, A. *The Pharmacological Basis of Therapeutics* (6th ed.). New York: Macmillan, 1980. Pp. 448–474.

Lander, C. M., et al. Plasma anticonvulsant concentration during pregnancy. *Neurology* 27:128, 1977.

Update: Drugs in breast milk. *Med. Lett. Drugs Ther.* 21:21, 1979.

Wilder, B. J., and Bruni, J. *Seizure Disorders: A Pharmacological Approach to Treatment.* New York: Raven, 1981.

Woodbury, D. M., Penry, J. K., and Pippenger, C. L. *Antiepileptic Drugs* (2nd ed.). New York: Raven, 1982.

Phenols (over-the-counter)

Indications and Recommendations

Phenols may be used safely during pregnancy in over-the-counter preparations containing dilute solutions. They should not be used in a strength greater than a 2% aqueous solution or on broken skin.

These drugs are used as an antiseptic in mouthwashes as well as in dermatologic and anorectal preparations. Hexylresorcinol is the phenol most commonly used in mouthwashes. Thymol, while used in mouthwashes, is more frequently employed as a remedy for acne, hemorrhoids, and tinea pedis. Phenols have also been used alone or in combination with calamine lotion as an antipruritic agent.

Special Considerations in Pregnancy

No unusual maternal effects have been described during pregnancy, and no mutagenic or teratogenic effects have been reported. Convulsions, hepatic toxicity, and bone marrow depression are possible problems if toxic levels were to reach the fetus.

Dosage

Hexylresorcinol is used in a 1:1,000 concentration in mouthwashes. The various phenols are utilized in different concentrations, with all being absorbed to some degree.

Adverse Effects

Significant skin penetration may occur when phenols are applied topically in solutions that are stronger than 2% aqueous or 4% in glycerin. This can result in tissue necrosis and systemic absorption. Erythema associated with some sloughing may occur. Cardiovascular effects include myocardial depression with secondary hypotension. Central nervous system action includes hypothermia. Ulceration of the stomach may occur if they are taken orally.

Mechanism of Action

Phenols are bacteriostatic as a 0.2% solution, bactericidal as a 1% solution, and fungicidal at 1.3% or greater. They combine with skin proteins to form a toxic substance. These drugs are more effective in an acid media, at higher temperatures, and in aqueous solution.

Absorption and Biotransformation

After being absorbed, about 80% is excreted by the kidney either unchanged or as a glucuronide. The remainder is oxidized to hydroquinone and pyrocatechol.

Recommended Reading

Gilman, A. G., Goodman, L. S., and Gilman, A. *The Pharmacological Basis of Therapeutics* (6th ed.). New York: Macmillan, 1980. P. 967.

Nelson, M. M., and Forfar, J. O. Associations between drugs administered during pregnancy and congenital abnormalities of the fetus. *Br. Med. J.* 1:523,1971.

Schenkel, B., and Vorherr, H. Non-prescription drugs during pregnancy: Potential teratogenic and toxic effects upon embryo and fetus. *J. Reprod. Med.* 12:27, 1974.

Phenothiazines: Chlorpromazine (Thorazine®), Fluphenazine (Prolixin®), Perphenazine (Trilafon®), Prochlorperazine (Compazine®), Promethazine (Phenergan®), Thioridazine (Mellaril®), Trifluoperazine (Stelazine®)

Indications and Recommendations

The use of phenothiazines during pregnancy should be limited to treatment of psychotic patients who require continued medication. They are also used in the treatment of anxiety and restlessness, but safer alternatives are available. Drug therapy with phenothiazines should be discontinued 1–2 weeks before delivery to avoid symptoms in the neonate.

Prochlorperazine and promethazine are widely used as antiemetics. During pregnancy these drugs should be reserved for the treatment of severe nausea and vomiting.

Special Considerations in Pregnancy

The phenothiazines theoretically pose a threat of maternal hypotension and consequent uteroplacental insufficiency. In sheep, maternally administered promazine was associated with both maternal and fetal tachycardia and hypotension. In addition, the fetal response to umbilical cord compression was augmented. There have been five reported cases of shock after the administration of phenothiazines to patients with pheochromocytomas, including one pregnant woman.

The Collaborative Perinatal Study evaluated 1,309 children exposed to phenothiazines during the first 4 months in utero. The overall rates of congenital malformations were similar among these exposed children and the 48,973 unexposed offspring. Although a slight excess of cardiovascular malformations (relative risk, 1.68) among phenothiazine-exposed individuals was suspected, this has not been validated and may simply be a statistical quirk due to the large number of comparisons made. Anecdotally, infants born to mothers who received phenothiazines during pregnancy have been reported to suffer from prolonged extrapyramidal effects, chromosomal anomalies, jaundice, mild sedation followed by motor excitement, agitation and hypertonicity, and depression. Phenothiazines have also been used intentionally to diminish the immune response in fetuses with erythroblastosis fetalis; the results have been inconclusive to date.

Several studies have documented the presence of phenothiazines in the breast milk of nursing mothers, but all state that no adverse effects have been noted in either the mother or infant. The quantities excreted in breast milk are very small, only 0.29 μg/ml having been measured 2 hours after a single 1,200-mg dose of chlorpromazine.

Dosage

Phenothiazine dosage should be individualized according to the severity of the condition, the patient's age, and the clinical response. It should be administered in divided doses during the first few weeks of therapy, but thereafter may be administered in a once-daily or twice-daily regimen. Fluphenazine is also available in injectable forms that may be administered every 2 weeks. Table 11 details the recommended dosages of some of the phenothiazines.

When used as an antiemetic, prochlorperazine may be given as an oral tablet (5 or 10 mg) q4–6h, or as a rectal suppository, 25 mg q12h. The intramuscular dose is 5–10 mg q6h. Promethazine is given orally or rectally, 25–50 mg/day, or intramuscularly, 12.5–25.0 mg q4–6h.

Adverse Effects

The most frequent side effects of the phenothiazines are drowsiness, postural hypotension, and anticholinergic effects, including dry mouth, constipation, mydriasis and cycloplegia, urinary retention, and tachycardia. These appear early in the treatment course, and patients usually develop a tolerance to them. Because phenothiazines depress the mechanism for heat regulation they may cause hyperthermia or hypothermia, depending on ambient temperature.

Table 11. Dosage range of phenothiazines[a] (for psychosis)

Drug	Usual daily dosage range PO or IM (mg)	Maximum daily dose (mg)
Chlorpromazine	50–800	2,000
Fluphenazine	2.5–20.0	40
Perphenazine	8–24	64
Thioridazine[b]	50–600	800
Trifluoperazine	2–15	64

[a] Prochlorperazine and promethazine are discussed in more detail in the text.
[b] Only given orally.

Parkinsonism, dystonia, galactorrhea, photosensitivity, menstrual changes, and blood dyscrasias have also been noted occasionally with their use.

Mechanism of Action

The mechanisms of action of the phenothiazines are only partly known. Their effects may be due to blockage of dopamine receptors and dopamine release in the caudate nucleus, and to inhibition of the dopamine activation of adenyl cyclase. In the brain stem, the inflow of stimuli to the reticular formation is selectively decreased. Most phenothiazine derivatives exert a depressant action on the chemoreceptor trigger zone, thereby suppressing emesis due to conditions in which this center is stimulated.

Antipsychotic agents have peripheral anticholinergic activity and alpha-adrenergic blocking activity. They can inhibit the release of growth hormone and may antagonize secretion of prolactin-release inhibiting hormone, producing galactorrhea. They can lower the convulsive threshold and may interfere with temperature regulation.

Absorption and Biotransformation

The phenothiazines are generally rapidly absorbed from the gastrointestinal tract and from parenteral injection sites. They are highly soluble and strongly bound to plasma proteins. Inactivation occurs largely through oxidation by hepatic microsomal enzymes.

Recommended Reading

AMA Drug Evaluations (5th ed.). Chicago: American Medical Association, 1983. Pp. 227–240.

Ananth, J. Side effects in the neonate from psychotropic agents excreted through breast-feeding. *Am. J. Psychiatry* 135:801, 1977.

Baldessarini, R. J. *Chemotherapy in Psychiatry.* Cambridge, Mass.: Harvard University, 1977. Pp. 12–56.

Cleary, M. F. Fluphenazine decanoate during pregnancy. *Am. J. Psychiatry* 134:7, 1977.

Cottle, M. K. W., Van Petten, G. R., and van Muyden, P. Maternal and fetal cardiovascular indices during fetal hypoxia due to cord compression in chronically cannulated sheep: II. Responses to promazine. *Am. J. Obstet. Gynecol.* 146:686, 1983.

Gilman, A. G., Goodman, L. S., and Gilman, A. *The Pharmacological Basis of Therapeutics* (6th ed.). New York: Macmillan, 1980. Pp. 395–418.

Montiminy, M., and Teres, D. Shock after phenothiazine administration in a pregnant patient with a pheochromocytoma. *J. Reprod. Med.* 28:159, 1983.

Slone, D., et al. Antenatal exposure to the phenothiazines in relation to congenital malformations, perinatal mortality rate, birth weight, and intelligence quotient score. *Am. J. Obstet. Gynecol.* 128:486, 1977.

Stenchever, M. A. Promethazine hydrochloride: Use in patients with Rh isoimmunization. *Am. J. Obstet. Gynecol.* 130:665, 1978.

Phenoxybenzamine (Dibenzyline®)

Indications and Recommendations

The use of phenoxybenzamine during pregnancy should be limited to the treatment of hypertension due to pheochromocytoma. Acute hypertensive *crises* associated with pheochromocytoma, however, should be controlled with intravenous phentolamine. Phenoxybenzamine then becomes the drug of choice for oral maintenance therapy. Control of blood pressure during cesarean section or during surgery to remove the tumor should also be maintained with intravenous phentolamine.

Special Considerations in Pregnancy

Untreated pheochromocytoma during pregnancy has been associated with maternal and fetal mortality rates of up to 48% and 47%, respectively. It is presumed that most of these deaths were due to maternal cardiovascular problems that led to fetal anoxia. Phenoxybenzamine has been used successfully in the last trimester of pregnancy for the treatment of hypertension secondary to pheochromocytoma.

One case of premature rupture of the membranes following 3 days of phenoxybenzamine therapy in the twenty-sixth week of pregnancy has been reported. The subsequent hypertensive crisis was controlled by phentolamine. A 640-g infant was born 21 hours later and died shortly thereafter. One instance of maternal and fetal tachycardia after parenteral administration of phenoxybenzamine has been reported. The child was normal at follow-up 8 years later.

Dosage

Only the oral form of phenoxybenzamine is currently available for use in the United States. The usual oral dose is 10 mg once a day initially; it can then be raised by 10-mg increments every 4 days until the desired response is obtained. At least 2 weeks are usually required to reach the optimal dosage.

Adverse Effects

The most frequently noticed side effects are due to alpha-adrenergic blockade and vary with the degree of blockade. These include postural hypotension, reflex tachycardia, miosis, and nasal congestion. Sedation, nausea, and vomiting are also seen. Patients with hypovolemia may suffer from a sharp fall in blood pressure when this drug is administered.

Mechanism of Action

Phenoxybenzamine produces alpha-adrenergic blockade by establishing stable bonds at receptor sites, thus reducing the total population of available alpha receptors and decreasing responses mediated by their excessive stimulation. Beta-adrenergic stimulation is consequently unopposed. Vasodilatation in various vascular beds depends in part on the degrees of alpha-adrenergic and beta-adrenergic control.

Normal subjects who are standing and receive phenoxybenzamine slowly by the intravenous route show little change in blood pressure, although diastolic values tend to fall; in normal recumbent subjects, however, a precipitous fall in blood pressure occurs. Cerebral and coronary vascular resistance is not altered greatly. Hypertension due to excessive catecholamine production in patients with pheochromocytoma can be controlled by the oral administration of phenoxybenzamine.

Absorption and Biotransformation

From 20–30% of an oral dose of phenoxybenzamine is absorbed from the gastrointestinal tract. The drug is primarily excreted in the urine, with 50% being eliminated in the first 12 hours and 80% being eliminated in 24 hours.

Recommended Reading

Brenner, W. E., et al. Pheochromocytoma: Serial studies during pregnancy. *Am. J. Obstet. Gynecol.* 113:779, 1972.

Gilman, A. G., Goodman, L. S., and Gilman, A. *The Pharmacological Basis of Therapeutics* (6th ed.). New York: Macmillan, 1980. Pp. 178–183.

Griffith, M. I., et al. Successful control of pheochromocytoma in pregnancy. *J.A.M.A.* 229:437, 1974.

Leak, D., et al. Management of pheochromocytoma during pregnancy. *Can. Med. Assoc. J.* 116:371, 1977.

Maughan, G. B., Shabanah, E. H., and Toth, A. Experiments with pharmacologic sympatholysis in the gravid. *Am. J. Obstet. Gynecol.* 97:764, 1967.

Phensuximide (Milontin®)

Indications and Recommendations

Phensuximide is contraindicated for use during pregnancy since other therapeutic agents are preferable. This drug is one of the succinimide group of anticonvulsants used in the treatment of absence seizures. It was the first of these compounds to be introduced for therapy, but low efficacy and toxic effects have relegated it to a secondary role. Experience with phensuximide in pregnancy is limited. In three cases in which other antiepileptic medications were also administered, fetal abnormalities including ambiguous genitalia, inguinal hernia, and pyloric stenosis were reported. When therapy for absence seizures is indicated during pregnancy, ethosuximide is the drug of choice.

Recommended Reading

Annegers, J. F., et al. Do anticonvulsants have a teratogenic effect? *Arch. Neurol.* 31:364, 1974.

Fabro, S., and Brown, N. A. Teratogenic potential of anticonvulsants. *N. Engl. J. Med.* 300:1280, 1979.

Fedrick, J. Epilepsy and pregnancy: A report from the Oxford record linkage study. *Br. Med. J.* 2:442, 1973.

Gilman, A. G., Goodman, L. S., and Gilman, A. *The Pharmacological Basis of Therapeutics* (6th ed.). New York: Macmillan, 1980. Pp. 460–465.

Heinonen, O. P., Slone, D., and Shapiro, S. *Birth Defects and Drugs in Pregnancy.* Littleton, Mass.: Publishing Sciences Group, 1977. Pp. 358–359.

McMullin, G. P. Teratogenic effects of anticonvulsants. *Br. Med. J.* 2:430, 1971.

National Institutes of Health. Anticonvulsants found to have teratogenic potential. *J.A.M.A.* 241:36, 1981.

Phentolamine (Regitine®)

Indications and Recommendations

The use of phentolamine during pregnancy should be limited to the treatment of acute hypertensive episodes in patients with pheochromocytoma and for the immediate preoperative and intraoperative management of such a patient undergoing cesarean section for delivery of the infant and removal of the tumor. Both mother and fetus should be monitored carefully during the procedure. It is not recommended as a diagnostic agent in, or for chronic management of, pheochromocytoma in pregnancy.

Special Considerations in Pregnancy

It is not recommended that phentolamine be used as a diagnostic agent for pheochromocytoma in the pregnant patient, since a severe drop in maternal blood pressure will cause decreased uterine blood flow and corresponding fetal anoxia. Safer diagnostic tests such as bioassays and chemical assays for catecholamines are available.

Phenoxybenzamine is the agent of choice for preoperative management of pheochromocytoma. Phentolamine, however, is given intravenously for the control of hypertension during delivery and tumor removal. One case of a baby born with "jitters" following treatment of the mother with phentolamine and guanethidine has been reported.

Dosage

For use in preoperative reduction of elevated blood pressure, 5 mg IV or IM is given 1–2 hours before surgery and repeated if necessary. During surgery, 5 mg may be administered intravenously to prevent or control paroxysms of hypertension, tachycardia, or other effects of epinephrine intoxication. The 5-mg dose is also used for treatment of acute hypertensive crises and may be repeated as necessary. Blood pressure should be monitored frequently for 10 minutes after injection. Norepinephrine should be on hand to reverse any hypotension.

Adverse Effects

The primary side effects of phentolamine are caused by gastrointestinal and cardiac stimulation. Gastrointestinal symptoms include pain, nausea, vomiting, diarrhea, and exacerbation of peptic ulcer. Cardiac stimulation may lead to tachycardia, angina, and cardiac arrhythmias, especially after parenteral administration. Death due to hypoglycemia has been observed with chronic overdosage.

Mechanism of Action

Phentolamine is a moderately effective alpha-adrenergic blocker; vasodilatation produced at dosages usually used in adults, however, results primarily from its direct effect on vascular smooth muscle. Only high dosages produce characteristic alpha-adrenergic blockade. The drug increases circulatory catecholamines in normal patients.

Clinical manifestations of pheochromocytoma result from the secretion of catecholamines. Vasodilatation produced by phentolamine causes a fall in blood pressure, especially in patients with pheochromocytoma. The hypotension may be potentially severe in such patients.

Absorption and Biotransformation

Phentolamine is absorbed after oral administration, but the drug is less than 20% as active when given orally than when given by parenteral administration. Approximately 10% of an intravenous dose is recovered unchanged in the urine. The fate of the remaining drug is unknown.

Recommended Reading

Brenner, W. E., et al. Pheochromocytoma: Serial studies during pregnancy. *Am. J. Obstet. Gynecol.*113:779, 1972.

Griffith, M. I., et al. Successful control of pheochromocytoma in pregnancy. *J.A.M.A.* 229:437, 1974.

Leak, D., Carroll, J. J., and Robinson, D. C. Management of pheochromocytoma during pregnancy. *Can. Med. Assoc. J.* 116:371, 1977.

Maughan, G. B., Shabanah, E. H., and Toth, A. Experiments with pharmacologic sympatholysis in the gravid. *Am. J. Obstet. Gynecol.* 97:764, 1967.

Phenylbutazone (Butazolidin®)

Indications and Recommendations

The use of phenylbutazone should be limited to a 4-day course of treatment for an attack of acute gouty arthritis. Gout is uncommon in women and rarely seen before menopause. If treatment of an acute attack becomes necessary during pregnancy, a *short* course of phenylbutazone is preferable to the use of colchicine or allopurinol. Monitoring blood counts, serum electrolytes, and fluid balance is mandatory. This drug is a potent antiinflammatory agent, a poor analgesic, and a weak antipyretic agent. It is contraindicated for the treatment of rheumatoid arthritis and allied disorders during pregnancy because aspirin or corticosteroids are preferable therapeutic agents.

Special Considerations in Pregnancy

Phenylbutazone causes marked sodium and water retention accompanied by decreased urinary output and increased plasma volume up to 50%. Since plasma volume in pregnancy is already expanded, cardiac decompensation could result from the administration of this drug. In addition, phenylbutazone, a prostaglandin synthetase inhibitor, could theoretically cause constriction of the ductus arteriosus in utero and can inhibit labor and prolong pregnancy (see *Nonsteroidal Antiinflammatory Agents*).

The risk of teratogenesis in humans is unknown. The package insert states that animal studies, though inconclusive thus far, exhibit evidence of embryotoxicity.

Dosage

The recommended dose to be used for an attack of gouty arthritis is 200 mg PO qid for the first day followed by 100 mg PO tid for 3 additional days.

Adverse Effects

Some type of side effect is noted in 10–45% of patients who take phenylbutazone. Side effects include nausea, vomiting, epigastric discomfort, skin rashes, diarrhea, vertigo, insomnia, euphoria, nervousness, and edema formation. More serious adverse sequelae include peptic ulceration with hemorrhage or perforation, serum sickness–like hypersensitivity reactions, hepatitis, nephritis, and the particularly dangerous possibility of bone marrow suppression with aplastic anemia, leukopenia, agranulocytosis, and/or thrombocytopenia. A number of patients have died from the aplastic anemia and agranulocytosis. There is also a well-documented increased risk of bleeding when phenylbutazone is given to a patient receiving warfarin anticoagulant therapy.

Mechanism of Action

The mechanism of action of the antiinflammatory effects of phenylbutazone is not known. Like the salicylates, this drug inhibits the biosynthesis of prostaglandins, uncouples oxidative phosphorylation, and inhibits the adenosine triphosphate (ATP)–dependent biosynthesis of mucopolysaccharide sulfates in cartilage. The uricosuric effect results from diminished tubular reabsorption of uric acid. Sodium and chloride retention also result from a direct effect on the renal tubules. The excretion of potassium is not changed. Phenylbutazone reduces iodine uptake by the thyroid gland by a direct action that inhibits the synthesis of organic iodine compounds.

Other antiinflammatory drugs, oral anticoagulants, oral hypoglycemic agents, sulfonamides, and some other drugs may be displaced from binding proteins by phenylbutazone. This can result in an increased pharmacologic or toxic effect of the displaced drug.

Absorption and Biotransformation

Phenylbutazone is rapidly absorbed from the gastrointestinal tract, and peak levels are reached in 2 hours. The drug is 98% bound to plasma proteins, and the serum half-life is 50–100 hours.

Phenylbutazone is almost entirely metabolized in the liver. Oxyphenbutazone, one of the two metabolites, has pharmacologic and toxic properties similar to the parent compound. Both phenylbutazone and oxyphenbutazone are slowly excreted in the urine, since binding to plasma proteins limits their glomerular filtration. Because of their slow metabolism and excretion, these compounds may accumulate in considerable quantities during long-term administration.

Recommended Reading

Burrow, G. N., and Ferris, T. F. (eds.). *Medical Complications During Pregnancy*. New York: Saunders, 1975, P. 805.

Gilman, A. G., Goodman, L. S., and Gilman, A. *The Pharmacological Basis of Therapeutics* (6th ed.). New York: Macmillan, 1980. Pp. 698–701.

Goldfinger, S. E. Treatment of gout. *N. Engl. J. Med.* 285:1303, 1971.

Phenytoin (Dilantin®)

Indications and Recommendations

The use of phenytoin during pregnancy should be limited to the treatment of those women who require anticonvulsant therapy. The following recommendations have been made in a bulletin published in 1979 by the American Academy of Pediatrics Committee on Drugs in collaboration with the American College of Obstetricians and Gynecologists (ACOG) Committee on Obstetrics: Maternal and Fetal Medicine.

> No woman should receive anticonvulsant medication unnecessarily. When possible, a woman who has been seizure free for many years should be withdrawn from her medication prior to pregnancy. When a woman who has epilepsy and requires medication asks about pregnancy, she should be advised that she has a 90% chance of having a normal child, but that the risk of congenital malformations and mental retardation is two to three times greater than average because of

her disease or its treatment. Women who seek advice later than the first trimester of pregnancy should be reassured with the foregoing figures rather than routinely urged to consider abortion. For these women, drug therapy should be continued throughout pregnancy because major anatomical malformations most likely would have taken place already, and the malformations associated with the hydantoin syndrome rarely have significant effect on the well-being of the child.

There is no reason at present to advise a woman to switch from phenytoin or phenobarbital to other anticonvulsants about which even less is known. Discontinuation of medication in a woman whose epilepsy is controlled by medicine may cause seizures, and prolonged seizures could cause serious sequelae to her and the fetus.*

Phenytoin is most commonly used as an anticonvulsant in the treatment of generalized tonic-clonic, simple complex, and partial seizures. It is ineffective against absence seizures and may even exacerbate them. It is also, more rarely, used as an intravenous antiarrhythmic agent in the treatment of ventricular arrhythmias, but alternative agents are preferred during pregnancy.

At delivery, measurement of cord blood calcium and prothrombin time followed by vitamin K administration is indicated. Neonatal glucose levels should be checked shortly after birth. Breast-feeding is not contraindicated.

Special Considerations in Pregnancy

Dosage requirements for phenytoin have been reported to increase during pregnancy and fall in the puerperium, although this remains controversial. Phenytoin readily crosses the placenta, and identical maternal and fetal plasma levels have been reported at delivery. Elimination of the drug by the full-term neonate has been shown to be similar to that of adults.

The risk of congenital heart disease and cleft palate is increased among the offspring of women with epilepsy and is highest in those women receiving anticonvulsant therapy. Part of this increase may be caused by phenytoin. The risk of these abnormalities in exposed infants is 4–5%, or approximately twice the rate of malformations in the general population. In addition, a combination of defects, termed the *fetal hydantoin syndrome*, has recently been described. This consists of craniofacial abnormalities, growth retardation, mental retardation, and nail and digital hypoplasia. This syndrome's degree of expression is variable. Its more serious consequences can be found in 10% of exposed neonates, while manifestations of its mildest form may be present in 30% of cases. Numerous case reports have also suggested a correlation between maternal phenytoin administration and fetal neuroblastoma, gastrointestinal and genitourinary defects, and melanotic neuroectodermal tumors. As with phenobarbital, phenytoin has been associated with a vitamin K–deficient coagulopathy in the neonate.

*Pediatrics 63:331, summary 333, February 1979. Copyright © 1979 by American Academy of Pediatrics.

Dosage

The usual adult maintenance dose of phenytoin in anticonvulsant therapy is about 300 mg/day. This dosage should produce serum levels in the therapeutic range of 10–20 μg/ml. As the half-life of phenytoin is relatively long, steady-state serum levels are reached in 6–10 days when no loading dose is given. These can be reached more quickly if a load of 1,000 mg in divided doses over 1–2 days is given before institution of maintenance therapy. Dosage alterations should await achievement of a plateau level and should be attempted in small stepwise increments. Since phenytoin exhibits dose-dependent kinetics, dosage increases may lead to larger than expected increases in serum levels.

Intravenous therapy is sometimes indicated when a patient is not able to take oral medications and in the treatment of status epilepticus. This drug must be given slowly at a rate of less than 50 mg/minute, preferably with concurrent maternal cardiac monitoring. Phenytoin should not be given intramuscularly since the drug is erratically absorbed from the site of administration.

Changes in the serum phenytoin level secondary to drug interactions may adversely affect the therapeutic response. Carbamazepine, folic acid, and alcohol may decrease steady-state phenytoin levels, whereas isoniazid, chloramphenicol, primidone, and warfarin (Coumadin®) may increase such levels. When phenobarbital is given concurrently, it may either increase or decrease phenytoin plasma concentrations by either increasing or competitively inhibiting its metabolism.

Adverse Effects

A variety of adverse effects have been reported, including nystagmus, ataxia, vertigo, diplopia, peripheral neuropathy, deterioration in intellect, hyperactivity, drowsiness, and hallucinations. Gastrointestinal symptoms, gingival hyperplasia, osteomalacia, megaloblastic anemia, hirsutism, and decreased insulin secretion with hyperglycemia can also occur. Some of these effects are dose related, but they may be seen with serum levels in the upper portion of the therapeutic range.

Idiosyncratic reactions include skin rash, Stevens-Johnson syndrome, systemic lupus erythematosus, aplastic anemia, hepatic necrosis, and nonspecific lymphadenopathy. With rapid intravenous administration, cardiovascular collapse and central nervous system depression can occur.

Mechanism of Action

Phenytoin blocks the spread of electrical activity from a seizure focus by stabilizing the neuronal membrane and preventing posttetanic potentiation. It is effective in the treatment of generalized tonic-clonic seizures, as well as simple complex and partial seizures. It is ineffective against absence seizures and may even exacerbate them.

Absorption and Biotransformation

Phenytoin is absorbed through the duodenum and is readily bound to albumin and alpha globulins. The plasma protein binding is not significantly altered in pregnancy. Phenytoin is hydroxylated to an inactive metabolite by the liver; the metabolite is excreted via the kidneys. The rate of metabolism is variable, with a half-life usually ranging from 17–56 hours.

Recommended Reading

Anticonvulsants and pregnancy. Prepared by the AAP Committee on Drugs in collaboration with the ACOG Committee on Obstetrics: Maternal and Fetal Medicine. January 1979.

Gilman, A. G., Goodman, L. S., and Gilman, A. *The Pharmacological Basis of Therapeutics* (6th ed.). New York: Macmillan, 1980. Pp. 448–474.

Kelly, T. E. Teratogenicity of anticonvulsant drugs. I. Review of the literature. *Am. J. Med. Genet.* 19:413, 1984.

Kochenour, N. K., Emery, M. G., and Sawchuk, R. J. Phenytoin metabolism in pregnancy. *Obstet. Gynecol.* 56:577, 1980.

Monson, R. R., et al.   Dilantin and selected congenital malformations. *N. Engl. J. Med.* 289:1049, 1973.

Wilder, B. J., and Bruni, J. *Seizure Disorders: A Pharmacological Approach to Treatment.* New York: Raven, 1981.

Woodbury, D. M., Penry, J. K., and Pippenger, C. E. *Antiepileptic Drugs* (2nd ed.). New York: Raven, 1982.

Piperazine (Antepar®)

Indications and Recommendations

Piperazine is contraindicated in pregnancy. It is an oral antiparasitic agent that is highly effective against *Ascaris lumbricoides* and *Enterobius vermicularis* infections. It paralyzes the parasite by blocking the response of the neuromuscular junction to acetylcholine, allowing the worm to be expelled by peristalsis. There are currently no studies of piperazine use in pregnancy. It is known to be absorbed into the maternal bloodstream, with 15–75% recoverable in the urine as active drug and metabolite, and may, therefore, have adverse effects on the fetus. As the infections for which piperazine is commonly used are not life-threatening and because treatment can safely be postponed, it is best to defer treatment until after delivery.

Recommended Reading

Gilman, A. G., Goodman, L. S., and Gilman, A. *The Pharmacological Basis of Therapeutics* (6th ed.). New York: Macmillan, 1980. Pp. 1023–1024.

Potassium Chloride, Oral (Kaochlor®, Kaon-Cl®, K-Lor®, Klotrix®, K-Lyte/Cl®, K-Tab®, Micro-K®, Slow-K®)

Indications and Recommendations

Oral potassium chloride is safe to use during pregnancy. It is indicated for treatment or prophylaxis of potassium deficiency. Serum potassium levels should be followed when this compound is administered. It will almost certainly be necessary to prescribe potassium chloride when a pregnant woman is taking thiazide diuretics for control of hypertension.

Special Considerations in Pregnancy

Fetal potassium levels are dependent on maternal potassium levels. Fetal bradycardia due to heart block has been reported in association with hypokalemia in the mother.

Dosage

The usual daily dose is 50 mEq over 24 hours. Oral potassium should be taken with a full glass of water or orange juice. Measurement of serial serum potassium levels should be used to monitor efficacy of therapy. The chloride salt of potassium should be given since failure to replace chloride will enhance the potassium loss in metabolic alkalosis.

Potassium chloride is available in a variety of dosage forms, including liquids in 10% (20 mEq/15 ml) and 20% (40 mEq/15 ml) strengths; powders providing 15 mEq, 20 mEq, and 25 mEq/dose; and wax matrix tablets in 8- or 10-mEq strengths. In addition there is a gelatin capsule containing 8 mEq potassium chloride embedded in polymer-coated crystalline particles. Although enteric-coated tablets are available, their use is not recommended as they are associated with an increased incidence of intestinal ulceration.

Adverse Effects

Side effects of excessive oral potassium supplementation include vomiting, diarrhea, nausea, and abdominal discomfort. Toxicity is most likely to occur in conditions such as oliguria, azotemia, acute dehydration, and untreated Addison's disease. Manifestations of toxicity include paresthesias of the extremities, flaccid paralysis, listlessness, mental confusion, weakness, and decrease in blood pressure. Electrocardiographic changes include loss of the P wave, widening of the QRS complex, ST-segment changes, and tall peaked T waves.

Mechanism of Action

The mechanism of action of potassium on skeletal, cardiac, and smooth muscle, and its renal and metabolic effects, are beyond the scope of this book. The reader is referred to a current textbook of physiology.

Causes of potassium deficiency include diarrhea, vomiting, decreased intake, increased renal excretion (as in diuresis, acidosis, or adrenocortical hyperactivity), increased cellular uptake (as in treatment of diabetic ketoacidosis), persistent alkalosis, and familial periodic paralysis.

Recommended Reading

Gilman, A. G., Goodman, L. S., and Gilman, A. *The Pharmacological Basis of Therapeutics* (6th ed.). New York: Macmillan, 1980. Pp. 877–878.

Micro-K potassium therapy. *Med. Lett. Drugs Ther.* 24:71, 1982.

Potassium Iodide

Indications and Recommendations

The use of potassium iodide, or any iodide, is contraindicated during pregnancy and lactation. Potassium iodide has been used as an expectorant in the form of a solution or pill. Iodides are contraindicated during pregnancy because of the potential for development of fetal goiter secondary to fetal thyroid trapping of the iodide. They are also contraindicated during lactation because inorganic iodine is preferentially concentrated in breast milk.

Recommended Reading

Carswell, F., Kerr, M. M., and Hutchison, J. H. Congenital goiter and hypothyroidism produced by maternal ingestion of iodides. *Lancet* 1:1241, 1970.

Postellon, D. C., and Aronow, R. Iodine in mother's milk. *J.A.M.A.* 247:463, 1982.

Prazosin (Minipress®)

Indications and Recommendations

Prazosin is relatively contraindicated in pregnancy because other drugs that seem to be equally effective have been studied far more extensively. It is used for the control of mild to moderate hypertension and is a quinazoline derivative that is chemically unrelated to any of the other existing antihypertensive drugs.

Prazosin functions principally as a direct vasodilator. It is an alpha-adrenergic blocking agent that acts on vascular smooth muscle. It is also a potent phosphodiesterase inhibitor and has some ganglionic blocking and anticholinergic activity. Its hemodynamic effects are similar to those of sodium nitroprusside in that both arterial resistance and venous tone are reduced. Since prazosin reduces peripheral vascular resistance without secondary reflex tachycardia, it rarely causes palpitations or tachycardia.

Experience with this drug in pregnant women is quite limited. One study of eight hypertensive women unresponsive to beta-adrenergic blockade in the third trimester revealed that this agent satisfactorily lowered both supine and standing blood pressure in six of the eight. The median prolongation of pregnancy in these cases was 22 days. Neonatal outcome was satisfactory, and all the infants were judged to have been developing normally at the time of the report. Pharmacokinetic analysis of these patients revealed that maternal absorption of the drug was delayed and its half-life prolonged when compared to healthy male control subjects of similar age.

Although prazosin appears attractive as a direct vasodilator without associated cardiac stimulating activity, experience with its use in pregnancy is too scant to recommend its use at this time. Until more is known about long-term fetal and neonatal effects as well as the drug's disposition in breast milk, more standard agents such as methyldopa or hydralazine should be used in hypertensive obstetric patients.

Recommended Reading

Gilman, A. G., Goodman, L. S., and Gilman, A. *The Pharmacological Basis of Therapeutics* (6th ed.). New York: Macmillan, 1980. Pp. 806–807.

Rutsen, P. C., et al. Clinical pharmacological studies with prazosin during pregnancy complicated by hypertension. *Br. J. Clin. Pharmacol.* 16:543, 1983.

Primaquine Phosphate

Indications and Recommendations

The use of primaquine phosphate during pregnancy is contraindicated. Primaquine, an 8-aminoquinoline derivative, is highly active against the primary exoerythrocytic forms of *Plasmodium vivax* and *Plasmodium falciparum*. It disrupts the parasite's mitochondria, creating major changes in its metabolic processes. In nonpregnant patients, primaquine is recommended specifically for the radical cure of vivax malaria, the prevention of relapse in vivax malaria, or after the termination of chloroquine phosphate suppressive therapy in an area where vivax malaria is endemic.

Its major side effects in the large majority of people is mild to moderate epigastric distress or, with larger dosages, mild anemia or cyanosis due to methemoglobinemia and leukocytosis. In susceptible patients whose red blood cells are deficient in glucose 6-phosphate dehydrogenase (G6PD), however, even small dosages of primaquine can be associated with severe hemolytic anemia. All patients with possible G6PD deficiency should be tested for adequate enzyme levels before therapy is instituted.

The effects of primaquine on the pregnant woman or fetus have not been studied. Chloroquine, a related 4-aminoquinoline derivative, is known to cross the placenta. The use of chloroquine in dosages greater than those necessary for malaria prophylaxis has been associated with spontaneous abortion and with retinal and vestibular damage in the fetus. As primaquine is chemically similar to chloroquine, it is most prudent to avoid primaquine therapy during pregnancy. When radical cure or terminal prophylaxis is indicated, the pregnant patient should receive chloroquine once weekly until delivery. Primaquine may be given after delivery.

Recommended Reading

Bruce-Chawatt, L. J. Malaria and pregnancy. *Br. Med. J.* 286:1457, 1983.
Gilman, A. G., Goodman, L. S., and Gilman, A. *The Pharmacological Basis of Therapeutics* (6th ed.). New York: Macmillan, 1980. Pp. 1052–1054.
Prevention of malaria in travelers. *M.M.W.R.* 31:19S, 22S, 1982.

Primidone (Mysoline®)

Indications and Recommendations

The use of primidone during pregnancy should be limited to the treatment of those women who require chronic anticonvulsant therapy. It is used alone or in combination with other anticonvulsants for the treatment of generalized tonic-clonic, simple partial, or complex partial seizures. Primidone may be given to breast-feeding mothers, but the nursing infant should be observed for drowsiness.

The following recommendations have been made in a bulletin published in 1979 by the American Academy of Pediatrics Committee on Drugs in collaboration with the American College of Obstetricians and Gynecologists (ACOG) Committee on Obstetrics: Maternal and Fetal Medicine.

> No woman should receive anticonvulsant medication unnecessarily. When possible, a woman who has been seizure free for many years should be withdrawn from her medication prior to pregnancy. When a woman who has epilepsy and requires medication asks about pregnancy, she should be advised that she has a 90% chance of having a normal child, but that the risk of congenital malformations and mental retardation is two to three times greater than average because of her disease or its treatment.*

Special Considerations in Pregnancy

Primidone crosses the placenta, and it has been cited as a possible cause of birth anomalies. Reported incidents in past years, however, have been inconclusive in light of the practice of multidrug therapy for epilepsy.

Offspring of pregnant mice receiving 25–150 mg/kg/day of primidone exhibited a high incidence of palatal defects, including full-length and submucosal clefts. No strong dose dependence was found in association with the abnormalities. The mice demonstrated the same metabolites as those found in humans. Administered doses were not much larger, on an mg/kg basis, than those used in humans.

The most commonly reported human fetal anomalies ascribed to primidone include cardiac malformations, nail or phalangeal hypo-

---

*Pediatrics 63:331, summary 333, February 1979. Copyright © 1979 by American Academy of Pediatrics.

plasia, craniofacial anomalies (hypertelorism, epicanthal folds, and a broad, depressed nasal bridge), growth retardation, and delayed development. In some of these reports, primidone was the only drug used by the mother during pregnancy, but in others, it was one of several agents prescribed. The latter fact is important since many of these anomalies are similar to those reported in fetuses who were exposed to phenytoin in utero.

In addition to the gross defects found at birth, a withdrawal-like syndrome has been reported in some otherwise normal infants born to mothers who received daily doses of primidone. In two reports, the infants were tremulous and irritable for 3 days, cord blood contained 8 μg/ml primidone, and the drug could be detected in the infants' urine for 10–11 days. In another report, tremulousness was also associated with neonatal hypocalcemia, which was refractory to therapy for 2 weeks. Hypoprothrombinemia has been reported in infants of mothers who received a combination of primidone and phenobarbital. It is not conclusive that primidone alone can decrease prothrombin levels, but because primidone is metabolized to phenobarbital, it is possible. The condition usually responds to vitamin K therapy.

The manufacturers recommend that mothers taking primidone discontinue nursing if the infant appears unusually drowsy.

Dosage

The usual adult oral dose is 500–1,500 mg/day given in divided doses. The dosage is adjusted on the basis of therapeutic results as well as the primidone and phenobarbital concentrations. The relationship between dosage and plasma concentrations is complex; both plasma primidone levels and phenobarbital levels should be measured. Primidone levels of 8–12 μg/ml and phenobarbital levels of 15–35 μg/ml are optimal. Increases in dosage must be undertaken slowly to minimize adverse effects, particularly if the patient has not been treated previously.

Adverse Effects

The side effects of primidone are similar to those of phenobarbital and include sedation, vertigo, dizziness, ataxia, diplopia, nystagmus, megaloblastic anemia, and possibly osteomalacia. Idiosyncratic reactions include skin rashes, leukopenia, thrombocytopenia, lymphadenopathy, and a systemic lupus erythematosus–like syndrome.

Mechanism of Action

The mechanism of action of primidone is complex due to the presence of two active metabolites, phenobarbital and phenylethylmalonamide (PEMA) in addition to the drug itself. In rat studies, PEMA has been shown to raise the thresholds for myoclonic jerks and clonic-tonic seizures induced by hexafluorodiethylether. In studies of electroconvulsion, in both humans and animals primidone appears more selective than phenobarbital alone in controlling certain phases of seizure activity. (See *Phenobarbital* for its actions.)

Primidone is useful in the control of generalized tonic-clonic, simple partial, or complex partial seizures. It can be used alone, particularly in the treatment of complex partial seizures, or in combination with other anticonvulsants, such as phenytoin, carbamazepine, or ethosuximide. Since primidone is metabolized to phenobarbital, these two drugs are rarely used together.

Absorption and Biotransformation

The drug is rapidly absorbed through the gastrointestinal tract and is metabolized in the liver to phenobarbital and PEMA, both of which are active compounds. Primidone's plasma half-life is 7–9 hours. Whereas PEMA appears within 24 hours and has a half-life of 24–48 hours, phenobarbital is measurable after 24–96 hours and has a half-life of 48–120 hours. Steady-state plasma levels of primidone are achieved within 2–4 days of initiating therapy or dosage adjustment. In children, over 90% of the drug is excreted by the kidneys as both unaltered primidone and its active metabolites.

Recommended Reading

Anticonvulsants and pregnancy. Prepared by the AAP Committee on Drugs in collaboration with the ACOG Committee on Obstetrics: Maternal and Fetal Medicine. January 1979.

Gilman, A. G., Goodman, L. S., and Gilman, A. *The Pharmacological Basis of Therapeutics* (6th ed.). New York: Macmillan, 1980. Pp. 458–471.

Mynre, S. A., and Williams, R. Teratogenic effects associated with maternal primidone therapy. *J. Pediatr.* 99:160, 1981.

Rating, G., et al. Teratogenic and pharmacokinetic studies of primidone during pregnancy and in the offspring of epileptic women. *Acta Paediatr. Scand.* 71:301, 1982.

Rudd, N. L., and Freedom, R. M. A possible primidone embryopathy. *J. Pediatr.* 94:835, 1979.

Wilder, B. J., and Bruni, J. *Seizure Disorders: A Pharmacologic Approach to Treatment.* New York: Raven, 1981.

Woodbury, D. M., Penry, J. K., and Pippenger, C. E. *Antiepileptic Drugs* (2nd ed.). New York: Raven, 1982.

Probenecid (Benemid®)

Indications and Recommendations

The use of probenecid during pregnancy should be limited to the treatment of gout or potentially symptomatic hyperuricemia. Since it has no analgesic or antiinflammatory activity, it is of no value in the treatment of acute attacks of gout; phenylbutazone may be used in these instances. Probenecid is commonly given before the administration of penicillin or ampicillin, especially in the treatment of gonorrheal infections, to increase blood levels of the antibiotics by inhibiting their renal excretion. It seems judicious to avoid using two drugs in pregnancy if one will suffice.

Special Considerations in Pregnancy

Probenecid is known to cross the placental barrier. With the exception of the death of one neonate not definitely related to probenecid therapy, the drug has been used in pregnancy without adverse effect to mother or child.

Dosage

Therapy should not be started until 2–3 weeks after an acute attack. The usual dose is 250 mg bid for 1 week followed by 500 mg bid. Daily dosage may be increased every 4 weeks by increments of 500 mg to a maximum of 2–3 g.

Adverse Effects

Frequently reported side effects include headache, anorexia, nausea, and vomiting. Dizziness, flushing, sore gums, urinary frequency, and anemia have also been reported. Probenecid therapy may exacerbate and prolong inflammation during the acute phase of gout. The frequency of attacks may also be increased during the first 6–12 weeks of therapy.

Mechanism of Action

Renal transport of organic acids is influenced by probenecid therapy. It is a competitive inhibitor to active reabsorption of uric acid at the proximal convoluted tubule. Urinary excretion of uric acid is therefore increased and serum urate levels are reduced. Subtherapeutic dosages may inhibit renal secretion of uric acid.

By decreasing serum urate levels, probenecid prevents or reduces chronic joint changes and tophi formation. It eventually reduces the frequency of attacks and may improve renal function in gouty patients. Serum urate levels usually reach a minimum within a few days after therapy is begun.

At the proximal and distal tubules, probenecid competitively inhibits secretion of many weak organic acids such as the penicillins. Plasma levels of acidic drugs primarily eliminated by tubular secretion can be substantially increased.

Absorption and Biotransformation

Probenecid is rapidly and completely absorbed from the gastrointestinal tract. After oral administration of 2 g, plasma half-life ranges from 4–17 hours and decreases as the dose decreases. Approximately 75% of the drug is bound to plasma proteins. Probenecid is metabolized in the liver.

Recommended Reading

American Hospital Formulary Service. Monographs for *Allopurinol* (1977), *Colchicine* (1973), and *Probenecid* (1977). Washington, D.C.: American Society of Hospital Pharmacists, 1973, 1977.
Gilman, A. G., Goodman, L. S., and Gilman, A. *The Pharmacological*

Basis of Therapeutics (6th ed.). New York: Macmillan, 1980. Pp. 722–723, 931–932.

Lee, F. I., and Loeffler, F. E. Gout and pregnancy. *J. Obstet. Gynaecol. Br. Commonw.* 69:299, 1962.

Procainamide (Pronestyl®)

Indications and Recommendations

The use of procainamide in pregnancy should be limited to the treatment of those patients with cardiac arrhythmias that are unresponsive to safer antiarrhythmic agents. Quinidine, with its similar electrophysiologic effects, is preferred during pregnancy because it has been studied more extensively.

Special Considerations in Pregnancy

Successful procainamide cardioversion of a supraventricular tachycardia in a 24-week-old fetus has recently been reported. Digoxin and propranolol had been given initially but no response was obtained. After procainamide was administered, fetal cardioversion occurred within 1 hour. The authors suggest that fetal blood, which is slightly more acidic than that of the mother, may trap procainamide and limit back-diffusion. However, a synergistic effect among digoxin, propranolol, and procainamide cannot be excluded. Therefore, until more is learned about procainamide's pharmacokinetics in pregnancy, other more familiar agents should be used in initial attempts at treating fetal arrhythmias.

Dosage

The usual oral maintenance dose is 6 mg/kg q3h. When given intravenously the dose is 200–500 mg administered at a rate not exceeding 25–50 mg/minute, followed by a maintenance infusion of 2 mg/kg/hour. The therapeutic range is 4–8 μg/ml.

Adverse Effects

The use of procainamide is often accompanied by prolongation of the QRS interval on electrocardiogram and by hypotension. Ventricular tachycardia and heart block may be seen with toxic doses (blood levels greater than 12 μg/ml). Besides these electrophysiologic side effects, chronic administration of procainamide is associated with a systemic lupus erythematosus–like syndrome. Most patients receiving long-term therapy develop a positive antinuclear antibody titer, although a few show a complete lupus syndrome. In a well-controlled age- and sex-matched study to characterize the autoimmune phenomena in patients receiving procainamide, there was a significant increase in the frequency of positive direct antiglobulin (Coombs') tests in those patients receiving the drug. The mechanism of red cell sensitization appears to be the production of red cell autoantibody, which is indistinguishable from that seen in warm autoimmune hemolytic anemia.

Mechanism of Action

Procainamide decreases cardiac membrane reponsiveness. Automaticity and speed of impulse conduction are therefore decreased, and the refractory period is increased.

Absorption and Biotransformation

Procainamide is rapidly and almost completely absorbed from the gastrointestinal tract. Maximal plasma concentration after oral administration occurs at about 60 minutes, and at 15–60 minutes after intramuscular administration. Procainamide has a half-life of 2.5–5.0 hours in patients with normal renal function. It is acetylated in the liver to N-acetylprocainamide (NAPA), a compound that also possesses antiarrhythmic activity. The rate of acetylation of procainamide is genetically determined and varies among individuals. The half-life of NAPA is 7 hours in patients with normal renal function. The total amount of unchanged procainamide excreted in the urine varies from 40–70% and depends on acetylator phenotype.

Recommended Reading

Avery, G. S. *Drug Treatment: Principles and Practice of Clinical Pharmacology and Therapeutics*. Sydney, Australia: Adis, 1976.

Gilman, A. G., Goodman, L. S., and Gilman, A. *The Pharmacological Basis of Therapeutics* (6th ed.). New York: Macmillan, 1980. Pp. 774–777.

Gwen, B. D., et al. Procainamide cardioversion of fetal supraventricular tachycardia. *Am. J. Cardiol.* 53:1460, 1984.

Kleinman, S., et al. Positive direct antiglobulin tests and immune hemolytic anemia in patients receiving procainamide. *N. Engl. J. Med.* 311:809, 1984.

Progestins

NATURAL PROGESTERONE AND ITS ESTERS (DELALUTIN®, PROVERA®)

Indications and Recommendations

The use of progesterone and its esters, 17-hydroxyprogesterone, medroxyprogesterone acetate (Provera®), and 17-hydroxyprogesterone caproate (Delalutin®), during pregnancy is controversial, and if used at all, they should be restricted to very specific situations.

Natural progesterone can probably be given safely during pregnancy for the treatment of an inadequate luteal phase, and along with its esters for the prevention of premature delivery. The efficacy of these agents is still open to question, however. There is no convincing evidence that progesterone in any form is useful in the management of threatened abortion or habitual abortion except in the specific case of inadequate luteal phase syndrome.

Special Considerations in Pregnancy

The effectiveness of progestins in preventing premature delivery remains controversial. Their use in preventing abortion (other than in the case of inadequate luteal phase) is unproved.

At least one random, prospective double-blind study has investigated the benefits of administering 17-hydroxyprogesterone caproate prophylactically to a group of women with histories of premature delivery. The group receiving this hormone exhibited a significantly lower prematurity rate than did a placebo-treated control group. The rationale for this therapy is based on the hypothesis that labor is at least partially a result of low or falling progesterone levels.

The use of natural progestins and their esterified derivatives during pregnancy has been associated with limb anomalies, but the literature is unclear as to whether any causal relationship exists. When 1,608 newborns whose mothers were treated with progestins (generally medroxyprogesterone acetate) for first-trimester bleeding were compared with 1,146 whose mothers bled during the first trimester but were not treated with progestins, the incidence of major congenital abnormalities was similar in both groups (6.3% vs. 7.2%). It may be that the previously reported increased anomaly rate was due not to the progestins but to the bleeding for which progestins were administered.

Dosage

In the maintenance of pregnancy with a luteal phase defect, the usual recommendation is to give progesterone vaginal suppositories, 25 mg bid, until the twelfth week, or progesterone in oil, 150 mg IM every other day, until the twelfth week. In the study mentioned previously in which 17-hydroxyprogesterone caproate was given to prevent premature labor, the dose was 250 mg IM every week from the eighteenth to thirty-seventh week of gestation.

Adverse Effects

Side effects of progesterone include weight gain and occasional episodes of depression. Because plasma progesterone levels are generally quite high in pregnancy, the addition of exogenous hormone should not cause noticeable side effects.

Mechanism of Action

Naturally occurring progesterone works at the intracellular level to produce many physiologic changes, among which is smooth muscle relaxation. This effect on the uterine musculature is probably critical for the maintenance of pregnancy. Exogenously administered progesterone may supplement that produced by the corpus luteum in early pregnancy and is therefore useful in the management of an inadequate luteal phase. In the absence of this condition, the prevailing evidence is that progestins are not useful in preventing first-trimester abortion.

Absorption and Biotransformation

These drugs are generally given parenterally and hydrolyzed in the liver to pregnanediol and pregnanediol derivatives that are excreted in the urine. Natural progesterone can be absorbed vaginally from suppositories. The progestins are secreted in breast milk at a concentration of 1–10% of their blood levels.

SYNTHETIC 19 NORTESTOSTERONE DERIVATIVES

Indications and Recommendations

Progestins derived from 19 nortestosterone are contraindicated during pregnancy. They are used as oral contraceptive agents and as pregnancy tests. These compounds have also been utilized in attempts to prevent abortion or premature delivery, or both. They are contraindicated because of reported associations between their use and cardiac anomalies, limb reduction defects, and masculinization of the female fetus. If progestin therapy is believed to be necessary during pregnancy, natural progesterone and its esters may be associated with less risk to the fetus.

If they are taken inadvertently during the first trimester, the patient should be told of the potential adverse sequelae. Although incidence figures are not available, the risk to the fetus appears to be small and elective termination of the pregnancy does not seem to be warranted.

Recommended Reading

Aarskog, D. Maternal progestins as a possible cause of hypospadias. *N. Engl. J. Med.* 300:75, 1979.

Chez, R. A. Proceedings of the symposium Progesterone, Progestins, and Fetal Development. *Fertil. Steril.* 30:16, 1978.

Ferre, F., et al. Oral administration of micronized natural progesterone in late human pregnancy. *Am. J. Obstet. Gynecol.* 148:26, 1984.

Hill, L. M., Johnson, C. E., and Lee, R. A. Prophylactic use of hydroxy-progesterone caproate in abdominal surgery during pregnancy. *Obstet. Gynecol.* 46:287, 1975.

Johnson, J. W. C., et al. Efficacy of 17 alpha-hydroxyprogesterone caproate in the prevention of premature labor. *N. Engl. J. Med.* 293:675, 1975.

Katz, Z., et al. Teratogenicity of progestogens given during the first trimester of pregnancy. *Obstet. Gynecol.* 65:775, 1985.

Keith, L., and Berger, G. S. The relationship between congenital defects and the use of exogenous progestational "contraceptive" hormones during pregnancy: A 20-year review. *Int. J. Gynecol. Obstet.* 15:115, 1977.

Nora, J. J., et al. Exogenous progestogen and estrogen implicated in birth defects. *J.A.M.A.* 240:837, 1978.

Yemini, M., et al. Prevention of premature labor by 17 alpha-hydroxyprogesterone caproate. *Am. J. Obstet. Gynecol.* 151:574, 1985.

Propoxyphene (Darvon®, Dolene®)

Indications and Recommendations

The use of propoxyphene is relatively contraindicated in pregnancy because other therapeutic agents are preferable. Propoxyphene is a synthetic analgesic structurally related to methadone. Its pharmacologic actions are similar to other narcotic analgesics; however, its clinical effects are no greater than those of aspirin or codeine. Chronic use can produce primarily psychologic but, with high dosages, also physical dependence. It is estimated that the incidence of propoxyphene abuse is equivalent to that of codeine. As with other narcotic analgesics, propoxyphene use during pregnancy has been associated with neonatal withdrawal syndromes. Because of its limited analgesic activity, it should not be used to treat minor pain in the pregnant woman. Acetaminophen is the drug of choice in these situations.

Recommended Reading

Gilman, A. G., Goodman, L. S., and Gilman, A. *The Pharmacological Basis of Therapeutics* (6th ed.). New York: Macmillan, 1980. Pp. 520–521.

Ringrose, C. A. D. The hazard of neurotropic drugs in the fertile years. *Can. Med. Assoc. J.* 106:1058, 1972.

Tyson, H. R. Neonatal withdrawal symptoms associated with maternal use of propoxyphene hydrochloride (Darvon). *J. Pediatr.* 85:684, 1974.

Protamine Sulfate

Indications and Recommendations

The use of protamine sulfate during pregnancy should be limited to the treatment of excessive anticoagulation due to an overdose of heparin. In this instance, the risk of maternal hemorrhage outweighs consideration of direct toxicity to the fetus.

Special Considerations in Pregnancy

No information is available regarding the safety of this drug in animals or humans during pregnancy.

Dosage

Each milligram of protamine sulfate neutralizes approximately 100 mg heparin. It should be given intravenously at a rate of no more than 50 mg over a 10-minute period. Protamine itself possesses anticoagulant properties, and it is therefore unwise to give more than 100 mg over a short period, unless there is certain knowledge of a larger requirement. This will avoid "overneutralization" of the heparin. Because of the rapid clearance of heparin, proportionately less protamine should be administered when more than a half-hour has passed following administration of the former.

Adverse Effects

Hypotension, the most common side effect of protamine, is usually associated with infusion at rates greater than 50 mg/10 minutes. Bradycardia, dyspnea, and transitory flushing may also be associated with rapid infusion. Allergic reactions have been reported after protamine administration to persons allergic to fish.

Mechanism of Action

The protamines are simple, low-molecular-weight, strongly basic proteins found in the sperm of certain fish. They are able to combine with the strongly acidic heparin to form a stable salt with loss of anticoagulant activity. The protamine-heparin complex is excreted in the kidney.

Recommended Reading

Caplan, S. N., and Berkman, E. M. Protamine sulfate and fish allergy (letter). *N. Engl. J. Med.* 295:172, 1976.

Gilman, A. G., Goodman, L. S., and Gilman, A. *The Pharmacological Basis of Therapeutics* (6th ed.). New York: Macmillan, 1980. P. 1352.

Goldstein, A., Aronow, L., and Kalman, S. M. *Principles of Drug Action.* New York: Harper & Row, 1968.

Pseudoephedrine (Sudafed®)

Indications and Recommendations

The use of pseudoephedrine in pregnancy should be limited to the treatment of allergic rhinitis when symptomatic relief is not afforded by other nonmedicinal treatments. Neither pseudoephedrine nor ephedrine significantly elevates blood pressure when given orally or topically in standard decongestant dosages, but they may cause cardiac stimulation and a redistribution of blood flow.

Special Considerations in Pregnancy

Pseudoephedrine is a sympathomimetic agent that is a common component of many proprietary compounds containing antihistamines and other ingredients. Although sympathomimetic amines are teratogenic in some animal species, human teratogenicity has never been proved.

The Collaborative Perinatal Project found an association between first-trimester sympathomimetic use and certain minor malformations such as inguinal hernia and clubfoot. Although these data do not serve as a specific indictment against the administration of pseudoephedrine in pregnancy, judicious use of this agent and other sympathomimetics is warranted.

Dosage

The usual oral dose of pseudoephedrine is 30–60 mg q4–6h for decongestion of mucous membranes.

Adverse Effects

Adverse effects include blanching of mucous membranes and "rebound" congestion when applied topically, dryness of mucous membranes, and occasional tachycardia and palpitations. These effects are usually mild and self-limited.

Mechanism of Action

Pseudoephedrine is predominantly an alpha-adrenergic stimulant that produces vasoconstriction in hyperemic nasal mucosa as well as in other vascular beds.

Absorption and Biotransformation

Pseudoephedrine is well absorbed when given orally. Most of the drug is metabolized by deamination and conjugation. Both metabolites and unchanged drug are excreted in the urine.

Recommended Reading

Gilman, A. G., Goodman, L. S., and Gilman, A. *The Pharmacological Basis of Therapeutics* (6th ed.). New York: Macmillan, 1980. Pp. 168–169.

Heinonen, O. P., Slone, D., and Shapiro, S. *Birth Defects and Drugs in Pregnancy*. Littleton, Mass.: Publishing Sciences Group, 1977. Pp. 345–356, 439.

Nishimura, H., and Tanimura, T. *Clinical Aspects of the Teratogenicity of Drugs*. Amsterdam: Excerpta Medica, 1976. P. 231.

Shepard, T. H. *Catalog of Teratogenetic Drugs* (3rd ed.). Baltimore: Johns Hopkins University, 1980. Pp. 134–135.

Pyrantel Pamoate (Antiminth®)

Indications and Recommendations

The use of pyrantel pamoate during pregnancy should be limited to treatment of infections due to susceptible helminths when the mother's well-being is compromised. It is a broad-spectrum antihelminthic agent useful in the treatment of hookworm, roundworm, pinworm, and (investigationally) *Trichostrongylus* infections. Since most parasitic infections are not life-threatening, it is safest to defer therapy until after delivery. Examples of infections that might be treated include a chronic hookworm infection that has produced a significant anemia and heavy roundworm infection with potential for intestinal obstruction.

Special Considerations in Pregnancy

Teratogenicity has not been described in animals, but no human data are available.

Dosage

For hookworm (*Ancyclostoma duodenale* or *Necator americanus*), roundworm (*Ascaris lumbricoides*), and *Trichostrongylus* species, 11 mg/kg (up to a maximum of 1 g) is given as a single oral dose. For pinworm (*Enterobius vermicularis*), the same dosage is given and repeated in 2 weeks.

Pyrantel pamoate is available as a suspension containing 50 mg base per milliliter.

Adverse Effects

Pyrantel has caused complete neuromuscular blockade in animals given the drug parenterally. Oral dosages in humans are relatively free of side effects, with the exception of occasional gastrointestinal disturbance, headache, dizziness, rash, or fever.

Mechanism of Action

Pyrantel is a depolarizing neuromuscular blocking agent that paralyzes the worm, allowing it to be eliminated in the feces. Pyrantel pamoate is 1,000 times more effective than piperazine, a hyperpolarizing agent, for *A. lumbricoides* infections. Pyrantel and piperazine are mutually antagonistic.

Absorption and Biotransformation

Pyrantel is poorly absorbed from the gastrointestinal tract with less than 15% of the parent compound or its metabolites recovered in the urine.

Recommended Reading

Drugs for parasitic infections. *Med. Lett. Drugs Ther.* 24:17, 1978.

Gilman, A. G., Goodman, L. S., and Gilman, A. *The Pharmacological Basis of Therapeutics* (6th ed.). New York: Macmillan, 1980. Pp. 1024–1025.

LaPorte, V. D., and Gibbs, R. S. Acute pancreatitis in pregnancy with *Ascaris* infestation. *Obstet. Gynecol.* 49(Suppl 1):84S, 1977.

Pitts, N. E., and Migliardi, J. R. Antiminth (pyrantel pamoate). *Clin. Pediatr.* 13:87, 1974.

Pyrvinium Pamoate (Povan®)

Indications and Recommendations

Pyrvinium is relatively contraindicated during pregnancy. This drug is used to treat enterobiasis (pinworm infection). It acts to inhibit oxygen uptake and respiration in aerobic organisms and also interferes with the absorption of exogenous glucose. No studies examining the use of pyrvinium in pregnancy have been performed, and therefore, its maternal and fetal effects are unknown. As enterobiasis is a non–life-threatening infection, it is best to defer treatment until after delivery. However, it is not absorbed from the gastrointestinal tract to any appreciable extent, and should treatment of enterobiasis be required, pyrvinium would appear to be safer to use than either piperazine or mebendazole. The tablets should be swallowed whole to avoid staining teeth; the drug colors stools and vomitus bright red.

Recommended Reading

Gilman, A. G., Goodman, L. S., and Gilman, A. *The Pharmacological Basis of Therapeutics* (6th ed.). New York: Macmillan, 1980. Pp. 1025–1026.

Quinacrine Hydrochloride (Atabrine®)

Indications and Recommendations

The use of quinacrine is contraindicated in pregnancy. Quinacrine couples with and fixes DNA so that DNA is unable to replicate or serve for transcription of RNA. It had been used in the treatment of malaria and tapeworm infections, but has been largely replaced for these indications by less toxic alternatives such as chloroquine. Its effective use in the treatment of malaria is limited by blood dyscrasias, urticaria, and exfoliative dermatitis. In addition, the drug tends to accumulate, causing yellow staining of the skin and blue or black pigmentation of the nails.

Currently, its primary indication is for the treatment of giardiasis. Because *Giardia* infestations are not life-threatening and because quinacrine is known to cross the placenta readily, it is recommended that therapy be deferred until after delivery.

Recommended Reading

Doberstyn, E. B. Resistance of *Plasmodium falciparum*. *Experientia* 40:1311, 1984.

Gilman, A. G., Goodman, L. S., and Gilman, A. *The Pharmacological Basis of Therapeutics* (6th ed.). New York: Macmillan, 1980. P. 1078.

Tanenbaum, L., and Taffanelli, D. L. Antimalarial agents. *Arch. Dermatol.* 116:587, 1980.

Quinidine (Cardioquin®, Quinaglute®)

Indications and Recommendations

Quinidine is safe to use during pregnancy. It is an antiarrhythmic agent used in both atrial and ventricular arrhythmias. It may be administered to pregnant women if it is believed to be the drug of choice for the particular arrhythmia encountered.

Special Considerations in Pregnancy

Although quinine, a compound related to quinidine, appears to have oxytocic properties and is reported to be an abortifacient, the oxytocic properties of quinidine itself are considered to be insignificant.

Quinidine has been shown to cross the placenta, with levels in the fetus being slightly lower than those in the mother. Neonatal thrombocytopenia has been reported. Although eighth nerve damage has also been reported, it was associated with much higher dosages than are ordinarily used.

Dosage

The usual maintenance dose of quinidine sulfate or quinidine gluconate is 200–300 mg PO q6h, or 300–600 mg PO q8–12h if the sustained-release forms are used. Serum levels should be monitored, the therapeutic range being 3–6 µg/ml. Intravenous administration of quinidine should only be undertaken in hospitalized patients who can have continuous electrocardiographic monitoring.

Adverse Effects

The most common toxic effects of quinidine are gastrointestinal. Cardiac effects include acceleration of existing atrial arrhythmias and ventricular tachycardia. Idiosyncratic reactions, such as angioedema and vascular collapse, may occur more commonly than with many other drugs.

Mechanism of Action

Quinidine increases the threshold for electrical excitation and decreases the conduction velocity in cardiac tissue. Other actions include an increase in the effective refractory period, and vagal blockade. Quinidine therapy is effective in the prevention or abolition of such cardiac arrhythmias as atrial fibrillation, atrial flutter, paroxysmal supraventricular and ventricular tachycardia, and premature systoles.

Absorption and Biotransformation

Quinidine salts are nearly completely absorbed after oral administration, with maximal effects occurring in 1–3 hours. Quinidine is 70–95% bound to plasma proteins, primarily albumin. It is metabolized in the liver, mainly to 2-hydroxy-quinidine. Within 24 hours, 10–50% of the administered drug is excreted unchanged in the urine.

An in vitro study comparing protein binding in blood obtained from three groups of infants of different ages disclosed that the binding of quinidine is diminished in neonates and young infants. This, of course, may result in enhanced drug activity. Analysis of six cord blood samples obtained at delivery, eight samples from infants aged 8–18 months, and 12 samples from children over the age of 2 demonstrated free quinidine levels of 39.2%, 24.4%, and 16.6%, respectively.

Recommended Reading

Aviado, D. M., and Salem, H. Drug action, reaction and interaction: I. Quinidine for cardiac arrhythmias. *J. Clin. Pharmacol.* 15:477, 1975.

Gilman, A. G., Goodman, L. S., and Gilman, A. *The Pharmacological Basis of Therapeutics* (6th ed.). New York: Macmillan, 1980. Pp. 768–774.

Hill, L. M., and Malkasian, G. D. The use of quinidine sulfate throughout pregnancy. *Obstet. Gynecol.* 54:366, 1979.

Pickoff, A. S., et al. Age-related differences in the protein binding of quinidine. *Dev. Pharmacol. Ther.* 3:108, 1981.

Quinine

Indications and Recommendations

The use of quinine during pregnancy should be limited to the treatment of attacks of chloroquine-resistant falciparum malaria. In this situation, the risk of teratogenicity is outweighed by that of congenital malaria. Its use is not warranted in the treatment of leg cramps in light of its oxytocic and possible teratogenic effects. Special counseling may be required because of quinine's availability without a prescription.

Special Considerations in Pregnancy

Quinine is known to have an oxytocic action in the pregnant woman. The nongravid human uterus is only slightly influenced, but as pregnancy proceeds, the oxytocic action of quinine becomes more noticeable. Toxic amounts of the drug may cause abortion.

Quinine crosses the placental barrier and causes toxicity in the fetus. Congenital anomalies of the eye and deafness have been attributed to quinine use during pregnancy.

Dosage

The dose of quinine given in the treatment of uncomplicated attacks of falciparum malaria is 650 mg tid for 10–14 days. It should be given in conjunction with pyrimethamine, sulfadiazine, or (in the nonpregnant patient) tetracycline.

Adverse Effects

Therapeutic dosages of quinine can produce cinchonism, a syndrome that includes tinnitus, headache, nausea, and visual disturbances. With continued treatment or large dosages, dermatologic, gastrointestinal, central nervous system, and cardiovascular symptoms may become prominent. Hematologic side effects are rare and include hemolytic anemia; hypoprothrombinemia, which can be reversed by vitamin K; and thrombocytopenia.

Mechanism of Action

Quinine has been described as a "general protoplasmic poison" affecting many enzyme systems. Its exact mechanism of action as an antimalarial is unknown. Quinine has analgesic activity and is a poor antipyretic. It exhibits cardiovascular effects similar to its isomer quinidine, oxytocic activity in late pregnancy, and curare-like effects on skeletal muscle.

Absorption and Biotransformation

Quinine is readily absorbed from the gastrointestinal tract. Peak levels are seen 1–3 hours after an oral dose. Approximately 70% of plasma quinine is bound to proteins. It is cleared primarily by the liver with less than 5% of the dose excreted unchanged in the urine.

Recommended Reading

Dannenberg, A. L., Dorfman, S. F., and Johnson, J. Use of quinine for self-induced abortion. *South. Med. J.* 76:846, 1983.

Drugs for parasitic infections. *Med. Lett. Drugs Ther.* 20:17, 1978.

Gilman, A. G., Goodman, L. S., and Gilman, A. *The Pharmacological Basis of Therapeutics* (6th ed.). New York: Macmillan, 1980. Pp. 1054–1057.

Heinonen, O. P., Slone, O., and Shapiro, S. (eds.). *Birth Defects and*

Drugs in Pregnancy. Littleton, Mass.: Publishing Sciences Group, 1977. Pp. 299–302, 313.

Lewis, R., Lauerson, N. H., and Birnbaum, S. Malaria associated with pregnancy. *Obstet. Gynecol.* 42:696, 1973.

Siroty, R. R. Purpura on the rocks—with a twist. *J.A.M.A.* 235:2521, 1976.

Sutherland, J. M., and Light, I. J. The effect of drugs upon the fetus. *Pediatr. Clin. North Am.* 12:781, 1965.

Rauwolfia Alkaloids: Reserpine (Sandril®, Serpasil®)

Indications and Recommendations

The rauwolfia alkaloids are relatively contraindicated during pregnancy because other therapeutic agents are preferable. Reserpine is one of approximately 20 related compounds that comprise this family of antihypertensive agents. They act by depleting the natural stores of biogenic amines in the brain, myocardium, adrenal medulla, and postganglionic nerve endings. The transport of norepinephrine into its storage granules is blocked and the reuptake of released catecholamines by the nerve endings is inhibited. The hypotensive action of these drugs is due to a reduction in sympathetic stimulation of the blood vessels and heart and is associated with a bradycardia as well as a decrease in vascular resistance.

Side effects include postural and exercise hypotension, although these are uncommon when the drug is taken orally in effective amounts. Unopposed parasympathetic stimulation may cause an increase in gastric acid secretion, peptic ulceration, frequent bowel movements or diarrhea, prolonged atrioventricular conduction, and enhanced second-degree heart block. Nasal arteriolar dilatation may result in nasal stuffiness. Brain amine and serotonin depletion can cause depression and behavioral changes, and these serve as limiting factors in the long-term administration of high enough dosages to cause major sympathoplegia.

The labeling of reserpine has been changed to reflect animal tumorigenicity from rodent studies. An increased incidence of mammary fibroadenomas in female mice, malignant tumors of the seminal vesicles in male mice, and malignant adrenal medullary tumors in male rats has been noted. The breast neoplasms are thought to be related to reserpine's prolactin-elevating effect. The extent to which these findings indicate a risk to humans is uncertain, but some epidemiologic studies suggest an association of reserpine therapy with breast cancer.

Reserpine crosses the placenta, and the major fetal complication is neonatal respiratory difficulty secondary to nasal congestion. Reserpine also appears in the breast milk. Although no case reports have been published, the same risks may exist for nursing infants as for neonates exposed in utero.

Although some authors recommend reserpine as an alternative drug in the therapy of chronic hypertension during pregnancy, the large number of maternal side effects makes this a less attractive choice than other agents that are currently available.

Recommended Reading

Armstrong, B., Stevens, N., and Doll, R. Retrospective study of the association between use of rauwolfia derivatives and breast cancer in English women. *Lancet* 2:672, 1974.

F.D.A. Drug Bull. 13:28, 1983.

Gilman, A. G., Goodman, L. S., and Gilman, A. *The Pharmacological Basis of Therapeutics* (6th ed.). New York: Macmillan, 1980. Pp. 202–204.

Lee, P. A., Kelly, M. R., and Wallin, J. D. Increased prolactin levels during reserpine treatment or hypertensive patients. *J.A.M.A.* 235:2316, 1976.

Reserpine. *Med. Lett. Drugs Ther.* 18:19, 1976.

Rifampin (Rifadin®, Rimactane®)

Indications and Recommendations

The use of rifampin in pregnancy should be limited to those cases of maternal tuberculosis in which the use of a third drug is necessary. It should be avoided in the treatment of nonmycobacterial infections for which other safer antibiotic therapy is available.

Special Considerations in Pregnancy

Experience with the use of rifampin in pregnancy is limited. It is known to cross the placenta and to cause malformations in both rats and mice. Although some anecdotal reports indicate that rifampin is not teratogenic, others suggest that rifampin use during pregnancy may be associated with complications. One retrospective review reports that of 229 conceptions in women who received rifampin during pregnancy, there were five intrauterine deaths; four deaths after live births; 9 infants with malformations including anencephaly, hydrocephaly, and limb and ear malformations; and 10 infants with hemorrhagic tendencies. The data are, however, difficult to evaluate because rifampin is often used in combination with other antitubercular agents.

Dosage

The usual dose given for chemotherapy of tuberculosis is 600 mg given once daily.

Adverse Effects

The most common side effects are rash, fever, and nausea and vomiting. Intermittent, high-dose administration is often associated with more frequent reactions including a flulike syndrome, thrombocytopenia, and rarely, acute reversible renal failure sometimes appearing with concomitant hepatic failure. Subclinical hepatitis is also seen, whereas clinical hepatitis is rare.

Mechanism of Action

Rifampin inhibits the action of DNA-dependent RNA polymerase in mycobacteria and other microorganisms, thus inhibiting RNA synthesis.

Absorption and Biotransformation

Rifampin is well absorbed from the gastrointestinal tract, but absorption may be delayed by food or such drugs as aminosalicylic acid. First-pass hepatic extraction is substantial. The primary pathway of elimination is deacetylation in the liver to a partially active metabolite that undergoes extensive enterohepatic circulation. About 50–60% of a dose is eventually excreted in the feces. The half-life is 1.5–5.0 hours and is increased by liver disease or biliary obstruction.

Recommended Reading

Gilman, A. G., Goodman, L. S., and Gilman, A. *The Pharmacological Basis of Therapeutics* (6th ed.). New York: Macmillan, 1980. Pp. 1203–1206.

Good, J. T., et al. Tuberculosis in association with pregnancy. *Am. J. Obstet. Gynecol.* 140:492, 1981.

Scheinhorn, D. J., and Angelillo, V. A. Antituberculosis therapy in pregnancy: Risks to the fetus. *West. J. Med.* 127:195, 1977.

Snider, D. E., et al. Treatment of tuberculosis during pregnancy. *Am. Rev. Respir. Dis.* 122:65, 1980.

Stein, J. S. M., and Stainton-Ellis, D. M. Rifampicin in pregnancy (letter). *Lancet* 2:604, 1977.

Ritodrine (Yutopar®)

Indications and Recommendations

Ritodrine is the first and only beta-adrenergic drug approved by the FDA for use as a tocolytic agent. It is a beta-2 adrenergic agonist that primarily acts on myometrial receptors.

Ritodrine's major usefulness is in the treatment of premature labor that is not due to an obvious cause. Premature labor accompanied by chorioamnionitis, fetal death, severe preeclampsia, life-threatening maternal complications, or severe third-trimester bleeding should be allowed to continue and is thus a contraindication to the use of a tocolytic agent. Women with cardiac disease may be adversely affected by the cardiovascular effects of ritodrine and diabetic control may be compromised by its effects on carbohydrate metabolism. Finally, great care must be exercised when ritodrine is used in combination with glucocorticoids, because of the possibility of causing pulmonary edema.

Special Considerations in Pregnancy

Ritodrine decreases the intensity and frequency of uterine contractions in women with spontaneous or induced labor. It has been found to be more effective than either placebo or ethanol. Prospective clinical trials comparing ritodrine with other selective beta-2 agonists are necessary in order to assess their relative effectiveness as tocolytic agents. The incidence of maternal cardiovascular side effects with ritodrine is reported to be lower than with less selective beta-2 agonists such as isoxsuprine.

Ritodrine is not indicated for use in the first half of pregnancy. Nevertheless, to date there are no reports of teratogenesis in humans associated with the use of this drug during embryogenesis. Ritodrine crosses the placenta but cord concentrations are lower than concomitant maternal values. Long-term follow-up study of children exposed to this drug in utero have thus far shown no adverse effects.

Uterine and placental blood flow is increased in women taking ritodrine, and fetal tachycardia may occur after maternal administration. It has also been shown to increase maternal and fetal serum glucose concentrations, as well as maternal insulin levels. Because neonatal hypoglycemia has been observed with maternal administration of ritodrine, infants who were exposed to this drug in utero should have their blood sugars carefully monitored. Diabetic mothers who take this drug may need increased dosages of insulin to maintain adequate glucose control.

Recent data suggest an acceleration of fetal lung maturation when ritodrine and other beta-2 agonists are administered to the mother.

Ritodrine has been used outside of the United States in the treatment of acute intrapartum fetal distress. It has not been approved for this use in the United States. The role of ritodrine in the prophylaxis of premature labor in multiple pregnancy requires further study.

No data exist concerning the secretion of ritodrine in breast milk, but since it is not indicated for use after delivery and the half-life is quite short, it is unlikely that ritodrine administered antenatally would cause significant problems in the nursing infant.

Dosage

Ritodrine is administered intravenously by constant infusion. The recommended starting dose is 100 μg/minute. This should be increased in 50-μg/minute increments every 10 minutes until a dose that provides satisfactory tocolytic action has been reached. Maternal cardiovascular side effects may be a limiting factor. The maximal recommended infusion rate is 350 μg/minute.

The intravenous infusion is maintained until satisfactory tocolysis has been achieved. Thirty minutes before termination of the intravenous infusion, oral ritodrine is begun. Oral dosage is 10 mg q2h. The initial oral dose is maintained for 24 hours and then reduced, if possible, to 10–20 mg q4–6h. Generally, oral therapy is continued until the pregnancy has reached term. Intramuscular ritodrine is not available for use in the United States.

Adverse Effects

In trials in the United States, intravenous ritodrine was associated with palpitations in 33% of patients; tremor, nausea, vomiting, headache, or erythema in 10–15%; and nervousness, restlessness, emotional upset, or anxiety in 5–6%. Cardiac symptoms including chest pain or tightness and arrhythmias were reported in 1–2% of patients. Other infrequently reported maternal effects included anaphylactic shock, rash, epigastric distress, ileus, bloating, constipation, diarrhea, dyspnea, hyperventilation, sweating, and weakness.

Maternal cardiac arrhythmias are due to ritodrine's chronotropic activity, and these include premature ventricular contractions as well as supraventricular tachycardias. This drug also increases stroke volume, and, therefore, systolic pressure. Peripheral vascular resistance, on the other hand, is decreased, and this reduces diastolic pressure and consequently widens the pulse pressure. Transient arrhythmias have been reported in newborns exposed to this drug in utero.

Maternal myocardial ischemia and corresponding electrocardiographic changes have been noted in women being treated with ritodrine. Some, but not all, of these patients were symptomatic. The changes usually reverted to normal when therapy was discontinued.

Ritodrine may cause hyperglycemia, which can lead to metabolic acidosis in poorly controlled diabetic women. In addition, the drug may cause hyperlactacidemia with secondary metabolic acidosis. Transient hypokalemia develops in most patients during ritodrine therapy. This is generally believed to be secondary to the hyperglycemia and hyperinsulinemia that drive serum potassium into the cells. Since there is no loss of potassium from the body, serum levels quickly return to baseline values after ritodrine is discontinued. When present, the hypokalemia is usually asymptomatic and rarely requires treatment.

Pulmonary edema has been reported with the use of ritodrine alone or in combination with glucocorticoids, but the incidence is higher with combined therapy. Pulmonary edema is also more likely to occur when ritodrine is administered to women with twin gestations. Whenever this drug is given, care should be taken to avoid iatrogenic fluid overloading.

All of these adverse effects occur primarily in association with intravenous administration of the drug. Oral therapy results in lower blood levels, and consequently, the incidence and severity of side effects are less.

Mechanism of Action

Ritodrine is a sympathomimetic agent with predominantly beta-2 activity. It is believed that such agents stimulate adenyl cyclase, the enzyme that catalyzes the conversion of adenosine triphosphate to cyclic AMP. Increased intracellular concentrations of cyclic AMP cause relaxation of the uterine musculature.

Absorption and Biotransformation

Orally administered ritodrine is rapidly absorbed in the gastrointestinal tract. Bioavailability of an oral dose is approximately 30%. The drug is conjugated in the liver, with a plasma half-life of 1.3–2.0 hours. Ninety percent of the drug may be recovered from the urine within 24 hours of administration.

Recommended Reading

Barden, T. P., Peter, J. B., and Merkatz, I. R. Ritodrine hydrochloride: A beta-mimetic agent for use in preterm labor. *Obstet. Gynecol.* 56:1, 1980.

Benedetti, T. J. Maternal complications of parenteral beta-sympathomimetic therapy for premature labor. *Am. J. Obstet. Gynecol.* 145:1, 1983.

Bieniarz, J., Ivankovich, A., and Scommegna, A. Cardiac output during ritodrine treatment in premature labor. *Am. J. Obstet. Gynecol.* 118:910, 1974.

Boog, G., Brahim, M. B., and Gandar, R. Beta-mimetic drugs and possible prevention of respiratory distress syndrome. *Br. J. Obstet. Gynaecol.* 82:285, 1975.

Brettes, J. P., Renand, R., and Gandar, R. A double-blind investigation into the effects of ritodrine on uterine blood flow during the third trimester of pregnancy. *Am. J. Obstet. Gynecol.* 124:164, 1976.

Caritis, S. N., et al. Pharmacodynamics of ritodrine in pregnant women during preterm labor. *Am. J. Obstet. Gynecol.* 147:752, 1983.

Hosenpud, J. D., Morton, M. J., and O'Grady, J. P. Cardiac stimulation during ritodrine hydrochloride tocolytic therapy. *Obstet. Gynecol.* 62:52, 1983.

Humphrey, M., et al. The effect of intravenous ritodrine on the acid-base status of the fetus during the second stage of labor. *Br. J. Obstet. Gynaecol.* 82:234, 1975.

Landesman, R., et al. The relaxant action of ritodrine, a sympathomimetic amine, on the uterus during term labor. *Am. J. Obstet. Gynecol.* 110:111, 1971.

Laurersen, N. H., et al. Inhibition of premature labor: A multicentric comparison of ritodrine and ethanol. *Am. J. Obstet. Gynecol.* 127:836, 1977.

Lipshitz, J. Beta adrenergic agonists. *Semin. Perinatol.* 5:252, 1981.

Nochimson, D. J., et al. The effects of ritodrine hydrochloride on uterine activity and the cardiovascular system. *Am. J. Obstet. Gynecol.* 118:523, 1974.

Wesselius-DeCasparis, A., et al. Results of a double-blind, multicentric study with ritodrine in premature labor. *Br. Med. J.* 3:144, 1971.

Salicylates: Acetylsalicylic Acid (Aspirin), Sodium Salicylate

Indications and Recommendations

The use of salicylates should be avoided, especially in the later stages of pregnancy. Salicylate use near term has been associated with prolonged labor, an increased blood loss during delivery, and an abnormally high incidence of stillbirths.

Salicylates may be used as antiinflammatory agents in the treatment of various forms of arthritis, but should be considered as second-line analgesic and antipyretic drugs since acetaminophen is an effective and potentially less toxic substitute. Long-term salicylate therapy may be necessary for treating arthritis during pregnancy; if so, prothrombin time and hemoglobin levels should be monitored closely.

Because of possible fetal sequelae, salicylates should not be used for their antiplatelet aggregation effect during pregnancy. Should anticoagulation be needed, heparin is the agent of choice.

Patients who take large doses of salicylates during pregnancy may have prolonged gestations. Any patient receiving such therapy whose pregnancy exceeds 42 weeks from her last menstrual period should be followed closely to rule out the postmaturity syndrome.

Because of the availability of salicylates in combination over-the-counter agents, those women who use these drugs as self-medications should be identified antenatally, advised of the potential adverse effects, and encouraged to stop.

Special Considerations in Pregnancy

Prolongation of the maternal bleeding time can occur after ingestion of only one 325-mg aspirin tablet while 650 mg, the usual dose, has been shown to double the mean bleeding time for 4–7 days. Although this would be of most concern in the third trimester, spontaneous abortion, premature labor, and placental hemorrhage make bleeding diatheses a potential problem at any time during pregnancy. Daily aspirin dosages of 3 g during the last months of pregnancy have been associated with increased length of gestation, prolonged labor, and increased blood loss during labor.

Potential fetal problems include increased bleeding time and jaundice (due to competition with bilirubin for albumin binding). Continuous administration of large doses to the pregnant woman has been associated with decreased birth weights and increased incidences of stillbirths, premature closure of the ductus arteriosus, and intracranial hemorrhage. The incidence of cephalhematoma and melena is reportedly increased in neonates exposed to salicylates in utero. Various severe birth defects have been anecdotally reported in the offspring of salicylate users, but no cause-and-effect relationship has been established.

Dosage

The usual analgesic-antipyretic dose for aspirin or sodium salicylate is 162–650 mg q4h. Higher doses, 3–6 g/day, are often used for severe arthritis.

Adverse Effects

Side effects of acetylsalicylic acid are numerous; they include nausea and vomiting, gastrointestinal irritation, and occult bleeding. Acute hemorrhage from gastric erosion is a rare occurrence. Iron deficiency anemia may occur with long-term use. Large dosages may prolong prothrombin time; a single analgesic dose may suppress platelet aggregation and lead to prolonged bleeding time.

Mild chronic salicylate intoxication (salicylism) consists chiefly of headache, dizziness, ringing in the ears, difficulty in hearing, blurred vision, and nausea and vomiting. Severe central nervous system disturbances (including restlessness, incoherent speech, tremor, delirium, and even convulsions, coma, and toxic encephalopathy) are associated with more severe intoxication. Initial hyperventilation may lead to respiratory alkalosis, but increased oxygen consumption and renal damage eventually produce a metabolic acidosis.

Mechanism of Action

Salicylates act peripherally by inhibiting prostaglandin synthesis in inflamed tissues. Pain receptors are thereby rendered insensitive to mechanical or chemical stimulation. Salicylates inhibit histamine release, render neutrophils unresponsive to chemotactic stimuli, and interfere with granulocyte adherence. At the high dosages used for arthritis therapy, they interfere with formation of antigen-antibody complexes and suppress lymphocyte function. The antipyretic action of salicylates is mediated via hypothalamic centers and may be due to inhibition of prostaglandin E release. Because acetylsalicylic acid preparations irreversibly reduce platelet aggregation by inhibiting the release of platelet adenosine diphosphate (ADP), they are sometimes prescribed as mild anticoagulants.

Physiologic effects include relief of low-intensity pain, antipyresis, antiinflammatory action, decreased urinary excretion of urates with low dosages, and increased urate excretion with high dosages.

Absorption and Biotransformation

Acetylsalicylic acid and sodium salicylate are the most commonly available salicylates. Oral administration results in rapid absorption from the stomach and upper small intestine. Therapeutic effects are observed 20–30 minutes after ingestion. Although absorption is fastest at low pH, solubility increases with rising pH such that "buffering" agents have little effect on absorption. Rectal administration is unreliable.

The absorbed drug is distributed to all tissues of the body, including cerebrospinal fluid. About 50–90% of salicylates are bound to serum albumin. Salicylates are metabolized in the liver to four main metabolites. Excretion of free drug and metabolites is mainly renal, and free drug excretion increases with alkalinization of the urine. The apparent half-life of salicylates is dependent on the serum concentration and ranges from 2–22 hours.

Recommended Reading

Collins, E. Maternal and fetal effects of acetaminophen and salicylates in pregnancy. *Obstet. Gynecol.* 58:57S, 1981.

Collins, E., and Turner, C. Maternal effects of regular salicylate ingestion in pregnancy. *Lancet* 2:335, 1975.

Collins, E., and Turner, C. Aspirin during pregnancy (letter). *Lancet* 2:797, 1976.

Gilman, A. G., Goodman, L. S., and Gilman, A. *The Pharmacological Basis of Therapeutics* (6th ed.) New York: Macmillan, 1980. Pp. 682–698.

Niederhoff, H., and Zahradnik, H. Analgesics during pregnancy. *Am. J. Med.* 75:117, 1983.

Rudolph, A. M. The effects of non-steroidal anti-inflammatory compounds on fetal circulation and pulmonary function. *Obstet. Gynecol.* 58:63S, 1981.

Rumack, C. M., et al. Neonatal intracranial hemorrhage and maternal use of aspirin. *Obstet. Gynecol.* 58:52S, 1981.

Scopolamine

Indications and Recommendations

Parenteral scopolamine administration is contraindicated during pregnancy. This drug is an anticholinergic agent used as a preanesthetic to decrease salivary secretions and produce amnesia. When given to laboring patients, it may cause outbursts of uncontrollable behavior, restlessness, hallucinations, or excitement.

Scopolamine readily crosses the placenta within 15 minutes of maternal administration. One report suggests that it may induce fetal tachycardia, decrease beat-to-beat variability, and mask decelerations in heart rate. Another report describes neonatal fever, tachycardia, and lethargy in an infant born to a mother who was treated with six doses of parenteral scopolamine along with meperidine and levallorphan tartrate during labor. Scopolamine toxicity was suspected and within 15 minutes of administration of 0.1 mg IM physostigmine, the neonatal heart rate fell from 200 to 140 beats/minute. The remainder of the infant's symptoms resolved completely over the following few hours.

The use of scopolamine in over-the-counter medications is discussed under *Belladonna Alkaloids*.

Recommended Reading

Ayromlooi, J., Tobias, M., and Berg, P. The effects of scopolamine and ancillary analgesics upon the fetal heart rate recording. *J. Reprod. Med.* 25:323, 1980.

Evens, R. P., and Leopold, J. C. Scopolamine toxicity in a newborn. *Pediatrics* 66:329, 1980.

Gilman, A. G., Goodman, L. S., and Gilman, A. *The Pharmacological Basis of Therapeutics* (6th ed.). New York: Macmillan, 1980. Pp. 121–136.

McDonald, J. S. Preanesthetic and intrapartal medications. *Clin. Obstet. Gynecol.* 20:447, 1977.

Simethicone (over-the-counter) (Mylicon®, Silain®)

Indications and Recommendations

Simethicone is safe to use during pregnancy. It is used for the relief of gaseous distention, bloating, or flatulence.

Special Considerations in Pregnancy

There are no special considerations related to pregnancy.

Dosage

The usual dose is 40–80 mg chewed thoroughly 3–4 times/day.

Adverse Effects

One study in rats has demonstrated a significant reduction in the absorption of phenytoin when simethicone was administered.

Mechanism of Action

Simethicone is a mixture of silica gel and dimethylpolysiloxanes. Its defoaming action relieves flatulence by dispersing and preventing the formation of mucus-surrounded gas pockets in the gastrointestinal tract. Simethicone changes the surface tension of gas bubbles in the stomach and intestine, allowing them to coalesce. The gas is freed and is eliminated easily by belching or passing flatus.

Absorption and Biotransformation

Simethicone is not absorbed to any extent.

Recommended Reading

Gilman, A. G., Goodman, L. S., and Gilman, A. *The Pharmacological Basis of Therapeutics* (6th ed.). New York: Macmillan, 1980. P. 954.

McElnay, J. C., and D'Arcy, P. F. Interaction of phenytoin with antacid constituents and kaolin. *Proc. Br. Phar. Soc.* 9:126P, 1980.

Schenkel, B., and Vorherr, H. Non-prescription drugs during pregnancy. Potential teratogenic and toxic effects upon embryo and fetus. *J. Reprod. Med.* 12:27, 1974.

Sodium Nitroprusside (Nipride®)

Indications and Recommendations

The use of sodium nitroprusside during pregnancy is controversial. It is the most potent and predictably effective drug available for hypertensive emergencies, but it has not been studied enough to define its safety before delivery. Animal data are worrisome because they suggest that cyanide toxicity could occur in the fetus while the mother remains asymptomatic. If used at all, sodium nitroprusside should be restricted to the treatment of an acute hypertensive emergency complicated by left ventricular failure and pulmonary edema unresponsive to intravenous hydralazine or diazoxide therapy. Nitroprusside should only be used to control the acute crisis, and delivery of the infant should be performed as quickly as possible thereafter.

Special Considerations in Pregnancy

No changes in umbilical or uterine blood flow have been observed in pregnant sheep when nitroprusside has been administered. In experiments with pregnant ewes, the administration of steadily increasing dosages of nitroprusside given to maintain a 20% reduction in mean arterial pressure was associated with marked accumulation of cyanide in the fetus. Cyanide levels in the fetus were significantly higher than those in the mother and were associated with death in utero. The placenta has therefore been shown to be readily permeable to the nitroprusside molecule and, at least in the sheep model, cyanide trapping seems to occur.

Human data include eight cases in which sodium nitroprusside was used to treat severe hypertension associated with cardiac failure and pulmonary edema during pregnancy. In these women, hypotensive effects were noted within 2 minutes of infusion and disappeared within 5 minutes of discontinuance of the drug. They were all monitored with balloon-tipped pulmonary artery (Swan-Ganz) catheters. This form of monitoring is necessary to assess left ventricular end-diastolic pressures and cardiac output. In all cases, the duration of drug infusion before delivery was kept as short as possible. Using infusion rates of less than $5-10$ $\mu g/kg/minute$, beneficial maternal antihypertensive effects were seen in each of these women, while the maternal and fetal cyanide and thiocyanate levels remained negligible.

Dosage

Nitroprusside is light sensitive and must be delivered in a system wrapped in a light-shielding material such as aluminum foil. It must be given by infusion pump while the patient's blood pressure is constantly monitored. Because its action is so evanescent, hypertension will recur almost immediately after the infusion is discontinued.

The dosage is variable and must be titrated against the individual patient's requirements. The dose range is $0.5-8.0$ $\mu g/kg/minute$ by constant intravenous infusion. The average dose required to sustain a $30-40\%$ decrease in diastolic pressure is 3 $\mu g/kg/minute$. The onset is immediate, and the duration of action is only as long as the infusion runs.

Adverse Effects

Side effects are usually minimal, but prolonged administration can result in cyanide or thiocyanate toxicity. Cyanide is liberated by direct combination of nitroprusside with sulfhydryl groups in red blood cells and tissue. Circulating cyanide is converted to thiocyanate in the liver. Principal manifestations of toxicity are fatigue, nausea, and anorexia followed by disorientation, psychotic behavior, and muscle spasm. Hypothyroidism has been reported following prolonged therapy.

The earliest manifestation of cellular hypoxia due to cyanide toxicity is metabolic acidosis, which is seen with cyanide levels of approximately 3 $\mu g/ml$. Twice this concentration is considered to be lethal. When cyanide toxicity has been diagnosed, intravenous sodium nitrite may be administered at a dose of 5 mg/kg. This will increase the rate of methemoglobin formation and bind cyanide ions, but will also further compromise oxygen delivery to the fetus. Alternatively, hydroxocobalamin (vitamin B_{12a}) can be utilized to treat cyanide toxicity. This compound binds cyanide to form cyanocobalamin. It is administered at a rate of 12.5 mg at 30-minute intervals up to a total dose of 100 mg.

Mechanism of Action

Nitroprusside acts specifically on both arteriolar and venous vascular smooth muscle. Its action is virtually immediate and evanescent, and therefore, it must be given through a carefully monitored intravenous infusion.

Nitroprusside causes variable effects on cardiac output and heart rate. These effects are related to the preexisting state of cardiac performance and are secondary to reductions in peripheral resistance and venous tone. In cases complicated by pulmonary edema, reduction of impedance to left ventricular outflow by dilating arterial resistance vessels (afterload reduction) and venous pooling aids in decreasing left ventricular end-diastolic volume and pressure. There are no demonstrable effects on the autonomic or central nervous system.

Absorption and Biotransformation

Sodium nitroprusside is a lipid-soluble, ferrocyanide compound of low molecular weight that does not bind to plasma proteins. As such, its physicochemical characteristics favor rapid and significant transplacental passage as well as potential entry into breast milk. It is metabolized to thiocyanate, which is excreted almost exclusively by the kidney. Its half-life is approximately 1 week in patients with normal renal function.

Recommended Reading

Goodlin, R. C. Fetal and maternal effects of sodium nitroprusside (letter). *Am. J. Obstet. Gynecol.* 146:350, 1983.

Goodlin, R. C. Safety of sodium nitroprusside (letter). *Obstet. Gynecol.* 62:270, 1983.

Kelly, J. V. Drugs used in the management of toxemia of pregnancy. *Clin. Obstet. Gynecol.* 20:395, 1977.

Lewis, P. E., et al. Placental transfer and fetal toxicity of sodium nitroprusside. *Gynecol. Invest.* 8:46, 1977.

Palmer, R. F., and Lasseter, K. C. Drug therapy: Sodium nitroprusside. *N. Engl. J. Med.* 292:294, 1975.

Shoemaker, C. T., and Meyers, M. Sodium nitroprusside for control of severe hypertensive disease of pregnancy: A case report and discussion of potential toxicity. *Am. J. Obstet. Gynecol.* 149:171, 1984.

Stempel, J. E., et al. Use of sodium nitroprusside in complications of gestational hypertension. *Obstet. Gynecol.* 60:533, 1982.

Spermicides

Indications and Recommendations

Spermicides are contraindicated during pregnancy, since they are used only as contraceptive agents. Those in most common use include nonoxynol-9 and octoxynol. Although it is unlikely that an individual would knowingly use a spermicide when already pregnant, it is also true that any contraceptive technique may fail, and it is thus possible to continue to use a spermicide during early pregnancy, before the contraceptive failure has been detected.

There is controversy as to the potential risk to a fetus from accidental exposure to spermicides around the time of conception. In a 1981 publication, Jick et al. reported a relative risk of 2.2 for major congenital anomalies among the offspring of 763 white women who had obtained a vaginal spermicide 600 or fewer days before delivery or abortion, compared to the offspring of 3,902 white women who had not obtained a spermicide. In particular, limb-reduction deformities, neoplasms, severe hypospadias, and chromosomal anomalies appeared to occur with increased frequency. This report was criticized for problems in ascertainment of actual spermicide use (thus, actual exposure of the fetus), for the absence of data regarding spermicide purchased outside of the health maintenance organization pharmacy involved, and for the extremely long time interval covered by 600 days between purchase and pregnancy outcomes. In addition, many critics found it significant that the incidence of these major birth defects was considerably lower among the unexposed pregnancies than would be predicted for the general population. The authors of this report considered it preliminary and suggested that further investigation would be appropriate.

In 1982, the original data from the Collaborative Perinatal Project were reanalyzed to investigate the relationship between spermicides and birth defects. Information about drug exposure was obtained by history taken before delivery. Among the 50,282 pregnant women enrolled, 462 mothers had used vaginal spermicides (other than phenylmercuric acetate, which is no longer available) during the first 16 weeks of pregnancy. Most of these mothers had also used spermicides during the month prior to conception. The relative risk for major malformations among the offspring of these spermicide users was 0.9, and they did not have an excess of the particular defects described in the Jick study. In that same year, Mills et al. reported a prospective study conducted at the Kaiser-Permanente Hospitals of northern California, in which all women registering for care over 3 years filled out a questionnaire at the first prenatal visit. Information about contraceptive use during each of the 12 months before conception was solicited. Of 34,660 women in the study, 3,146 had used spermicides before, but not after, their last menstrual period, and 2,282 had used spermicides after their last menstrual period. When the 3,146 women who used spermicides only before the last menstrual period were compared with 13,148 women who had used other forms of contraception before the last menstrual period, the relative risk for malformations was 1.04. When the 2,282 women who had used spermicides after the last menstrual period were compared with 2,831 who had used other methods, the relative risk was 1.01. Thus, again, no increased risk was associated with spermicide use. Similarly, there was no increased risk for the particular anomalies described in the Jick study.

Authors of a recent publication reviewed the 10 studies in the literature in which the relationship between spermicides and congenital malformations was explored, and concluded that the available evidence does not support an etiologic role for these agents. Nevertheless, it remains possible that a small increase in risk may exist, although this remains unconfirmed at present. From a practical perspective, since most questions will center around patients who have inadvertently used spermicides while already pregnant, it is reasonable to advise such couples that the risk, if any, is quite small compared to the general population background rate for congenital anomalies, usually quoted as upward of 3%.

Recommended Reading

Bracken, M. B. Spermicidal contraceptives and poor reproductive outcomes: The epidemiologic evidence against an association. *Am. J. Obstet. Gynecol.* 151:552, 1985.

Bracken, M. B., and Vita, K. Frequency of non-hormonal contraception around conception and association with congenital malformations in offspring. *Am. J. Epidemiol.* 117:281, 1983.

Cordero, J. F., and Layde, P. M. Vaginal spermicides, chromosomal abnormalities and limb reduction defects. *Fam. Plan. Perspec.* 15:16, 1983.

Jick, H., et al. Vaginal spermicides and congenital disorders. *J.A.M.A.* 245:1329, 1981.

Mills, J. L., et al. Are spermicides teratogenic? *J.A.M.A.* 248:2148, 1982.

Oakley, G. P., Jr. Spermicides and birth defects. *J.A.M.A.* 247:2405, 1982.

Shapiro, S., et al. Birth defects and vaginal spermicides. *J.A.M.A.* 247:2381, 1982.

Spironolactone (Aldactone®)

Indications and Recommendations

Spironolactone is contraindicated during pregnancy. If diuretics are necessary at that time, a thiazide or furosemide is preferable. Serum potassium levels should be followed closely whenever pregnant women are given diuretics. If hypokalemia develops, oral potassium supplementation will effectively correct this problem. There is, therefore, no important advantage of spironolactone over these other agents, whose effects in pregnancy are better known.

Spironolactone is a competitive antagonist of aldosterone at receptor sites in the distal renal tubules. Aldosterone normally acts to augment renal tubular reabsorption of sodium and chloride and to increase the excretion of potassium. Spironolactone has been used for the treatment of primary and secondary hyperaldosteronism and low renin level hypertension.

It also has antiandrogenic effects, probably through competitive inhibition at the level of testosterone, dihydrotestosterone (DHT), and androstenedione receptors. The drug has, therefore, been used to treat idiopathic hirsutism in females, as well as prostate carcinoma and precocious puberty in males. Messina and coworkers have shown that daily administration of 40-mg doses of spironolactone to pregnant rats between the thirteenth and twenty-first day of gestation produced anomalies of the external genitalia in male fetuses. The defects observed included reduction of the anogenital distance, urethral malformations, and altered prostate development.

The effects of this drug on uterine blood flow and the human fetus have not been well studied. Metabolic products may appear in breast milk.

Recommended Reading

Gifford, R. W., Jr. A guide to the practical use of diuretics. *J.A.M.A.* 235:1890, 1976.

Gilman, A. G., Goodman, L. S., and Gilman, A. *The Pharmacological Basis of Therapeutics* (6th ed.). New York: Macmillan, 1980. Pp. 907–908.

Messina, M., et al. Possible contraindications of spironolactone during pregnancy (letter). *J. Endocrinol. Invest.* 2:222, 1979.

Molinatti, G. M. Can the anti-androgenic effect of spironolactone contraindicate its use in pregnancy? *Minerva Ginecol.* 32:239, 1980.

Streptokinase (Streptase®)

Indications and Recommendations

The use of streptokinase for thrombolysis during pregnancy is contraindicated. Streptokinase is used primarily in the treatment of extensive pulmonary emboli, coronary venous thrombosis, deep venous thrombosis, and occluded arteriovenous cannulae. It acts to stimulate the conversion of plasminogen to plasmin, a proteolytic enzyme that hydrolyzes fibrin. Because of its ability to alter hemostasis profoundly and thereby to cause both internal and superficial bleeding, it must be used in all patients with great care. This risk of bleeding may be of particular significance in the pregnant patient. If anticoagulant therapy is required during pregnancy, heparin should be used.

In one report, a patient who received streptokinase for 41 hours through labor and delivery developed a slow but persistent postpartum hemorrhage associated with failure of the uterus to remain firmly contracted despite large doses of oxytocics. It was, therefore, recommended by the authors that if streptokinase is used near term, it should be discontinued 4–6 hours before delivery.

Streptokinase does not cross the placenta in significant amounts and infants exposed to streptokinase in utero do not exhibit evidence of fibrinolytic activation. However, streptokinase antibodies can be detected in cord and neonatal blood immediately after birth. These antibodies may cause passive sensitization of the fetus as a result of antepartum maternal therapy. Such sensitization is of no clinical importance unless the neonate later requires streptokinase therapy.

Recommended Reading

Bell, W. R., and Meek, A. G. Guidelines for the use of thrombolytic agents. *N. Engl. J. Med.* 301:1206, 1979.

Gilman, A. G., Goodman, L. S., and Gilman, A. *The Pharmacological Basis of Therapeutics* (6th ed.). New York: Macmillan, 1980. P. 1362.

Hall, R. J. C., et al. Treatment of acute massive pulmonary embolism by streptokinase during labour and delivery. *Br. Med. J.* 4:647, 1972.

Ludwig, H. Results of streptokinase therapy in deep venous thrombosis during pregnancy. *Postgrad. Med. J.* (Suppl. 5):65, 1973.

Pfeifer, G. W. Distribution and placental transfer of 131-I streptokinase. *Australas. Ann. Med.* 19(Suppl.):17, 1970.

Sulfonamides: Sulfadiazine, Sulfamethizole (Thiosulfil Forte®), Sulfamethoxazole (Gantanol®), Sulfisoxazole (Gantrisin®)

Indications and Recommendations

Sulfonamides are contraindicated during the last 3 months of pregnancy but may be administered earlier in pregnancy to treat urinary tract infections. These agents are antibiotics with a wide range of activity against both gram-positive and gram-negative organisms. They should not be used during the last 3 months of pregnancy because of the danger of kernicterus to the neonate. If premature delivery is anticipated, these agents should not be administered at any time during the third trimester.

Special Considerations in Pregnancy

There are no unusual maternal effects of sulfonamides during pregnancy. These drugs rapidly cross the placenta and appear in amniotic fluid at a slower rate than in fetal blood. They compete with bilirubin for binding with albumin. In utero the fetus can clear free bilirubin through the placental circulation, but in the neonatal period this route of clearance no longer exists. In the neonate elevated levels of free bilirubin traverse the blood-brain barrier, where binding to the basal ganglia, with subsequent kernicterus, may occur.

Sulfonamides appear in breast milk. Infants with glucose 6-phosphate dehydrogenase (G6PD) deficiency might develop hemolytic anemia if nursed by mothers taking sulfonamides. Theoretically, the chance of kernicterus might also be increased in babies with an Rh or ABO incompatibility.

Dosage

Table 12 details recommended dosages.

Adverse Effects

Frequent side effects consist of allergic reactions that include rash, photosensitivity, and drug fever. Rarely, these drugs can cause hepatic damage; vasculitis, hemolytic anemia, especially in those with G6PD deficiency; and other blood dyscrasias. The long-acting sulfonamides may be associated with the Stevens-Johnson syndrome and can increase the effects of oral anticoagulants. Renal damage may occur as a result of crystalluria, the risk of which, however, may be diminished by maintaining a high urine output.

Mechanism of Action

The relative antibacterial differences in this group are insignificant and preferences for one agent over another are based on pharmacologic or toxicologic considerations. They compete with the para-

Table 12. Dosage chart for sulfonamides

Drug	Oral Dosage (g)	Interval	Usual maximum dose/day (g)
Sulfadiazine	0.5–1.0	q4–6h	8
Sulfisoxazole	0.5–1.0	q4–6h	8
Sulfamethizole	0.5–1.0	q4–6h	8
Sulfamethoxazole	1.0	q8–12h	8

aminobenzoic acid utilized by bacteria for the synthesis of folic acid and act as bacteriostatic agents. They are used primarily to treat urinary tract infections due to susceptible organisms. Other indications for their use include chancroid, trachoma, inclusion conjunctivitis, and nocardiosis.

Absorption and Biotransformation

Sulfonamides are rapidly absorbed from the small intestine and stomach. They quickly bind to albumin and are distributed throughout all the tissues of the body. About 10–40% is metabolized by acetylation to the inactive form. Both free and acetylated metabolites are excreted in the urine.

Recommended Reading

Davies, D. M. *Textbook of Adverse Drug Reactions*. Oxford, Engl.: Oxford University, 1977. P. 70.

Gilman, A. G., Goodman, L. S., and Gilman, A. *The Pharmacological Basis of Therapeutics* (6th ed.). New York: Macmillan, 1980.

Handbook of Antimicrobial Therapy. The Medical Letter on Drugs and Therapeutics (rev. ed.). New Rochelle, N.Y.: The Medical Letter, 1978.

Landers, D. V., Green, J. R., and Sweet, R. L. Antibiotic use during pregnancy and the postpartum period. *Clin. Obstet. Gynecol.* 26:391, 1983.

Update: Drugs in breast milk. *Med. Lett. Drugs Ther.* 21:21, 1979.

Sulfonylureas: Acetohexamide (Dymelor®), Chlorpropamide (Diabinese®), Glipizide (Glucotrol®), Glyburide (DiaBeta®, Micronase®), Tolazamide (Tolinase®), Tolbutamide (Orinase®)

Indications and Recommendations

Sulfonylureas are relatively contraindicated during pregnancy because other therapeutic agents are preferable. These drugs are orally administered to lower the blood glucose in mild nonketosis-prone (type II) diabetics. Their mechanism of action includes stimulation of pancreatic beta cells with increased release of endogenous insulin, and a presumed effect on both hepatic and peripheral insulin sensitivity.

Some studies have shown increased perinatal mortality when pregnant diabetics were treated with sulfonylureas rather than insulin, while other series have not borne out this finding. There is evidence of teratogenicity in laboratory animals given high doses of some of the sulfonylureas, and case reports of birth defects among offspring of sulfonylurea-treated human pregnancies have been published. However, it should be remembered that maternal diabetes is a powerful teratogen, and there are no well-controlled human studies implicating sulfonylureas in congenital malformations.

It is known that tolbutamide and chlorpropamide cross the placenta easily. Less is known about the other agents. Since it is widely believed that fetal hyperinsulinemia is the primary cause of the various manifestations of diabetic fetopathy, it would be illogical to treat maternal diabetes with drugs that would be expected to stimulate fetal insulin secretion. Although a number of investigators have used oral hypoglycemic agents in series of diabetic pregnancies without obvious ill effects on the fetus or neonate, there have been a number of isolated case reports of prolonged neonatal hypoglycemia when the mothers were taking these drugs. A case of transient neonatal diabetes insipidus (as well as hypoglycemia) was reported in the offspring of a mother taking chlorpropamide.

It is recommended that sulfonylureas not be used during pregnancy because of the relative lack of data regarding their safety and efficacy. When diabetes is present during pregnancy, insulin is the drug of choice.

Recommended Reading

Adam, P. A. J., and Schwartz, R. Diagnosis and treatment: Should oral hypoglycemic agents be used in pediatric and pregnant patients? *Pediatrics* 42:819, 1968.

Coetzee, E. J., and Jackson, W. P. U. Metformin in management of pregnant insulin-independent diabetics. *Diabetologia* 16:241, 1979.

Douglas, C. P., and Richards, R. Use of chlorpropamide in the treatment of diabetes in pregnancy. *Diabetes* 16:60, 1967.

Kemball, M. L., et al. Neonatal hypoglycaemia in infants of diabetic mothers given sulphonylurea drugs in pregnancy. *Arch. Dis. Child.* 45:696, 1970.

Kolterman, O. G., et al. The acute and chronic effects of sulfonylurea therapy in type II diabetic subjects. *Diabetes* 33:346, 1984.

Notelovitz, M., and James, S. Tolbutamide-induced insulin release in pregnant diabetics. *Horm. Metab. Res.* 9:167, 1977.

Sutherland, H. W., et al. Evaluation of chlorpropamide in chemical diabetes diagnosed during pregnancy. *Br. Med. J.* 3:9, 1973.

Uhrig, J. D., and Hurley, R. M. Chlorpropamide in pregnancy and transient neonatal diabetes insipidus. *Can. Med. Assoc. J.* 128:368, 1983.

Sympathomimetics (over-the-counter): Ephedrine, Phenylephrine, Phenylpropanolamine

Indications and Recommendations

Sympathomimetics are generally safe to use during pregnancy, although they should be avoided in patients with essential hypertension or toxemia because of their potential for elevating systemic blood pressure. They should also be avoided in situations in which there is poor fetal reserve, as distress in utero could be precipitated.

Members of this group of drugs are used in expectorants, decongestants, cough and cold medications, antiasthmatic combinations, and ophthalmic decongestants and vasoconstrictors. As a general policy, it is wise to avoid all medications during the first trimester whenever possible. These drugs should therefore not be used indiscriminately for upper respiratory symptoms during the period of embryogenesis, but should be reserved for conditions that create significant maternal discomfort.

Special Considerations in Pregnancy

There are no maternal side effects unique to pregnancy. These substances cross the placental and blood-brain barriers, and fetal central nervous system effects may include hyperactivity and irritability following maternal ingestion. The fetus may also develop a tachycardia. Maternal hypertension could stress a compromised fetus. Congenital anomalies have not been associated with the use of sympathomimetics in over-the-counter (OTC) preparations.

The Collaborative Perinatal Project found no evidence of an increase in major or minor anomalies when ephedrine was taken in the first trimester. Phenylephrine and phenylpropanolamine were associated with a slight increase in the incidence of minor abnormalities such as clubfoot and inguinal hernia, as well as eye or ear deformities, when taken in the first trimester. It should be noted, however, that quite often more than one compound was used in the same preparation. Furthermore, it was impossible to determine whether viral infections were present and possibly responsible for the associations observed.

Dosage

The dosage varies with the preparation being used. This group of drugs is most effective when administered orally. Their onset of action is rapid, and they are effective for hours because of their resistance to inactivating enzymes.

Adverse Effects

Side effects from sympathomimetics include insomnia, anxiety, headache, tremor, dizziness, palpitations, anorexia, nausea, vomiting, abdominal cramps, and diarrhea.

Mechanism of Action

The sympathomimetic drugs used in OTC preparations are primarily noncatecholamines. They may act directly on effector cells or act indirectly by stimulating the release of norepinephrine from adrenergic nerve endings. The structure of each substance determines its predominant mode of action.

Ephedrine causes norepinephrine release and has alpha-receptor effects. It also has a direct effect on beta receptors in the bronchial tree, resulting in a relaxation of bronchospasm. Phenylephrine acts directly on alpha receptors, especially in the heart; it has little effect on beta receptors, however.

Ephedrine and phenylpropanolamine may cause an increase in systolic and diastolic blood pressures as well as cardiac output. They may also increase alertness, decrease fatigue, and cause mild mood elevation. Phenylephrine can elevate both systolic and diastolic blood pressures and increase circulation time and venous pressure. It may also be associated with a reflex bradycardia.

Absorption and Biotransformation

The sympathomimetics included in OTC preparations are generally well absorbed from the gastrointestinal tract. Their metabolic pathways include hydroxylation, N-demethylation, deamination, and conjugation in the liver, followed by urinary excretion. They may also be excreted unchanged by the kidneys, the amount depending on urinary pH.

Recommended Reading

Gilman, A. G., Goodman, L. S., and Gilman, A. *The Pharmacological Basis of Therapeutics* (6th ed.). New York: Macmillan, 1980. Pp. 163–175.

Heinonen, O. P., Slone, D., and Shapiro, S. *Birth Defects and Drugs in Pregnancy.* Littleton, Mass.: Publishing Sciences Group, 1977. Pp. 345–356, 439.

Jick, H., Aselton, P., and Hunter, J. R. Phenylpropanolamine and cerebral hemorrhage. *Lancet* 1:1017, 1984.

Lasagna, L. Phenylpropanolamine and blood pressure (letters). *J.A.M.A.* 253:2491, 1985.

Nelson, M. M., and Forfar, J. O. Associations between drugs administered during pregnancy and congenital abnormalities of the fetus. *Br. Med. J.* 1:523, 1971.

Noble, R. E. Phenylpropanolamine and blood pressure. *Lancet* 1:1419, 1982.

Pentel, P. Toxicity of over-the-counter stimulants. *J.A.M.A.* 252:1898, 1984.

Schenkel, B., and Vorherr, H. Non-prescription drugs during pregnancy: Potential teratogenic and toxic effects upon embryo and fetus. *J. Reprod. Med.* 12:27, 1974.

Terbutaline (Brethine®)

Indications and Recommendations

The use of terbutaline as an antiasthmatic agent during pregnancy should be limited to the treatment of those patients who remain symptomatic though receiving maximum dosages of theophylline. Patients who take terbutaline orally may use an aerosol form of another beta-2 adrenergic agent at the same time. Concurrent use of other *systemic* beta-2 sympathomimetics should be avoided because of the unpleasant side effects associated with excessive adrenergic stimulation.

Terbutaline has been extensively used to arrest premature labor; however, it has not yet been approved by the FDA for this purpose. Ritodrine, another beta-2 sympathomimetic agent with equal effectiveness, is the only drug currently approved for the treatment of premature labor.

Special Considerations in Pregnancy

There are no published reports of teratogenesis in humans who use terbutaline, although controlled studies establishing its safety early in gestation are not available.

The effectiveness of terbutaline in inhibiting premature labor has been demonstrated in several clinical trials. One double-blind controlled study found that 80% of patients' premature labor was arrested with terbutaline as compared to 20% in the control group. In addition, this drug has been shown to decrease both spontaneous and oxytocin-stimulated labor at full term. This effect was seen even in the second stage of labor. Terbutaline has been used to treat acute intrapartum fetal distress, but reports are limited in this area.

Various beta-sympathomimetic agents, including ritodrine and terbutaline, have been reported to cause pulmonary edema when used in the treatment of premature labor. The precise mechanism for this adverse effect is in dispute. Katz et al., in a retrospective analysis of 160 patients, found an incidence of severe cardiovascular complications of 5% when intravenous terbutaline was used to treat premature labor. The most common problems encountered were pulmonary edema and/or electrocardiographic (ECG) changes indicative of myocardial ischemia. All of these incidents occurred after at least 24 hours of terbutaline infusion, and the majority of patients had pulse rates in excess of 140 beats/minute. Administration of corticosteroids and the presence of a multiple gestation increased the risk of complications, although pulmonary edema *did* occur in three patients who did not receive steroids.

On the other hand, Ingemarsson and Bengtsson, in an analysis of 330 patients treated with intravenous terbutaline as a tocolytic agent, found no cases of pulmonary edema or any other serious cardiovascular complication. Sixty-five of these patients also were given corticosteroids. In this study, however, intravenous fluid administration was carefully monitored, dextrose in water was used instead of normal saline, and the infusion rate of the drug was not increased further if the maternal pulse exceeded 120 beats/minute. Only 2.7% of the patients developed side effects that led to discontinuation of terbutaline therapy. The most common problems in this small group were nausea, vomiting, and tachycardia. It, therefore, seems that terbutaline can be used safely in the treatment of premature labor if careful attention is paid to the amount of fluid infused and the maternal pulse rate. In addition, maternal potassium and glucose levels should be monitored and a baseline ECG obtained. Diabetic mothers who take this drug may need increased dosages of insulin to maintain adequate diabetic control.

Wagner and coworkers studied pregnant patients with echocardiography during terbutaline administration and found increased chronotropic and isotropic activity. This was evidenced by increased heart rate, ejection fraction, and cardiac output as well as decreased end-systolic volume. In addition, terbutaline caused a decrease in systemic vascular resistance.

Terbutaline has been reported to cross the placenta readily after a single injection before delivery. Average cord blood–maternal vein concentration ratios range between 0.36 and 0.64. An increase in fetal heart rate has been observed after parenteral administration of the drug to pregnant women. Follow-up study of infants exposed to terbutaline in the second half of pregnancy reveals a modest rise in the incidence of postnatal hypoglycemia, but no other short- or long-term sequelae. Therefore, newborns exposed to this drug in utero should be observed for hypoglycemia.

The breast milk concentrations of terbutaline in a small number of nursing mothers treated for asthma were found to be similar or higher than maternal plasma concentrations. However, the drug was not detectable in the nursing infants' plasma, and no symptoms of beta-adrenoreceptor stimulation could be found in any of the babies.

Dosage

For treatment of asthma, the oral dose is 2.5–5.0 mg q6–8h, with onset of action in about 30 minutes. Peak effect occurs in 2–3 hours, and the duration of action is usually 4–6 hours. The subcutaneous dose is 0.25 mg, which may be repeated in 30 minutes if no clinical response occurs. If there is still no clinical response within the next half-hour, other measures should be taken to treat the bronchospasm. The onset of action of subcutaneous terbutaline is about 15 minutes, peak effect occurs in 30–60 minutes, and the duration of action is 1.5–4.0 hours.

Terbutaline aerosols are marketed elsewhere but are not currently available in the United States.

Terbutaline has not been approved by the FDA for the treatment of premature labor, but because of the extensive experience in Europe and the United States, many centers do use it for this purpose. The recommended intravenous dose is 10–25 μg/minute. The subcutaneous dose is 0.25 mg q6h for 3 days. Once premature labor is arrested, oral treatment can be commenced with 2.5–7.5 mg q6h. This regimen is continued up to 36–37 weeks' gestation.

Adverse Effects

Side effects include tachycardia, palpitations, headache, nausea, vomiting, anxiety, sweating, tremor, and tinnitus. These side effects are generally transient and do not require treatment.

Other common sequelae include maternal hyperglycemia, hypokalemia, mild anemia, increased free fatty acids and glycerol, and fetal tachycardia. Hypokalemia is generally believed to be secondary to the hyperglycemia and hyperinsulinemia that drive serum potassium into the cells. Since there is no loss of potassium from the body, serum levels quickly return to baseline values after terbutaline is discontinued. When present, the hypokalemia is usually asymptomatic and rarely requires treatment.

Mechanism of Action

Terbutaline is a sympathomimetic agent with predominantly beta-2 activity. It is believed that sympathomimetics work by stimulating adenyl cyclase, the enzyme that catalyzes the conversion of adenosine triphosphate to cyclic AMP.

Terbutaline produces significant bronchodilatation, which may result in an increased vital capacity, forced expiratory volume in 1 second (FEV_1), peak expiratory flow (PEF), and maximum expiratory flow (MEF) in asthmatic patients. It is also effective in decreasing uterine activity during the second and third trimesters. In pregnant ewes and baboons, uterine blood flow is not decreased by the dosages required to inhibit premature labor.

Absorption and Biotransformation

Approximately 30–55% of an oral dose is absorbed from the gastrointestinal tract. Terbutaline is metabolized in the liver, primarily to an inactive sulfated conjugate, and after being metabolized is excreted in the urine. Only 1% of a subcutaneously administered dose is recovered from bile, indicating the absence of a significant enterohepatic circulation. Excretion of the drug and its metabolites is essentially complete within 72–96 hours after the administration of a single parenteral or oral dose.

Recommended Reading

Andersson, K. E., et al. The relaxing effect of terbutaline on the human uterus during term labor. *Am. J. Obstet. Gynecol.* 121:602, 1975.

Andersson, K. E., Bengtsson, L. P., and Ingemarsson, I. Terbutaline inhibition of midtrimester uterine activity induced by prostaglandin $F_{2\alpha}$ and hypertonic saline. *Br. J. Obstet. Gynaecol.* 82:745, 1975.

Arner, B. A comparative clinical trial of different subcutaneous doses of terbutaline and orciprenaline in bronchial asthma. *Acta Med. Scand.* 512(Suppl.):45, 1970.

Arner, B., et al. Circulatory effects of orciprenaline, adrenaline and a new sympathomimetic β-receptor–stimulating agent, terbutaline, in normal human subjects. *Acta Med. Scand.* 512(Suppl.):25, 1970.

Carlstrom, S., and Westling, H. Metabolic, circulatory and respiratory effects of a new sympathomimetic β-receptor–stimulating agent, terbutaline, compared with those of orciprenaline. *Acta Med. Scand.* 512(Suppl.):33, 1970.

Ingemarsson, I. Effects of terbutaline on premature labor. A double-blind placebo-controlled study. *Am. J. Obstet. Gynecol.* 125:520, 1976.

Ingemarsson, I., and Bengtsson, B. A five-year experience with terbutaline for preterm labor: Low rate of severe side effects. *Obstet. Gynecol.* 66:176, 1985.

Katz, M., Robertson, P. A., and Creasy, R. K. Cardiovascular complications associated with terbutaline treatment for preterm labor. *Am. J. Obstet. Gynecol.* 139:605, 1981.

Sackner, M. A., et al. Hemodynamic effects of epinephrine and terbutaline in normal man. *Chest* 68:616, 1975.

Svenningsen, N. W. Followup studies on preterm infants after maternal beta receptor agonist treatment. *Acta Obstet. Gynecol. Scand.* 108:67, 1982.

Wagner, J. M., et al. Terbutaline and maternal cardiac function. *J.A.M.A.* 246:2697, 1981.

Tetracyclines: Demeclocycline (Declomycin®), Oxytetracycline (Terramycin®), Tetracycline (Achromycin®, Sumycin®)

Indications and Recommendations

Tetracyclines are contraindicated during pregnancy. These broad-spectrum antibiotics cross the placenta and are deposited in fetal teeth and bones. Because of adverse effects on these fetal organs, and potential maternal hepatotoxicity, other antibiotics should be used in the pregnant woman.

The deciduous teeth begin to mineralize at approximately 14 weeks of gestation. This process continues until 2–3 months after birth. Staining of deciduous teeth is most likely when tetracyclines are administered after the twenty-fifth week.

In one study, when tetracycline was administered to premature newborns a 40% depression of normal skeletal growth resulted. Although this process was rapidly reversed by discontinuing the drug, chronic tetracycline use by a pregnant woman in the third trimester can be expected to have an effect on fetal bone growth.

Hepatotoxicity in the form of acute fatty liver, leading to death in some cases, has been reported in pregnant women treated with tetracyclines in large dosages. In most of these women, the drug was administered intravenously for treatment of pyelonephritis. In addition, low-dose chronic therapy before conception has been reported to result in fatal hepatotoxicity. It is speculated that with chronic use, tetracyclines are deposited in bone and are released during periods of bone turnover, including pregnancy, at which time they damage the liver.

Occasionally tetracyclines are inadvertently taken during the first trimester. Although these drugs have been associated with congenital anomalies in rats, the data pertaining to humans are, at best, anecdotal. While tetracycline is not recommended for the pregnant woman, the data currently available do not support a recommendation for abortion if inadvertent first-trimester exposure occurs.

Recommended Reading

Carter, M. P., and Wilson, F. Antibiotics and congenital malformations. *Lancet* 1:2367, 1963.

Cohlan, S. Q., Bevelander, G., and Tiamsie, T. Growth inhibition of prematures receiving tetracycline. *Am. J. Dis. Child.* 103:453, 1963.

Gilman, A. G., Goodman, L. S., and Gilman, A. *The Pharmacological Basis of Therapeutics* (6th ed.). New York: Macmillan, 1980. Pp. 1181–1191.

Harley, J. D., et al. Aromatic drugs and congenital cataracts. *Lancet* 1:472, 1964.

Kucers, A., and Bennett, N. McK. *The Use of Antibiotics* (2nd ed.). London: William Heinemann, 1975. Pp. 381–416.

Kunelis, C. T., Peters, J. L., and Edmondson, H. A. Fatty liver of pregnancy and its relationship to tetracycline therapy. *Am. J. Med.* 38:359, 1967.

Wenk, R. E., Gebhart, F. C., and Bhagavan, B. S. Tetracycline-associated fatty liver of pregnancy, including possible pregnancy risk after chronic dermatologic use of tetracycline. *J. Reprod. Med.* 26:135, 1981.

Whalley, P. J., Adams, R. H., and Combes, B. Tetracycline toxicity in pregnancy. *J.A.M.A.* 189:357, 1964.

Wilson, W. R., and Cockerill, F. R. Tetracyclines, chloramphenicol, erythromycin, and clindamycin. *Mayo Clin. Proc.* 58:92, 1983.

Theophylline and Aminophylline (Aminodur®, Elixophyllin®, Slo-Phyllin®, Somophyllin®, Theo-Dur®)

Indications and Recommendations

Theophylline is safe to use during pregnancy. It is a bronchodilator and the drug of choice for the treatment of asthma in pregnant patients. Theophylline may also be used as an adjunctive agent in the therapy of acute pulmonary edema and in some cases of Cheyne-Stokes respirations.

Blood levels should be monitored in patients receiving theophylline by any route, but clinical response should be the main guide to therapy. When the drug is administered orally, peak and trough levels should be monitored. Patients given the drug intravenously should undergo cardiac monitoring. Appropriate adjustment of dosage should be made in patients with congestive heart failure and severe liver impairment.

Neonates exposed to theophylline in utero as well as those ingesting it in breast milk should be observed for evidence of toxicity. Breast-feeding women should nurse their infants just before taking the drug in order to decrease the quantity of drug passing over to the neonate.

Special Considerations in Pregnancy

In pregnant women and newborn infants, the binding affinity of plasma protein for many drugs is decreased. Since only the unbound drugs in plasma are generally considered to be pharmacologically active, an enhanced response may be obtained in pregnant women when compared to their nonpregnant counterparts at similar total plasma theophylline concentrations. On the other hand, because of a larger volume of distribution, pregnant women may require a higher dosage to reach a given plasma concentration.

When two mother-neonate pairs were investigated, cord serum theophylline levels were equal to, or slightly higher than, maternal levels at delivery. Neonatal theophylline levels remained near or within the therapeutic range for at least 18 hours after birth, but fell to minimal levels at 30 hours. One of the two infants was noted to be jittery, but no other toxic effects were observed. In a second report, 12 newborns of asthmatic mothers were found to have cord blood theophylline levels similar to the levels in their mothers, with a few infants manifesting tachycardia and transient jitteriness. As in the previous report, neonatal heelstick theophylline levels tended to be higher than maternal levels.

Theophylline appears to be mutagenic only in lower organisms. This may be due to the inability of those animals to demethylate this compound, a process that takes place readily in humans. A single case report describes chromosomal abnormalities in association with ingestion of theophylline by the mother, but this remains an isolated occurrence to date. The limited data available appear to support the impression that teratogenesis with theophylline is unlikely.

In a randomized trial of maternal aminophylline therapy (250 mg IM q12h for 3 days), 70 neonates of treated mothers who delivered before 34 weeks' gestation were compared to 78 born to untreated control mothers. The infants of aminophylline-treated mothers had a significantly lower incidence of perinatal death and respiratory distress syndrome. Confirmatory studies are not available.

Toxicity can occur by transplacental passage of the drug or in breast-fed infants. Toxic levels have not been well defined and vary from one infant to another. Symptoms may include vomiting, feeding difficulties, jitteriness, tachycardia, cardiac arrhythmias, and transient hyperglycemia. Theophylline concentration in breast milk reaches its peak 1–3 hours after an oral dose. The milk concentration parallels the serum concentration at a mean milk-serum ratio of 0.73. The drug is not bound to protein in breast milk.

Dosage

The therapeutic range for theophylline in plasma is 10–20 µg/ml in the nonpregnant woman. Lower levels may possibly suffice during pregnancy. Dosages should be adjusted downward for patients with liver disease or congestive heart failure.

The only intravenous preparation available is aminophylline (theophylline ethylenediamine), which is 86% theophylline by weight. It has been recommended that in the treatment of status asthmaticus a loading dose of 6 mg/kg given over 20 minutes be followed by a maintenance infusion of 0.7 mg/kg/hour aminophylline (equivalent to 0.6 mg/kg/hour anhydrous theophylline) in nonsmokers and 1.0 mg/kg/hour (equivalent to 0.85 mg/kg/hour theophylline) in smokers. If the patient continues to have bronchospasm and does not have signs of toxicity, a further increase can be attempted if plasma levels are not in the therapeutic range. After a bolus dose of 3 mg/kg given over 20 minutes, the maintenance infusion rate may be increased to 1.3–1.5 mg/kg/hour depending on the plasma level. If the patient has been taking theophylline orally in adequate amounts, half the loading dose described previously and the same maintenance dosage should be administered. If she has been taking the drug erratically, it is probably best to proceed as if she were not taking it at all.

Oral theophylline is used for the long-term treatment of bronchospasm. Plain, enteric-coated, and sustained-release preparations are available. The use of enteric-coated preparations is not recommended as absorption is unpredictable. Plain theophylline or aminophylline tablets or liquids are usually taken q6h. Sustained-release preparations have the advantage of an 8- to 12-hour dose interval.

Theophylline can be given rectally as either a suppository or a solution. The use of suppositories is not recommended as they tend to be absorbed erratically and can produce unpredictable and dangerous blood levels. Rectal solutions are more predictably absorbed and produce less proctitis. Rectal solutions may be administered as follows: aminophylline solution, 300 mg/5 ml, q8–12h, or theophylline monoethanolamine, 250 mg/30 ml or 500 mg/30 ml, q8–12h.

Adverse Effects

Side effects and toxicity are related in most cases to plasma concentrations of the drug. They are usually of minor significance when the drug is maintained within the usual therapeutic range. Side effects include anorexia, nausea, vomiting, diuresis, and abdominal distention. Palpitations and sinus and atrial tachycardias may occur. Precordial pain and hypotension have been reported with rapid intravenous administration of aminophylline. Excitation, anxiety, insomnia, diaphoresis, tremor, and even convulsions may occur. The latter is a toxic phenomenon and is usually seen with plasma levels close to 60 μg/ml.

Mechanism of Action

The actions of theophylline are mediated through its inhibition of phosphodiesterase, the enzyme responsible for the degradation of cyclic AMP. Increase in the intracellular concentration of cyclic AMP produces smooth muscle relaxation.

The primary action of theophylline is to relax bronchiolar smooth muscle, especially during muscle spasm. It also sensitizes the respiratory center to carbon dioxide, causing an increase in both respiratory rate and depth. It has both inotropic and chronotropic effects on the myocardium and causes vasodilatation in the pulmonary, coronary, and systemic circulations. Cardiac output is increased and venous filling pressure is reduced. Theophylline is a central nervous system stimulant and has been used to treat apnea in the premature infant. It also increases gastric secretion and decreases small and large bowel motility. In addition, catecholamine release may be stimulated.

Absorption and Biotransformation

Ninety percent of an oral dose reaches the circulation, and absorption is better in the fasting state. Peak concentrations are achieved between 1 and 3 hours after administration of uncoated tablets and in 30 minutes with elixir and solutions. Theophylline is metabolized by the liver and excreted in the urine. Sixty percent of the drug is bound to plasma proteins at therapeutic concentrations. It does not displace bilirubin from albumin. The half-life is usually 4–5 hours in adults but may be elevated in patients with liver disease or congestive failure.

Recommended Reading

Arwood, L. L., Dasta, J. D., and Friedman, C. Placental transfer of theophylline: Two case reports. *Pediatrics* 63:844, 1979.

Hadjigeorgiou, E., et al. Antepartum aminophylline treatment for prevention of the respiratory distress syndrome in premature infants. *Am. J. Obstet. Gynecol.* 135:257, 1979.

I.V. dosage guidelines for theophylline products. *F.D.A. Drug Bull.* 10:4, 1980.

Labovitz, E., and Specter, S. Placental theophylline transfer in pregnant asthmatics. *J.A.M.A.* 247:786, 1982.

Mitenko, P. A., and Ogilvie, R. I. Pharmacokinetics of intravenous theophylline. *Clin. Pharmacol. Ther.* 14:509, 1973.

Mitenko, P. A., and Ogilvie, R. I. Rational intravenous doses of theophylline *N. Engl. J. Med.* 289:600, 1973.

Mitenko, P. A., and Oglivie, R. I. Bioavailability and efficacy of a sustained release theophylline tablet. *Clin. Pharmacol. Ther.* 16:720, 1974.

Pollowitz, J. A. Theophylline therapy during pregnancy. *J.A.M.A.* 243:651, 1980.

Salem, H., and Jackson, R. H. Oral theophylline preparations–a review of their clinical efficacy in the treatment of bronchial asthma. *Ann. Allergy* 32:189, 1974.

Timson, J. Theobromine-theophylline. *Mutat. Res.* 32:169, 1975.

Yeh, T. F., and Pildes, R. S. Transplacental aminophylline toxicity in a neonate (letter). *Lancet* 1:910, 1977.

Yurchak, A. M., and Jusko, W. J. Theophylline secretion into breast milk. *Pediatrics* 57:518, 1976.

Thioamides: Carbimazole, Methimazole (Tapazole®), Propylthiouracil

Indications and Recommendations

The thioamides, carbimazole, propylthiouracil (PTU), and methimazole, are antithyroid drugs used in the treatment of hyperthyroidism. Although these drugs cross the placenta and may cause fetal goiter, they are generally regarded as the treatment of choice for hyperthyroidism during pregnancy. They should be used in the lowest dosage compatible with treatment goals, and it is usually possible to reduce the dosage during the third trimester. There is currently no documented advantage to using totally suppressive dosages of these drugs combined with thyroid replacement therapy.

Special Considerations in Pregnancy

Since thioamides cross the placenta, fetal thyroid suppression may result, with increased thyroid-stimulating hormone (TSH) levels resulting in stimulation of the fetal thyroid gland. This stimulation may rarely result in fetal goiter, which, in turn, can cause hyperextension of the fetal head leading to dystocia during labor. Modest doses of PTU (100–200 mg/day) given to 11 hyperthyroid mothers were associated with chemical evidence of hypothyroidism (i.e., low T4 and reverse T3 levels, elevated TSH) in the offspring, compared to 40 control neonates. One of the newborns met the clinical criteria for hypothyroidism, but the condition lasted less than 2 weeks.

If a pregnant woman has autoimmune hyperthyroidism, thyroid-stimulating immunoglobulin G (IgG) may cross the placenta and cause fetal and neonatal thyrotoxicosis. If such a patient is treated with a thioamide, the resulting transient neonatal hypothyroidism may temporarily mask thyrotoxicosis until the effects of the thioamide have dissipated. Unfortunately, such a neonate may be discharged from the hospital before the thyrotoxicosis is manifested, with a resultant delay in diagnosis. Awareness of this problem will permit appropriate short-term follow-up studies to be scheduled.

In one long-term follow-up study, 18 children born to PTU-treated mothers were compared to 17 siblings born at a time when the mothers were not taking PTU. There were no differences in intellectual or motor function between the two groups.

Intrauterine fetal therapy (PTU given to the mother) has been successfully used to prevent fetal hyperthyroidism and growth retardation in a patient with Hashimoto's thyroiditis. This woman was hypothyroid, but had high levels of thyroid-stimulating immunoglobulins diagnosed because of the previous delivery of a hyperthyroid growth-retarded baby.

Both PTU and methimazole inhibit thyroid hormone synthesis but only the former blocks the conversion of T4 to T3. Furthermore, methimazole administration during pregnancy has been associated with aplasia cutis in the offspring. For these reasons, PTU is the more widely used of the two drugs in obstetric patients.

Although old data on thiouracil suggested that significant amounts of this compound appeared in breast milk, a more recent report on nine mother-infant pairs showed breast milk concentrations of PTU 1.5 hours after the ingestion of 400 mg to be only 10% of maternal serum concentrations. The total amount of PTU appearing in breast milk during the 4 hours after maternal ingestion was 0.025% of the administered dose. No abnormalities in thyroid function tests were found in a suckling baby followed for 5 months, during which time the mother took 200–300 mg PTU daily. Methimazole, on the other hand, has been found in approximately equal concentrations in breast milk and maternal serum, with 0.18% of the maternal dose appearing in the milk over 8 hours. Thus, PTU appears to be safer than methimazole for treatment of nursing mothers.

Dosage

Propylthiouracil is available in 50-mg tablets that can be broken in half. Methimazole is manufactured in 5- and 10-mg tablets. Carbimazole, available mainly in Europe, comes as 5- and 10-mg tablets. The usual starting dose is 100 mg PTU, or 5–10 mg methimazole, taken q8h. Because PTU has such a short half-life, a single daily dose of 300 mg is usually not effective.

Although serum PTU levels of 3 $\mu g/ml$ have been shown to halve thyroid function, it is currently impractical to monitor this drug by measurement of serum levels. Thus, its efficacy is titrated by the patient's clinical response and by measurement of serum thyroid hormone levels. It should be borne in mind that many symptoms are common to both hyperthyroidism and pregnancy, and that the total T4 level is increased during normal pregnancy due to increased protein binding. Thus, an estimate of the free thyroxine level is the most useful parameter to follow. The goal of therapy should be maintenance of the free thyroxine level in the high-normal or slightly elevated range. It is sometimes necessary to use doses as high as 1,000 mg/day PTU in order to achieve euthyroidism. Although the hyperthyroid patient may begin to feel improvement within a week of starting thioamide therapy, it may be as long as 4 weeks before a full effect has occurred, depending on the amount of colloid stored in the thyroid gland.

It is most practical to measure thyroid function monthly. Once the therapeutic goal has been attained, a reduction in the dose of PTU or methimazole should be instituted, usually down to 50–150 mg/day PTU (5–15 mg methimazole) after 4–6 weeks. Thyroid function should continue to be monitored, since hyperthyroidism often spontaneously improves during the third trimester and it is sometimes possible to eliminate treatment entirely. Recrudescence post partum should be anticipated.

Adverse Effects

Frequently noted side effects (1–5% of patients) include fever, rash, urticaria, arthralgias, and arthritis, all apparently dose related. Transient leukopenia ($<4,000/mm^3$) occurs in up to 12% of adults and is benign. This leukopenia is not an antecedent of agranulocytosis and its occurrence does not necessitate stopping the medication. The incidence of cross-sensitivity between PTU and methimazole is approximately 50%, so although the appearance of any of these side effects may prompt substitution of the other thioamide, the unwanted sequelae may recur.

Both PTU and methimazole are associated with agranulocytosis in approximately 0.5% of patients. This potentially life-threatening complication almost always develops during the first 3 months of treatment and is characterized by fever, systemic toxicity, bacterial pharyngitis, and an absolute granulocyte count below $250/mm^3$. Because the onset is sudden, routine monitoring of the white cell count is not helpful. When thioamides are discontinued, clinical improvement usually occurs over days to weeks, but fatalities have occurred. This complication tends to be seen most frequently in patients over 40 years of age, and seems to be dose related for methimazole but not for PTU. Patients who take thioamides should be instructed to discontinue them if fever, pharyngitis, or other signs of infection develop, and to report this to their physician.

Drug-related toxic hepatitis has been associated with PTU and may occasionally be life-threatening; this may have an immune basis. Cholestatic jaundice has been associated with methimazole. Vasculitis and a lupuslike syndrome have also been reported and should be treated with corticosteroids and discontinuation of the thioamide. The appearance of circulating antibodies to insulin or glucagon has been reported with methimazole. Extremely rare complications include aplastic anemia (either PTU or methimazole), nephrotic syndrome (methimazole), loss of taste (methimazole), and hypoprothrombinemia (PTU).

Mechanism of Action

The thioamides act directly on the thyroid gland and also have systemic effects. Within the thyroid gland, these drugs inhibit thyroglobulin formation by diverting iodide away from tyrosine residues. They also inhibit the coupling of iodotyrosines to form iodothyronines. Futhermore, they may alter the structure of thyroglobulin and inhibit thyroglobulin synthesis, but these effects have not been proved. Systemically, PTU inhibits the conversion of T4 to T3, the more active thyroid hormone. There is also some evidence to support a role of these agents in altering the immune system, perhaps contributing to remission of immune thyroid disease.

Absorption and Biotransformation

The thioamides are well absorbed from the gastrointestinal tract, with peak serum levels reached 1–2 hours after dosing. The serum half-life of PTU is approximately 1 hour, while that of methimazole is approximately 5 hours. Hepatic and renal disease may prolong the half-lives of these drugs.

Thioamides are concentrated by the thyroid gland within minutes of dosing, peak intrathyroid levels occurring in 1 hour. Intrathyroidal concentrations are about 100 times serum levels, unless high dosages are given, at which point the active transport system evidently becomes saturated.

The action of these drugs is relatively short, with a 100-mg dose of PTU beginning to wane within 2–3 hours. Methimazole has a longer half-life, but even with this agent, a single dose of 10–25 mg is needed to obtain a therapeutic effect lasting 24 hours. Carbimazole is metabolized to methimazole.

The thioamides and their metabolites are excreted in the urine.

Recommended Reading

Burrow, G. N. The Thyroid Gland in Pregnancy. In *Major Problems in Obstetrics and Gynecology*. Philadelphia: Saunders, 1972. Vol. 3.

Burrow, G. N. Thyroid Diseases. In G. N. Burrow and T. F. Ferris (eds.), *Medical Complications During Pregnancy*. Philadelphia: Saunders, 1982.

Burrow, G. N., et al. Children exposed in utero to propylthiouracil. Subsequent intellectual and physical development. *Am. J. Dis. Child.* 116:161, 1968.

Check, J. H., et al. Prenatal treatment of thyrotoxicosis to prevent intrauterine growth retardation. *Obstet. Gynecol.* 60:122, 1982.

Cheron, R. G., et al. Neonatal thyroid function after propylthiouracil for maternal Graves' disease. *N. Engl. J. Med.* 304:525, 1981.

Cooper, D. S. Antithyroid drugs. *N. Engl. J. Med.* 311:1353, 1984.

Cooper, D. S., et al. Methimazole pharmacology in man: Studies using a newly developed radioimmunoassay for methimazole. *J. Clin. Endocrinol. Metab.* 58:473, 1984.

Gilman, A. G., Goodman, L. S., and Gilman, A. *The Pharmacological Basis of Therapeutics* (6th ed.). New York: Macmillan, 1980. Pp. 1408–1412.

Kampmann, J. P., et al. Propylthiouracil in human milk: Revision of a dogma. *Lancet* 1:736, 1980.

Mujtaba, Q., and Burrow, G. N. Treatment of hyperthyroidism in pregnancy with propylthiouracil and methimazole. *Obstet. Gynecol.* 46:282, 1975.

Tegler, L., and Lindstrom, B. Antithyroid drugs in milk. *Lancet* 2:591, 1980.

Tobacco

Indications and Recommendations

The use of tobacco is contraindicated during pregnancy. This drug is the dried leaf of the *Nicotiana tabacum* plant and a widely used agent that is smoked by approximately one-third of American women of childbearing age. An estimated 20–25% of women smoke throughout pregnancy. Tobacco has no known therapeutic uses.

Cigarette smoking should be actively discouraged in anyone, but particularly in pregnant women. Even if a habituated person cannot stop smoking completely, there is good evidence to show that she should try to decrease her cigarette consumption to less than seven cigarettes/day.

Lactating women also should be discouraged from smoking and should smoke as little as possible if they cannot achieve complete abstinence.

Special Considerations in Pregnancy

Nicotine, carbon monoxide, and probably other components of cigarette smoke cross the placenta and appear in fetal blood in higher concentrations than in maternal blood. Nicotine is also present in amniotic fluid and placental tissues in higher concentrations than in maternal serum.

Evidence linking cigarette smoking to complications of pregnancy has continued to accumulate. Every investigator who has looked at the relationship of birth weight to cigarette smoking has confirmed that offspring of smoking mothers have lower birth weights than those of nonsmokers. Although the actual difference in birth weight is only in the range of a few hundred grams, each study has shown a statistically significant difference in these weights. Not only have smokers been shown to have smaller offspring than nonsmokers, but over 30 investigations have indicated that they also have twice the number of growth-retarded babies.

This effect of smoking appears to be dose related, as well as related to the stage of pregnancy in which smoking occurs. If a woman stops smoking before the end of the fourth month of pregnancy, it is probable that her offspring will not differ significantly in weight from that of a nonsmoker. In a recent prospective clinical trial, smokers randomly assigned to a smoking cessation intervention program prior to the eighteenth week of gestation delivered babies who were, on average, 92 g heavier and 0.6 cm longer than those of control smokers. Women who smoke fewer than 7–10 cigarettes/day tend to have children whose birth weights do not differ significantly from those of nonsmokers. The direct causative factor in cigarette smoke that leads to decreased birth weight is not clear, although animal studies show that prolonged exposure to elevated levels of carbon monoxide will cause lowering of birth weight.

Retrospective and prospective studies of the relationship between cigarette smoking and spontaneous abortions have been suggestive of, but not conclusive for, such an association. While many of these studies do not adequately control for confounding variables, those of Kline et al. and Hemminki and associates attempted to do so. The former study revealed a nearly twofold greater risk of spontaneous abortion in smokers, whereas the latter was unable to demonstrate a significant difference in abortion incidence between 2,313 nonsmokers and 389 smokers.

Cigarette smoking is most obviously related to stillbirth in women with other complicating problems, including low socioeconomic status and poor obstetric history. In the United States, for example, black women have more stillbirths than white women, and cigarette smoking magnifies this difference. Animal studies have shown that nicotine and some other cigarette components may significantly increase the incidence of stillbirths.

In large studies from both Canada and England, the perinatal mortality for infants of smokers was significantly higher than that for infants of nonsmokers. The Canadian study showed a highly significant dose-response relationship. In addition, the British study demonstrated a significant relationship between smoking after the fourth month of pregnancy and increased perinatal mortality. Patients who gave up smoking by the fourth month were found to reduce the risk of perinatal mortality to that of nonsmokers. In addition, this study showed that smoking in patients of low socioeconomic status caused an even higher than expected increase in perinatal mortality. The same association has been made with regard to poor obstetric history combined with smoking.

A recent prospective epidemiologic study of 30,596 pregnant women in northern California demonstrated a significant association between maternal cigarette smoking and preterm birth. Potential confounding variables were controlled: Thus, this effect is probably a real one.

Paradoxically, the perinatal mortality for infants under 2,500 g born to smokers is less than that of nonsmokers. The reason seems to be that these infants are primarily small for gestational age rather than premature. However, for infants of comparable gestational age, the mortality is higher for the offspring of smokers than nonsmokers. In a collaborative randomized trial of antenatal steroid therapy for the prevention of respiratory distress syndrome, it was found that premature infants of smokers had a significantly lower incidence of respiratory distress syndrome when compared to infants of nonsmokers born at similar gestational ages. The investigators interpreted this finding as evidence of accelerated pulmonary maturation caused by chronic fetal stress produced by maternal smoking.

Several epidemiologic studies reveal a significant decrease in the incidence of preeclampsia in smokers. This appears to be inversely proportional to the amount the woman smokes. However, there are data to show that if a smoker does develop preeclampsia, her infant is at higher risk than that of a preeclamptic nonsmoker.

Nicotine is present in higher concentrations in breast milk than in maternal serum. However, in one study in which both breast milk and infant serum were analyzed, infant blood contained very little nicotine despite high breast milk levels. Nevertheless, several cases of nicotine poisoning in infants of mothers who smoke 20–40 cigarettes/day have been reported. In addition, smoking mothers expose their children to the dangers of passive smoking. In one longitudinal study of 1,156 children, there was a 10% reduction in pulmonary function below expected levels among the 1- and 2-year-old children of smokers. Another long-term study showed a higher incidence of mild cognitive and behavioral abnormalities among children of smokers compared to children of nonsmokers.

Adverse Effects

Among the many medical conditions clearly associated with ingestion of cigarette smoke are mucosal epitheliomas; lung cancer; cancers of the oropharyngeal cavity, esophagus, and larynx; emphysema; "smoker's respiratory syndrome"; coronary artery disease;

cerebrovascular disease; cardiac arrhythmias; and peripheral vascular disease.

Nicotine has parasympathetic effects on the gastrointestinal tract, occasionally resulting in diarrhea and often leading to decreased intestinal motility. It can cause respiratory depression and arrest by its action of blocking the neuromuscular junction of respiratory muscles. Furthermore, a minor central nervous system (CNS) paralysis may occur. Other CNS effects such as tremors (at low dosages) and convulsions (at higher dosages) can be reversed with antiparkinsonian drugs, curariform drugs, adrenergic blockers, hypnotics, and anticonvulsants. Nicotine also has an antidiuretic effect mediated through release of antidiuretic hormone (ADH).

Mechanism of Action

Nearly 500 compounds have been isolated from tobacco smoke. These include several chemicals irritating to mucous membranes; polonium-210 and nickel, which have been implicated in lung cancer; and carbon monoxide, which makes up approximately 1% of cigarette smoke by volume. The major active component of tobacco, however, is nicotine, which averages 6–8 mg/cigarette. Approximately 90% of the nicotine in inhaled tobacco smoke is systemically absorbed.

Nicotine, a toxic substance that acts on a variety of neuroeffector junctions, has both stimulant and depressant phases of action. Its net effect therefore is the algebriac summation of those actions. These are usually dose related and depend on time since ingestion. An initial stimulatory effect is usually followed by a depressant effect. This pattern occurs in all autonomic ganglia and is responsible for many if not most of the effects of nicotine.

In general, nicotine will increase heart rate and blood pressure and its cardiovascular effects parallel those of sympathetic stimulation. The sympathomimetic effects can be negated by catecholamine blockers, which implies that they are mediated through the adrenal glands and other catecholamine-releasing organs.

Absorption and Biotransformation

Nicotine, the major component of tobacco smoke, is absorbed from oral and gastrointestinal mucosa, the respiratory tract, and skin. Between 80 and 90% is detoxified by the liver, kidney, and lungs; the remainder plus the detoxification products are excreted through the kidney. This occurs most expeditiously in acidified urine. Nicotine is also excreted in the milk of lactating women in direct proportion to the amount of tobacco consumed. The milk may contain as much as 0.5 mg/liter.

Recommended Reading

American College of Obstetricians and Gynecologists. Cigarette Smoking and Pregnancy. *Tech. Bull.* No. 53, 1979.

Coles, C. D., et al. Neonatal ethanol withdrawal: Characteristics in clinically normal, nondysmorphic neonates. *J. Pediatr.* 105:445, 1984.

Curet, L. B., et al. Maternal smoking and respiratory distress syndrome. *Am. J. Obstet. Gynecol.* 147:446, 1983.

Gilman, A. G., Goodman, L. S., and Gilman, A. *The Pharmacological Basis of Therapeutics* (6th ed.). New York: Macmillan, 1980. Pp. 557–560.

Hemminki, K., Mutanen, P., and Saloniemi, I. Smoking and the occurrence of congenital malformations and spontaneous abortions: Multivariate analysis. *Am. J. Obstet. Gynecol.* 145:61, 1983.

Kline, J., Stein, Z. A., and Susser, M. Smoking: A risk factor for spontaneous abortion. *N. Engl. J. Med.* 297:793, 1977.

Luck, W., and Nau, H. Exposure of the fetus, neonate, and nursed infant to nicotine and cotinine from maternal smoking. *N. Engl. J. Med.* 311:672, 1984.

Meyer, M. B., and Tonascia, J. A. Maternal smoking, pregnancy complications, and perinatal mortality. *Am. J. Obstet. Gynecol.* 128:494, 1977.

Naeye, R. L., and Peters, E. C. Mental development of children whose mothers smoked during pregnancy. *Obstet. Gynecol.* 64:601, 1984.

Sexton, M., and Hebel, J. R. A clinical trial of change in maternal smoking and its effect on birth weight. *J.A.M.A.* 251:911, 1984.

Shiono, P. H., et al. Smoking and drinking during pregnancy: Their effects on preterm birth. *J.A.M.A.* 255:82, 1986.

Tager, I. B., et al. Longitudinal study of the effects of maternal smoking on pulmonary function in children. *N. Engl. J. Med.* 309:699, 1983.

Tolazoline (Priscoline®)

Indications and Recommendations

Tolazoline is relatively contraindicated during pregnancy because other therapeutic agents are preferable. Tolazoline, like phentolamine, is an alpha-adrenergic blocker. In addition to its alpha-blocking effects, it has a variety of nonrelated sympathomimetic, parasympathomimetic, and histaminic actions. There are no clear-cut indications for its use during pregnancy.

Tolazoline produces vasodilatation and cardiac stimulation, which usually result in a rise in systemic blood pressure. It can produce tachycardia and arrhythmias. Although the drug has been used to treat neonates for pulmonary hypertension, little is known of its effects when administered during pregnancy. In one study, neonates given tolazoline showed complications of gastrointestinal hemorrhage, thrombocytopenia, and transient renal failure.

There are few documented indications for the use of tolazoline. The most favorable clinical responses have been described with early Raynaud's syndrome. However, because tolazoline has had limited use in pregnancy, it cannot be recommended.

Recommended Reading

Gilman, A. G., Goodman, L. S., and Gilman, A. *The Pharmacological Basis of Therapeutics* (6th ed.). New York: Macmillan, 1980. Pp. 183–184.

Goetzman, B. W., et al. Neonatal hypoxia and pulmonary vasospasm response to tolazoline. *J. Pediatr.* 89:617, 1976.

Triamterene (Dyrenium®)

Indications and Recommendations

Triamterene is relatively contraindicated during pregnancy because other therapeutic agents are preferable. It is a potassium-sparing diuretic that acts directly on tubular transport in the distal tubule. It is not an aldosterone antagonist.

The effects of the drug on uterine blood flow and the fetus have not been well studied.

If diuretics are necessary during pregnancy, a thiazide or furosemide is preferable to triamterene. Serum potassium levels should be followed closely whenever pregnant women are given diuretics. If hypokalemia develops, oral potassium supplementation will effectively correct this problem. This drug, therefore, has no important advantage over others whose effects in pregnancy are better known.

Recommended Reading

Christianson, R., and Page, E. W. Diuretic drugs and pregnancy. *Obstet. Gynecol.* 48:647, 1976.

Gifford, R. W., Jr. A guide to the practical use of diuretics. *J.A.M.A.* 235:1890, 1976.

Gilman, A. G., Goodman, L. S., and Gilman, A. *The Pharmacological Basis of Therapeutics* (6th ed.). New York: Macmillan, 1980. Pp. 908–909.

Pruitt, A.W., McNay, J. L., and Dayton, P. G. Transfer characteristics of triamterene and its analogs. Central nervous system, placenta, and kidney. *Drug Metab. Dispos.* 3:30, 1975.

Tricyclic Antidepressants:
Amitriptyline (Elavil®), Desipramine (Norpramin®), Doxepin (Sinequan®), Imipramine (Tofranil®), Nortriptyline (Aventyl®, Pamelor®), Protriptyline (Vivactil®)

Indications and Recommendations

The use of tricyclic antidepressants during pregnancy should be limited to the treatment of those women who clearly require the medication for psychiatric indications, especially endogenous depression of abrupt onset. Reactive depression and depression accompanied by anxiety are less likely to be relieved by these drugs and therefore do not indicate their use during pregnancy. It does not appear that any member of this family of drugs is the agent of choice for use during pregnancy.

Special Considerations in Pregnancy

Animal studies have shown that the tricyclic antidepressants cross the placenta. Congenital malformations, including limb-reduction deformities, have been reported in infants whose mothers used tricyclic antidepressants during pregnancy, but a causal relationship has not been demonstrated. The Finnish Registry of Congenital Malformations contains 2,784 cases of birth defects for the years 1964–1972, which were matched with an equal number of controls. Four of the mothers of malformed infants had taken tricyclics during the first trimester, as opposed to one of the control mothers. No increase in the incidence of birth defects occurred in the 41 exposed pregnancies reported by the Collaborative Perinatal Project. Neither was there an increased incidence of exposure to such drugs in utero among hundreds of children with limb-reduction defects. Similarly, in an uncontrolled series from England, none of 81 mothers treated with imipramine, 50 mg tid, delivered babies with anomalies. In the Royal College of General Practitioners' survey of 10,000 pregnancies in 1964, none of the 47 fetuses exposed to tricyclic antidepressants in utero had congenital malformations.

Cases have been reported of infants born to women who received tricyclic antidepressants immediately before delivery who have suffered from heart failure, tachycardia, myoclonus, respiratory distress, and urinary retention. Withdrawal symptoms have been observed in infants whose mothers were treated with imipramine during the antenatal period.

Very small amounts of this drug are excreted in breast milk. Such doses have not been shown to have an effect on the neonate. When serum samples from nursing infants whose mothers were taking tricyclics have been tested, levels of the drugs were not detectable.

Dosage

Dosages of the tricyclic antidepressants must be individualized. After an initial dose has been given, dosage is gradually increased over 1–2 weeks to the maintenance dosage that will provide maximal efficacy and minimal side effects. Table 13 details recommended dosages of these antidepressants.

Adverse Effects

Sedation is the most prominent initial effect of the tricyclic antidepressants, the magnitude of which depends on the individual agent. Other side effects include tachycardia and orthostatic hypotension.

Table 13. Recommended dosages of the tricyclic antidepressants

Drug	Usual daily starting dose (mg)	Usual daily maintenance dosage range (mg)
Amitriptyline	50–75	75–300
Desipramine	50–75	75–300
Doxepin	50–75	75–300
Imipramine	50–75	75–300
Nortriptyline	75	40–100
Protriptyline	10	10–40

These agents have potent anticholinergic activity and commonly cause dry mouth, blurred vision, urinary retention, and constipation. Allergic reactions, inappropriate secretion of antidiuretic hormone, and galactorrhea are only encountered rarely. Toxicity due to acute overdosage is characterized by hyperpyrexia, hypertension, seizures, and coma.

Mechanism of Action

The tricyclic antidepressants block the reuptake of neurotransmitters, including norepinephrine and serotonin, in adrenergic nerve endings. The resulting increased concentration of neurotransmitter at the receptor is postulated to be responsible for the therapeutic effects of these agents. Nortriptyline is a metabolite of amitriptyline, while desipramine is a metabolite of imipramine.

Absorption and Biotransformation

The tricyclic antidepressants are well absorbed from the gastrointestinal tract; they are metabolized in the liver. They and their metabolites are excreted in urine and feces.

Recommended Reading

Australian Drug Evaluation Committee. Tricyclic antidepressants and limb reduction deformities. *Med. J. Aust.* 1:768, 1973.

Bader, T. F., and Newman, K. Amitriptyline in human breast milk and the nursing infant's serum. *Am. J. Psychiatry* 137:855, 1980.

Banister, P., et al. Possible teratogenicity of tricyclic antidepressants. *Lancet* 1:838, 1972.

Bourke, G. M. Antidepressant teratogenicity. *Lancet* 1:98, 1974.

Crombie, D. L., Pinsent, R. J. F. H., and Fleming, D. Imipramine in pregnancy. *Br. Med. J.* 1:745, 1972.

Douglas, B. H., and Hume, A. S. Placental transfer of imipramine, a basic, lipid-soluble drug. *Am. J. Obstet. Gynecol.* 99:573, 1967.

Erickson, S. H., Smith, G. H., and Heidrich, F. Tricyclics and breast feeding. *Am. J. Psychiatry* 136:1483, 1979.

Gilman, A. G., Goodman, L. S., and Gilman, A. *The Pharmacological Basis of Therapeutics* (6th ed.). New York: Macmillan, 1980. Pp. 418–427.

Heinonen, O. P., Slone, D., and Shapiro, S. *Birth Defects and Drugs in Pregnancy.* Boston: John Wright PSG, 1977.

Hollister, L. E. Doxepin hydrochloride. *Ann. Intern. Med.* 81:360, 1974.

Idanpaan-Heikkila, J., and Saxen, L. Possible teratogenicity of imipramine/chloropyramine. *Lancet* 2:282, 1973.

McBride, W. G. Limb deformities associated with iminodibenzyl hydrochloride. *Med. J. Aust.* 1:492, 1972.

The Neuropharmacology of Depression. Merrell-National Laboratories, Cincinnati, Ohio, July 1977.

Rachelefsky, G. S., et al. Possible teratogenicity of tricyclic antidepressants. *Lancet* 1:838, 1972.

Scanlon, F. J. Use of antidepressant drugs during the first trimester. *Med. J. Aust.* 2:1077, 1969.

Shearer, W. T., Schreiner, R. L., and Marshall, R. E. Urinary retention in a neonate secondary to maternal ingestion of nortriptyline. *J. Pediatr.* 81:570, 1972.

Sim, M. Imipramine and pregnancy. *Br. Med. J.* 2:45, 1972.

Sovner, R., and Orsulak, P. J. Excretion of imipramine and desipramine in human breast milk. *Am. J. Psychiatry* 136:451, 1979.

Webster, P. A. Withdrawal symptoms in neonates associated with maternal antidepressant therapy. *Lancet* 2:318, 1973.

Trimethadione (Tridione®)

Indications and Recommendations

Trimethadione is contraindicated during pregnancy because other therapeutic agents are preferable. It is an anticonvulsant used in the treatment of petit mal epilepsy and has largely been replaced by newer, less toxic agents. It has been associated with teratogenic effects in the human fetus. A fetal trimethadione syndrome has been described, consisting of mild mental retardation, V-shaped eyebrows, speech difficulties, developmental delay, cleft lip or palate, abnormal ears, and epicanthus. In addition, intrauterine growth retardation (IUGR), cardiac anomalies, and urogenital and skeletal malformations have been reported, with many of these abnormalities being serious enough to result in neonatal death. If treatment for petit mal epilepsy is required during pregnancy, ethosuximide is preferred.

Recommended Reading

Feldman, G. L., Weaver, D. D., and Lovrien, E. W. The fetal trimethadione syndrome: Report of an additional family and further delineation of this syndrome. *Am. J. Dis. Child.* 131:1389, 1977.

German, J., Kowal, A., and Ehlers, K. H. Trimethadione and human teratogenesis. *Teratology* 3:349, 1970.

Gilman, A. G., Goodman, L. S., and Gilman, A. *The Pharmacological Basis of Therapeutics* (6th ed.). New York: Macmillan, 1980. Pp. 464–471.

Goldman, A. S., and Yaffe, S. J. Fetal trimethadione syndrome. *Teratology* 17:103, 1978.

Rosen, R. C., and Lightner, E. S. Phenotypic malformations in association with maternal trimethadione therapy. *J. Pediatr.* 92:240, 1978.

Zackai, E. H., et al. The fetal trimethadione syndrome. *J. Pediatr.* 87:280, 1975.

Trimethaphan (Arfonad®)

Indications and Recommendations

The use of trimethaphan is relatively contraindicated during pregnancy because other therapeutic agents are preferable. It is a ganglionic blocker that acts almost immediately as an antihypertensive agent. Its therapeutic action is so evanescent that it must be given by continuous infusion.

Trimethaphan prevents the attachment of acetylcholine released by the preganglionic neuron to the receptor sites of the postganglionic axon. This results in the inhibition of both sympathetic and parasympathetic impulses.

Prolonged apnea after succinylcholine administration to a severely preeclamptic primigravida undergoing emergency cesarean section has been reported. The patient was concurrently receiving trimethaphan by continuous infusion. At the end of the operation, peripheral nerve stimulation demonstrated a profound depolarization type of neuromuscular blockade. The authors believe that this was due to trimethaphan's noncompetitive inhibition of plasma cholinesterase activity.

Decreased intravascular volume or any drug that inhibits sympathetic activity will augment the antihypertensive action of this drug. Furthermore, the hypotensive action of trimethaphan is accompanied by a decrease in glomerular filtration rate.

Side effects include the many problems that accompany ganglionic blockade, most importantly obstipation and urinary retention. In addition, administration of ganglionic blockers to the mother has been associated with meconium ileus in the neonate.

Trimethaphan should not be used during pregnancy unless other more acceptable agents have proved unsuccessful.

Recommended Reading

Koch-Weser, J. Hypertensive emergencies. *N. Engl. J. Med.* 290:211, 1974.

Martin, J. D. A critical survey of drugs used in the treatment of hypertensive crises of pregnancy. *Med. J. Aust.* 2:252, 1974.

Poulton, T. J., James, F. M., III, and Lockridge, O. Prolonged apnea following trimethaphan and succinylcholine. *Anesthesiology* 50:54, 1979.

Sklar, G. S., and Lanks, K. W. Effects of trimethaphan and nitroprusside on hydrolysis of succinylcholine. *Anesthesiology* 47:31, 1977.

The treatment of malignant hypertension and hypertensive emergencies. A statement by the AMA Committee on Hypertension. *J.A.M.A.* 228:1673, 1974.

Trimethobenzamide (Tigan®)

Indications and Recommendations

Trimethobenzamide is safe to use during pregnancy. The usual therapeutic dosages may be used for treatment of nausea and vomiting during pregnancy.

Special Considerations in Pregnancy

Large-scale prospective studies assessing the use of trimethobenzamide in pregnancy have failed to show an increased risk of malformation in the fetus at normal dosages.

Dosage

The usual adult oral dose of trimethobenzamide is 250 mg 2–3 times/day. The intramuscular and rectal dose is 200 mg 3–4 times/day.

Adverse Effects

At recommended dosages, side effects are relatively uncommon; they include drowsiness and dizziness, and local irritation if the intramuscular or rectal route is used.

Mechanism of Action

The exact mechanism of action of trimethobenzamide as an anti-emetic is obscure. It is thought to depress the chemoreceptor trigger zone. It does not suppress the vomiting center or block visceral impulses to the vomiting center. It is structurally related to the antihistamines but has only weak antihistaminic activity.

Absorption and Biotransformation

Trimethobenzamide is well absorbed after oral administration. Measurable blood levels may persist for as long as 24 hours. Within 72 hours, 30–50% of the administered dose is excreted unchanged in the urine. Trimethobenzamide may also be metabolized in the liver and its metabolites excreted in bile and urine.

Recommended Reading

Heinonen, D., Slone, D., and Shapiro, S. (eds.). *Birth Defects and Drugs in Pregnancy*. Littleton, Mass.: Publishing Sciences Group, 1977. Pp. 323–330.

Long, J. W. *Essential Guide to Prescription Drugs*. New York: Harper & Row, 1977. Pp. 641–643.

Milkovich, L. and van den Berg, B. J. An evaluation of the teratogenicity of certain antinauseant drugs. *Am. J. Obstet. Gynecol.* 125:244, 1976.

Pearlman, D. S. Antihistamines: Pharmacology and clinical use. *Drugs* 12:258, 1976.

Tripelennamine (PBZ®, Pyribenzamine®)

Indications and Recommendations

The use of tripelennamine during pregnancy should be limited to the treatment of allergic symptoms caused by histamine release, including urticaria, rhinitis, and pruritus. Whenever possible, however, the primary treatment for such symptoms should be avoidance of the allergen. This drug should be avoided by breast-feeding women.

Special Considerations in Pregnancy

No prospective studies that evaluate the safety of tripelennamine's use during pregnancy have been conducted. One large retrospective study, however, found no evidence incriminating tripelennamine as a teratogenic agent.

Because of its anticholinergic properties, tripelennamine may inhibit lactation. In addition, small amounts may be secreted into breast milk. This and all antihistamines should therefore be avoided by the lactating mother.

Dosage

The adult dose of tripelennamine hydrochloride is 50–100 mg q4–6h. An extended-release preparation is available and may be prescribed in a dose of 100 mg q8–12h. Tripelennamine citrate is available in an elixir; 37.5 mg of the citrate is equivalent to 25 mg of the hydrochloride.

Adverse Effects

Anticholinergic side effects are the most common. These include dry mouth and eyes, and rarely, blurred vision. Drowsiness, anorexia, nausea, epigastric distress, and dizziness also may be seen.

Mechanism of Action

Tripelennamine is a competitive antagonist of histamine that decreases edema formation by diminishing capillary dilatation and permeability. It merely provides palliative, not curative, therapy for allergic symptoms. It has anticholinergic activity, produces drowsiness, and possesses local anesthetic activity when applied topically.

Absorption and Biotransformation

The drug is primarily metabolized in the liver, probably by hydroxylation followed by glucuronidation. Excretion is via the kidney.

Recommended Reading

Gilman, A. G., Goodman, L. S., and Gilman, A. *The Pharmacological Basis of Therapeutics* (6th ed.). New York: Macmillan, 1980. P. 628.

Greenberger, P., and Patterson, R. Safety of therapy for allergic symptoms during pregnancy. *Ann. Intern. Med.* 89:234, 1978.

Heinonen, O. P., Slone, D., and Shapiro, S. *Birth Defects and Drugs in Pregnancy*. Littleton, Mass.: Publishing Sciences Group, 1977. Pp. 323–324.

Nishimura, H., and Tanimura, T. *Clinical Aspects of the Teratogenicity of Drugs*. Amsterdam: Excerpta Medica, 1976.

Valproic Acid (Depakene®)

Indications and Recommendations

The use of valproic acid is contraindicated during pregnancy because alternative agents that seem to be safer for the fetus are available. This drug is a second-line agent for the treatment of absence seizures, which are rare among women of childbearing age. It is also effective in the treatment of myoclonic and grand mal seizures, and its use in this setting is expanding.

Valproic acid readily crosses the placenta and is present in fetal serum at levels equal to or greater than maternal serum levels. The neonate metabolizes the drug slowly and its plasma half-life is 30–60 hours, compared to 8–12 hours in the adult.

From data collected at birth defects registries in several countries, an association between neural tube defects and exposure to valproic acid is emerging. Although this has yet to be confirmed in collaborative cohort studies, the estimated risk to exposed fetuses is 1%. An increased incidence of congenital heart disease has also been suggested in these fetuses although this is less well characterized. Finally, a fetal valproate syndrome may exist. In a study of seven children exposed in utero, all had consistent facial changes including epicanthal folds connecting with an infraorbital crease, flat nasal bridge, small nose and mouth, and a long upper lip with a shallow philtrum. Three of these children had developmental delays and one had congenital heart disease.

The drug is found in very small quantities in breast milk, and breast-feeding is therefore considered safe.

Recommended Reading

Bjerkedal, T., et al. Valproic acid and spina bifida. *Lancet* 2:1096, 1982.

Diliberti, J. H., et al. The fetal valproate syndrome. *Am. J. Med. Genet.* 19:473, 1984.

Gilman, A. G., Goodman, L. S., and Gilman, A. *The Pharmacological Basis of Therapeutics* (6th ed.). New York: Macmillan, 1980. Pp. 462–464.

Lindhout, D., and Meinordi, H. Spina bifida and in-utero exposure to valproate. *Lancet* 2:396, 1984.

Nau, H., et al. Valproic acid and its metabolites: Placental transfer, neonatal pharmacokinetics, transfer in a mother's milk, and clinical status in neonates of epileptic mothers. *J. Pharmacol. Exp. Ther.* 219:768, 1981.

Pinder, R. M., et al. Sodium valproate: A review of its pharmacologic properties and therapeutic efficacy in epilepsy. *Drugs* 13:81, 1977.

Robert, E., and Rosa, F. Valproate and birth defects. *Lancet* 2:1142, 1983.

Wilder, B. V., and Bruni, J. *Seizure Disorders: A Pharmacological Approach to Treatment.* New York: Raven, 1981.

Vancomycin (Vancocin®)

Indications and Recommendations

The use of intravenous vancomycin during pregnancy should be limited to the treatment of life-threatening infections in patients allergic to penicillin, or to treatment of serious staphylococcal infections caused by strains resistant to penicillinase-resistant penicillins or cephalosporins. Oral vancomycin may be used in the treatment of antibiotic-induced *Clostridium difficile* colitis.

Special Considerations in Pregnancy

Because of potential ototoxicity to the fetus, vancomycin should be used only when specifically indicated.

Dosage

The usual intravenous dose is 2 g/day, divided into doses given q6–12h. The dose should be given in 100–200 ml of 5% D/W to reduce hypersensitivity reactions. If creatinine clearance is 50–80 ml/minute, the dose should be given every 1–3 days. If the creatinine clearance is 10–50 ml/minute, the dose is given every 3–10 days. If the creatinine clearance is less than 10 ml/minute, only 1 g is given every 7 days.

The oral dose for treatment of *C. difficile* colitis is 500 mg qid.

Adverse Effects

The most common side effect of intravenous vancomycin is a histaminelike reaction occurring shortly after infusion and consisting of fever, chills, paresthesias, and erythema at the base of the neck and upper back. This reaction is minimized by administering the drug slowly in a large volume (100–200 ml) of fluid. Neurotoxicity is the most serious complication of vancomycin therapy. Damage to the auditory nerve, with possible deafness, is associated with serum levels of 60–80 µg/ml and is a problem primarily in patients with diminished renal function.

The nephrotoxicity previously ascribed to vancomycin use has been attributed to impurities found in earlier preparations. As purified preparations have become available, it is now uncommon.

Mechanism of Action

Vancomycin is a bactericidal antibiotic that acts primarily by inhibiting cell wall synthesis. In addition, it has a small effect on inhibiting RNA synthesis in bacterial cytoplasmic membranes. At clinically achievable concentrations, vancomycin is only active against gram-positive organisms.

Absorption and Biotransformation

Vancomycin is almost negligibly absorbed from the gastrointestinal tract, achieving serum levels of <1 µg/ml in normal subjects and slightly higher levels in patients with inflammatory bowel disease. When administered intravenously to patients with normal renal function, its half-life is 4–8 hours, and it is almost completely excreted in the urine. In the presence of renal insufficiency, dangerously high blood concentrations may occur.

Recommended Reading

Cunha, B. A., and Ristaccia, A. M. Clinical usefulness of vancomycin. *Clin. Pharmacol.* 2:417, 1983.

Davis, D. M. *Textbook of Adverse Drug Reactions*. Oxford, Engl.: Oxford University, 1977. P. 70.

Gilman, A. G., Goodman, L. S., and Gilman, A. *The Pharmacological Basis of Therapeutics* (6th ed.). New York: Macmillan, 1980. Pp. 1230–1231.

Handbook of Antimicrobial Therapy. The Medical Letter on Drugs and Therapeutics (rev. ed.). New Rochelle, N.Y.: The Medical Letter, 1978.

McHenry, M. C., and Gavan, T. L. Vancomycin. *Pediatr. Clin. North Am.* 30:31, 1983.

Xanthines (over-the-counter): Caffeine, Theobromine, Theophylline

Indications and Recommendations

Xanthines in the quantities present in coffee, tea, cocoa, and cola-flavored drinks are probably safe during pregnancy if consumed in moderation in the absence of peptic ulcer or hypertensive heart disease. In 1980, the FDA cautioned pregnant women to avoid excessive caffeine intake. This warning was based on a study linking large dosages of caffeine (human equivalent of 20–24 cups of coffee daily), administered as a bolus via nasogastric tube to pregnant rats, with missing digits in the offspring. Teratogenicity has not been associated with the ingestion of beverages containing xanthines during human pregnancy.

It is recommended that nursing mothers limit their intake of coffee or tea to two cups per day or less.

Special Considerations in Pregnancy

The xanthines produce no unique effects in the mother during pregnancy. In pregnant sheep, slight reductions in uterine blood flow were demonstrated with intravenous infusion of 24–35 mg/kg caffeine (equivalent to more than 10 cups of coffee in the human). Maternal and fetal oxygenation and acid-base levels were unaffected. At lower dosages, the results were less clear-cut. In a study of 20 third-trimester human pregnancies, Finnish investigators using xenon clearance methodology detected a slight decrease in intervillous blood flow after the ingestion of two cups of coffee. There were no changes in umbilical venous blood flow, maternal or fetal pulse rates, or maternal blood pressure, despite a doubling of maternal serum caffeine levels.

Human studies have demonstrated that caffeine elimination is significantly prolonged in pregnant women as compared to nonpregnant individuals.

Caffeine has been shown to cross the placenta, with peak fetal levels approaching 75% of peak maternal levels. The fetus may be subject to stimulation of its central nervous system, skeletal musculature, or both, which could result in an increase in activity in utero. Fetal cardiac stimulation may cause tachycardia or premature contractions. In a study performed in Hungary, human fetal hearts were shown to increase in their contraction rates when exposed to caffeine in vitro.

Xanthines have caused chromosomal breakage in some microorganisms and in fruit flies. Breakages in human chromosomes, however, have only been observed with dosages far greater than those obtainable from drinking coffee or tea.

Three cases of hand anomalies in offspring of women who drank large amounts of coffee (8–25 cups/day) were collected in response to the FDA's warning stemming from the previously mentioned association with limb anomalies in rats. Unfortunately, no denominator information is available, so that these three cases may have occurred by chance in heavy coffee drinkers. An epidemiologic study of 12,205 pregnancies failed to uncover any association between caffeine consumption and malformations, low birth weight, or premature delivery after smoking and multiple other variables had been controlled. In a case-control study of 2,030 malformed infants, caffeine ingestion during pregnancy was not associated with any of the defects being considered. However, only 22 infants with limb-reduction defects were included in this study. Therefore, an association with caffeine ingestion could not be ruled out, despite the similarity of these 22 mothers' caffeine habits to those of the control mothers.

A recent prospective cohort study of 3,135 pregnant women demonstrated a significantly increased risk for late first-trimester and second-trimester spontaneous abortions (relative risk, 1.73) among moderate to heavy caffeine users (> 1.5 cups of coffee/day). Until more data are available, it is probably best for pregnant women to limit their caffeine intake, although no threshold dosage has been defined.

Caffeine reaches detectable levels in the blood of nursing infants. Jitteriness has been reported in an infant whose mother had a history of heavy caffeine use. Children and infants are more sensitive to the effects of xanthines than adults.

Dosage

1. Coffee and tea contain 100–150 mg caffeine per average cup.
2. Nondietetic cola drinks contain 35–55 mg caffeine per 12-ounce glass.
3. Dietetic drinks in some cases contain unstated amounts of caffeine.
4. Cocoa contains approximately 200 mg theobromine per cup.
5. Tea contains theophylline in varying amounts.

Adverse Effects

The fatal dose of caffeine is 10 g. It is quite unlikely that this amount will be ingested, however, because reactions usually begin after 1 g has been consumed. Central nervous system (CNS) side effects include restlessness and disturbed sleep patterns, tremor, tinnitus, and excitement, which may progress to delirium. Tachycardia and arrhythmias may occur. Other side effects include diuresis, dyspepsia, and nausea and vomiting. Theophylline may be fatal to adults, but only if administered intravenously. Children, however, have been fatally intoxicated by pharmacologic preparations of theophylline administered orally, rectally, or parenterally. In adults, theophylline may cause headaches, palpitations, nausea, and hypotension.

Mechanism of Action

The xanthines affect many systems in the body by increasing intracellular cyclic AMP, altering ionic calcium levels, and potentiating the action of catecholamines. Central nervous system, respiratory, and skeletal muscle effects are greatest for caffeine, less for theophylline and least for theobromine. Smooth muscle relaxation, coronary artery dilatation, myocardial stimulation, and diuresis, on the other hand, are related to theophylline, theobromine, and caffeine, in decreasing order of potency. Excitation of the CNS on all levels results from ingestion of 150–250 mg caffeine (1–2 cups of coffee). This is manifested by reduced drowsiness, increased motor activity, a reflex excitability, and awareness of sensory stimuli, as well as stimulation of respiratory, vasomotor, and vagal centers. Theophylline increases reflex excitability and the rate and depth of respirations.

The xanthines directly stimulate the myocardium and increase cardiac output. Heart rate may be slowed secondary to medullary vagal center stimulation but is increased with large dosages. Blood vessels are usually dilated by these agents, but there may be an increase in cerebrovascular resistance. Although bronchial and bile duct musculature are relaxed, there is an increase in the strength of skeletal muscle contraction. Glomerular filtration rate and renal blood flow are increased, with a resultant diuresis and increase in sodium and chloride excretion. Caffeine may increase the amount of gastric acid secretion and aggravate peptic ulcers. The xanthines also cause a slight increase in the basal metabolic rate and in higher concentrations stimulate lipolysis, glycogenolysis, and gluconeogenesis.

Absorption and Biotransformation

The xanthines are absorbed after oral, parenteral, or rectal administration. Because caffeine and theophylline have poor aqueous solubility, absorption from the gastrointestinal tract may be erratic, but when taken orally, their onset of action is usually within 30 minutes. The xanthines are metabolized by partial demethylation and oxidation, but about 10% is excreted unchanged in the urine.

Recommended Reading

Anderson, P. O. Drugs in breast feeding—a review. *Drug. Intell. Clin. Pharm.* 11:208, 1977.

Conover, W. B., Key, T. C., and Resnik, R. Maternal cardiovascular response to caffeine infusion in the pregnant ewe. *Am. J. Obstet. Gynecol.* 145:534, 1983.

Gilman, A. G., Goodman, L. S., and Gilman, A. *The Pharmacological Basis of Therapeutics* (6th ed.). New York: Macmillan, 1980. Pp. 592–607.

Goyan, J. E. Food and Drug Administration News Release No. P80–36, September 4, 1980.

Jacobson, M. F., Goldman, A. S., and Syme, R. H. Coffee and birth defects. *Lancet* 1:1415, 1981.

Kirkinen, P., et al. The effect of caffeine on placental and fetal blood flow in human pregnancy. *Am. J. Obstet. Gynecol.* 147:939, 1983.

Knutti, R., Rothweiler, H., and Schlatter, C. Effect of pregnancy on the pharmacokinetics of caffeine. *Eur. J. Clin. Pharmacol.* 21:121, 1981.

Linn, S., et al. No association between coffee consumption and adverse outcomes of pregnancy. *N. Engl. J. Med.* 306:141, 1982.

Morris, M. B., and Weinstein, L. Caffeine and the fetus: Is trouble brewing? *Am. J. Obstet. Gynecol.* 140:607, 1981.

Parsons, W. D., and Pelletier, J. G. Delayed elimination of caffeine by women in the last 2 weeks of pregnancy. *Can. Med. Assoc. J.* 127:377, 1982.

Resch, B. A., and Papp, J. G. Effects of caffeine on the fetal heart. *Am. J. Obstet. Gynecol.* 146:231, 1983.

Rosenberg, L., et al. Selected birth defects in relation to caffeine-containing beverages. *J.A.M.A.* 247:1429, 1982.

Srisuphan, W., and Bracken, M. B. Caffeine consumption during pregnancy and association with late spontaneous abortion. *Am. J. Obstet. Gynecol.* 154:14, 1986.

Wilson, S. J., Ayromlooi, J., and Errick, J. K. Pharmacokinetic and hemodynamic effects of caffeine in the pregnant sheep. *Obstet. Gynecol.* 61:486, 1983.

Appendixes

Appendix A
Vitamins and Minerals

Vitamins

WATER-SOLUBLE VITAMINS

Folic Acid

Folate and folic acid are nutrients required for pyrimidine metabolism. Folic acid is also used in a number of other reactions in intermediary metabolism, including the conversion of homocysteine to methionine and the metabolism of the histidine nucleus.

Since the blockage of DNA synthesis is the major consequence of folate deficiency, the most rapidly dividing cells are those primarily affected. Bone marrow cells develop megaloblastic changes. The peripheral manifestation of this change is a macrocytic anemia, moderate leukopenia (with hypersegmented neutrophils), and thrombocytopenia.

Folates are present in large quantities in peanuts, liver, kidney, and green leafy vegetables. Cereal and dairy products contain low quantities. These folates are usually supplied as polyglutamates that are cleaved in the intestinal lumen. The monoglutamate form is believed to be absorbed into the bloodstream. Oral contraceptives and phenytoin may affect this metabolism and account, at least in part, for the alterations in folate levels when these medications are used.

Folic acid deficiency is rare except in malabsorption conditions, infancy, and pregnancy. The fetus can apparently extract adequate amounts of folate even in the presence of megaloblastic anemia in the mother. This extraction and possibly the reduced availability of folate produced by intestinal flora account for decompensation in pregnant women who have a long history of poor dietary intake.

There is evidence, from a large (but nonrandomized) controlled trial and a smaller randomized study, that daily periconceptional supplementation with folic acid (0.4 mg) plus multivitamins is associated with a reduction in the recurrence risk for neural tube defects among pregnancies in mothers with previously affected children. Because of problems of possible selection bias in the larger nonrandomized study and insignificance due to small numbers in the smaller randomized trial, a large-scale randomized trial is currently in progress in the United Kingdom. If the results from this trial are similar to those from the previous studies, folic acid and multivitamin supplementation *before* conception may become a reasonable recommendation.

As noted previously, there appears to be an interaction between folic acid and anticonvulsants, most notably phenytoin and phenobarbital. A number of studies have reported an association between low maternal folate levels and congenital malformations. Although prospective studies have failed to confirm this as a causal relationship, it has been implicated as the etiology of teratogenicity in phenytoin-associated malformations. Clinical decision-making is made more difficult by the ability of folic acid supplementation to lower phenytoin blood levels. In some instances, a significant rise in the number of seizures has been reported when folate has been given to a patient receiving phenytoin. Therefore, in gravid patients on antiepileptic medications, it is suggested that blood levels of folic acid and anticonvulsants be carefully followed and changes in dosage made accordingly.

Tissue stores of folate are in the range of 5–10 mg. Nonpregnant women require 50 μg folate daily, and during pregnancy, this rises to 450 μg. A daily dose of 500 μg and 1.0 mg for singleton and twin gestation, respectively, will provide an adequate prophylactic dose of folic acid for mother and fetus during gestation. For treatment of folate deficiency anemia, a daily dose of 1.0 mg with or without a parenteral loading dose is recommended.

Thiamine (Vitamin B₁)

Thiamine functions as a coenzyme in carbohydrate metabolism. Dietary deficiency leads to beriberi. Pregnant women being treated with parenteral feeding for severe hyperemesis gravidarum have been reported to develop Wernicke's encephalopathy, which responded rapidly to thiamine repletion. Studies have revealed an increased requirement for thiamine during pregnancy if serum levels are to be maintained. One study revealed a 25% incidence of deficiency in biochemical parameters requiring thiamine. The significance of these findings is unclear, however, in that the fetus is able to achieve a higher serum level than the mother.

In view of these studies, the recommended dietary allowance (RDA) of thiamine in pregnancy is 0.1 mg/1,000 kcal greater than the 0.5 mg/1,000 kcal needed by a nonpregnant woman.

Riboflavin (Vitamin B₂)

Riboflavin acts as a coenzyme required for the flavoproteins involved in oxidative metabolism. Moderate degrees of deficiency have caused fetal malformations in rodents. No association between deficiency and malformations in humans has been noted.

Recent studies have used levels of erythrocyte glutathione reductase as a measure of riboflavin deficiency. This test measures flavin-adenine-dinucleotide, the major riboflavin coenzyme. These studies have revealed an increasing requirement as pregnancy progresses. This has been clinically confirmed by the manifestations of deficiency (i.e., glossitis, angular stomatitis, cheilosis, and corneal vascularization) in the third trimester in mothers with low riboflavin intake.

Despite symptoms in the mother, however, no influence on the outcome of pregnancy could be detected. This maternal-fetal discrepancy may be related to the active transport of riboflavin across the placenta. Cord levels have been reported to be as high as 4 times those in the mother's serum.

In view of these studies, the RDA includes an intake of 0.3 mg/day during pregnancy above the baseline of 0.6 mg/1,000 kcal/day.

Niacin

Niacin is the generic name for nicotinic acid and nicotinamide. Nicotinamide functions in coenzymes concerned with glycolysis, fat synthesis, and tissue respiration.

Although pellagra has been found to be associated with dietary deficiency of niacin in areas in which corn is the major source of protein, the relationship between the two is not linear. Some dietary tryptophan can be converted to niacin, and a ratio of 60 mg tryptophan to 1 mg niacin has been proposed.

The RDA includes an increase for pregnant women of 2 mg above the basal allowance of 6.6 mg/1,000 kcal. This accounts for the increased allowance of calories during gestation. There have been no controlled studies regarding the influence of dietary deficiency during pregnancy.

Pyridoxine (Vitamin B_6)

Vitamin B_6 is a group of interrelated substances: pyridoxine, pyridoxamine, pyridoxal, and pyridoxal phosphate. Phosphorylated pyridoxal is required as a coenzyme in amino acid metabolism. A number of conditions have been related to B_6 deficiency; dietary deprivation can result in seizures, hypochromic microcytic anemia, abdominal distress, vomiting, depression, and confusion. The use of certain medications such as penicillamine, isoniazid, and oral contraceptives has been shown to increase the excretion of B_6.

Vitamin B_6 was first administered in 1942 as a treatment for hyperemesis gravidarum. Since that time much controversy has arisen regarding B_6 supplementation during pregnancy. All studies reveal a lower level of B_6-dependent activities during pregnancy. Serum levels fall late in the first trimester and remain depressed throughout pregnancy. A rise to the normal values for nonpregnant women has been noted by the fourth postpartum day.

The placenta actively transports B_6, and studies have revealed high placental levels of pyridoxal kinase. Levels in the fetus are 2–3 times higher than those in the mother, but they rise further with increases in the mother's levels. Umbilical vein levels are higher than those in the umbilical artery, indicating fetal utilization.

Attempts at normalization of biochemical and excretion indices, as well as serum levels, in pregnant women have suggested that supplementation of 10–15 mg/day is needed. No controlled trials have suggested benefits to the mother or fetus by this type of supplementation. The use of megadose pyridoxine (2,000–6,000 mg/day) has been associated with a form of sensory neuropathy consisting of sensory ataxia and profound distal limb impairment of position and vibration sense in human adults.

In view of these difficulties, the RDA includes an increase of 0.5 mg/day above the basal requirements of 2.5 mg/day.

Pyridoxine in doses of 200–600 mg/day has been shown to be effective in reversing hyperprolactinemia in women with amenorrhea-galactorrhea syndromes and in suppressing postpartum lactation in normal individuals. For this reason, high dosages should not be taken by breast-feeding mothers.

Cyanocobalamin (Vitamin B_{12})

Vitamin B_{12} is present in all cells of mammalian tissue. It is essential in nucleic acid metabolism because of its role in allowing 5-methyltetrahydrofolate to return to the utilizable folate pool. Deficiency results in megaloblastosis of the bone marrow and gastrointestinal mucosa as well as in neuronal dysfunction.

The average diet contains 5–15 μg vitamin B_{12} daily. Absorption via intrinsic factor is quite efficient, and dietary deficiency is very rare, except in strict vegetarians. An infant has been reported with megaloblastic anemia, coma, and hyperpigmentation of the extremities who manifested methylmalonic aciduria and homocystinuria. This child's mother, who was exclusively breast-feeding him, was a strict vegetarian who was taking no vitamin B_{12} supplements. The infant's problems completely resolved with vitamin B_{12} therapy.

Studies have revealed a progressive decline in serum vitamin B_{12} levels during pregnancy. It is unlikely that this is a true deficiency state; rather, it is a physiologic alteration. The fetus has been shown to concentrate vitamin B_{12} and fetal cord serum levels are about 3 times maternal values.

In view of a demonstrated increase in urinary excretion of vitamin B_{12} during pregnancy, the RDA includes the addition of 1 μg/day during pregnancy above the basal requirement of 3 μg/day.

Pantothenic Acid

Pantothenic acid is a portion of coenzyme A, an integral link in the acetylation processes of intermediary metabolism. It is widely distributed in nature, and dietary deficiency has not been demonstrated.

A study in pregnant teenage women found a daily intake of 4.7 mg. This is lower than the average American daily ingestion of 5–20 mg. Blood and urinary excretion levels were also found to be lower in the pregnant teenagers.

Ingestion of 10 mg daily is suggested for pregnant and lactating women. Supplementation with 5–10 mg daily during pregnancy may be required to meet these needs.

Ascorbic Acid (Vitamin C)

Humans and other primates, when deprived of vitamin C, develop scurvy, a fatal disease characterized by weakening of collagen. Scurvy still occurs in infants who are fed only cow's milk and in malnourished and alcoholic adults. Although levels in the fetus are 2–3 times higher than those in the mother, congenital scurvy has occurred in children born to mothers with the disease. Deficiency of vitamin C has been associated with impaired wound healing. This vitamin is involved in the synthesis of epinephrine and the adrenal steroids.

Ascorbic acid levels progressively decline during pregnancy. Increased levels in the fetus appear to be due to "trapping." The placenta allows passive transfer of dehydroascorbic acid, and conversion to the impermeable ascorbic acid in the fetus allows higher concentrations to accumulate.

A great deal of controversy has arisen regarding the intake of large doses of vitamin C to prevent the common cold. Studies have not consistently shown this practice to be effective. Theoretic risks include the oxidant effect of large amounts of ascorbic acid in the fetus, and the possibility that prenatal conditioning of the fetus to large amounts of this substance could lead to the development of infantile scurvy despite a diet that contains adequate amounts of ascorbic acid. In view of these considerations, large doses of vitamin C are not recommended during pregnancy. The RDA includes an intake of 60 mg/day in pregnant women and 80 mg/day in lactating women.

FAT-SOLUBLE VITAMINS

Vitamin A

Dietary vitamin A (retinol) is in the form of preformed vitamin A and carotenoids, especially beta-carotene. Carotenoids must be converted to retinol in order to be useful to the body. Retinol is required for mucous membrane maintenance and as an essential link in the conversion of light energy to nervous activity in the visual process. The chronic intake of large amounts of vitamin A ($\geq$ 50,000 units/day) has been associated with hypervitaminosis A, which includes headache, nausea, stiff neck, elevated intracranial pressure, papilledema, and elevated serum glutamic oxaloacetic transaminase (SGOT) levels.

Serum vitamin A levels fall in early pregnancy, with a subsequent rise early in the second trimester. Levels at midpregnancy exceed those of nonpregnant women and rise to approximately 150% of baseline values. A slight fall is noted before the onset of labor.

The placenta seems to be much more permeable to carotene than to retinol. Levels of retinol of mother and fetus are similar. Lower levels of carotene in the fetus occur with fetal conversion of carotene to retinol, causing trapping of the vitamin.

No effects on the fetus from low levels of vitamin A have been reported. Conversely, experimental hypervitaminosis A has been associated with a variety of congenital anomalies. Although these have been principally seen in experimental animals, a recent report has documented ureteral anomalies in a patient whose mother consumed large doses of vitamin A. In a study of 56 mothers of babies with central nervous system malformations, postpartum serum levels of vitamin A were found to be higher than those of normal control mothers. Isotretinoin, a vitamin A isomer, has been clearly associated with teratogenesis in humans. This drug is covered separately (see *Isotretinoin*).

The RDA is 1,000 retinol units during pregnancy. This rise of 20% above the requirement for nonpregnant women allows for fetal storage. In view of the higher dosages recommended in some popular literature, vitamin A intake in the pregnant woman should be carefully monitored by the physician.

Vitamin D

The physiologic importance of vitamin D resides in its regulatory role in calcium hemostasis. Vitamin D accelerates intestinal absorption of calcium against an electrochemical gradient and is required for proper bone formation. A deficiency results in rickets in children and osteomalacia in adults.

Vitamin D exists in two forms: D_2 (ergocalciferol) and D_3 (cholecalciferol). D_2 is synthetically produced by the ultraviolet irradiation of the plant sterol ergosterol. D_3 is naturally formed in animal tissue by the exposure of 7-dehydrocholesterol to sunlight. Both forms are equally effective in humans. Activity requires conversion of these substrates to the 1,25-dihydroxycholecalciferol form sequentially in the liver and kidney.

The level of active forms of vitamin D during pregnancy appears to be related to dietary intake. Values in the fetus seem to reflect the mother's levels, but some regulation via facilitated diffusion probably occurs. This mechanism has been suggested because high maternal levels have been associated with values in the fetus of 68–90% of those in the mother, while levels in the fetus of 108% of the mother's values have been noted with low maternal levels.

The importance of proper vitamin D intake during pregnancy has been documented by the finding of hypocalcemia with low 25-hydroxycholecalciferol levels in premature infants born to mothers with little prenatal care and low serum levels.

Excessive levels of vitamin D intake may contribute to the production of severe maternal and neonatal hypercalcemia. This is especially hazardous with concomitant antacid ingestion. A syndrome of supravalvular aortic stenosis, as well as cranial and facial anomalies, has been reported in animal species and in humans exposed to large amounts of vitamin D in utero. For this reason, excessive dosages should not be ingested by pregnant women.

The RDA does not include an increase during pregnancy above the basal requirement of 400 IU/day. This quantity of vitamin D is present in 1 quart of fortified milk.

Vitamin E

Vitamin E has not been shown to be essential for humans. Plasma levels of full-term newborns are about one-third those of adults, and lower levels are found in premature infants. Values in the mother rise during pregnancy to 60% above nonpregnant levels. Since the bulk of plasma vitamin E is carried by serum lipoproteins, the relative concentrations of these substances probably account for these differences.

Although various symptoms have developed in laboratory animals deprived of vitamin E, the only condition associated with deficiency in humans is decreased red blood cell survival time in infants with low birth weight. Studies attempting to raise levels in the fetus to normal adult levels have required increases of 150–500% over the values of nonpregnant women to achieve this goal. Supplementation has been found to be more effective in the newborn period.

In view of the sparsity of data, the suggested RDA is an intake of 10–20 IU/day since this is present in the average American diet. The increase in caloric intake for pregnant and lactating women should account for any additional quantities required by the fetus.

Vitamin K

The synthesis of coagulation factors II, VII, IX, and X by the liver requires the presence of vitamin K. This vitamin exists in two forms, K_1 (phylloquinone) and K_2 (menaquinone). The former is produced by plants, the latter by bacteria. Menadione, a fat-soluble synthetic product, has approximately twice the biologic activity of the natural forms. In view of the production of K_2 by intestinal bacteria, dietary deficiency does not exist in the absence of suppression of gut flora.

The newborn intestine contains few bacteria, and the neonate is subject to hemorrhagic tendencies due to relative vitamin K deficiency as well as hepatic immaturity. To a large extent the prolonged prothrombin time seen in the neonate can be normalized by the administration of vitamin K.

In an effort to influence coagulation in the early postnatal period, several investigators have given vitamin K prenatally. The use of large dosages of menadione has produced hemolytic anemia in rats and kernicterus in infants of low birth weight. Oral but not intramuscular administration of water-soluble vitamin K_1 over the last month of pregnancy has been most effective in improving the neonate's coagulation status.

The current recommendation is 0.5–1.0 mg vitamin K_1 administered intramuscularly to the neonate immediately after birth.

Minerals

Iron

Iron is absorbed primarily in the duodenum and jejunum. Mucosal absorption is affected by gastric juice and gastroferrin, an iron-binding mucoprotein. It is also affected by dietary and pharmacologic substances such as phosphates, and oxalates, which may bind iron in nonabsorbable complexes. In the mucosal cell the excess iron absorbed by the intestine is bound as ferritin and shed. This regulatory mechanism usually prevents excess iron accumulation when dietary intake increases.

Approximately 0.5–2.0 mg iron daily is transported into the bloodstream, where it is bound by transferrin. The transferrin-iron complex circulates, allowing the iron to reach the normoblasts of the bone marrow. In the normoblast, through the action of the enzyme ferrochetolase, an atom of iron is added to protoporphyrin, forming heme. The combination of four globin and four heme molecules forms hemoglobin. Iron is also used in the production of myoglobin, cytochromes, and catalases.

Nature has provided an efficient method of conserving iron in the absence of blood loss. Despite an average red blood cell (RBC) life span of 120 days, loss of iron is prevented by reutilization. The hemoglobin molecule is broken down in the reticuloendothelial system. The iron molecule is then transferred via transferrin back to the normoblasts in the marrow.

A normal 60-kg woman has about 2.1 g iron in her body. A nonpregnant woman has a menstrual loss of 0.5–1.5 mg iron/month as well as a daily loss of about 0.6 mg from the gastrointestinal tract and skin. A pregnant woman continues to have the same daily loss. In addition, the average fetus at term contains approximately 200–250 mg iron while the placenta and cord have another 50 mg. The physiologic increase in maternal RBC volume requires an additional 500–600 mg iron. This leads to a requirement of about 750–900 mg iron over the course of a pregnancy.

An average American diet contains approximately 6 mg iron/1,000 kcal. Of this iron, approximately 10–20% is absorbed, depending on body requirements. Although it would seem that the availability of 0.6–1.2 mg iron/1,000 kcal is sufficient to meet daily requirements, the demands of growth in adolescence and poor nutrition have led to an incidence of iron deficiency of between 10 and 60% in teenage women.

Observations that utilized bone marrow samples stained for iron stores have shown that 30 mg oral iron taken every day in the second and third trimesters prevents the depletion of stores during pregnancy.

Most authorities believe that higher dosages are justified in order to obtain normal levels of hemoglobin in those patients with iron-deficiency anemia. Since 34 mg absorbed iron per day results in a maximal response in these patients, the recommendation is for 180 mg of oral elemental iron supplementation daily in three divided doses.

Many oral iron preparations exist. Standard forms include ferrous sulfate (20% elemental iron), ferrous gluconate (12% elemental iron), and ferrous fumarate (33% elemental iron). Generally the quantity of elemental iron absorbed in iron-deficient states from these inorganic preparations is higher than that from foods. Although prenatal multivitamin preparations often contain iron, inhibition of iron absorption has been demonstrated to be directly related to the amounts of calcium carbonate and magnesium oxide in these preparations.

The most prominent side effects of oral medicinal iron are related to gastrointestinal intolerance. These include nausea, vomiting, diarrhea, and constipation. Melena, unrelated to gastrointestinal hemorrhage, may develop. It has been recommended that these effects can be minimized with a gradual increase of iron dosage up to the amount desired.

Parenteral iron is sometimes prescribed when an iron-deficiency anemia is initially discovered during the last few weeks of pregnancy or when the patient cannot be relied on to take oral iron. It is important to realize when administering parenteral iron that the rapidity of response is essentially the same as with the oral preparations. The major advantage of using parenteral preparations is that the total estimated dose required can be delivered to the patient within a few days and one can be assured that the patient has actually received the iron.

The use of parenteral forms of iron must be undertaken with great caution. Anaphylactic reactions, sometimes fatal, occur in association with both intramuscular and intravenous use. There is no evidence that such reactions occur less frequently with intramuscular administration. Other adverse effects that have been reported with use of iron dextran (Imferon®) include severe febrile reactions, reactivation of quiescent rheumatoid arthritis, and phlebitis at the intravenous infusion site.

Intramuscular injections of iron dextran may be less preferable than slow intravenous infusion, as the former often causes pain at the site of injection as well as severe skin discoloration. Intramuscular administration may also be associated with sarcoma formation at the injection sites.

Iron dextran is given in a total dosage of 10–40 ml (500–2,000 mg), according to the patient's calculated needs. The total dosage may be diluted in a liter of intravenous fluid and administered slowly for the first 15–30 minutes to detect any allergic reactions, and then more rapidly over 2–6 hours. Alternatively, 0.5 ml may be given intravenously over a 1-minute period, with the remainder of the dose administered slowly after 15–20 minutes. In the latter method, the total dose may be given at one time or it may be divided into 5- to 10-ml increments over several injections.

Calcium

The body of the human adult contains 1,100–1,200 g calcium, 99% of which is present in bone. Bone calcium is complexed with phosphate as hydroxyapatite. There is a diurnal flux of about 700 mg daily.

The level of ionized serum calcium is controlled by hormonal and nutritional factors and is maintained in a narrow range. At physiologic conditions, approximately 7% of calcium is complexed with citrates and phosphates. The remainder is divided approximately evenly between free forms and protein-bound forms. Only the free ionized calcium exerts its physiologic effects and is hormonally governed.

The major influences on serum calcium concentration and phosphorus concentration are their solubility products, vitamin D intake and metabolism, and secretion of the hormones parathormone and calcitonin.

Parathormone is released in response to low or falling levels of ionized calcium. It then acts to increase this level by increasing osteoclast activity, decreasing the renal tubular absorption of phosphate, and augmenting the action of vitamin D in facilitating calcium absorption. High serum levels of ionized calcium cause release of calcitonin, and this hormone inhibits release of calcium from bone.

Vitamin D in its physiologic forms, 1-hydroxycholecalciferol and 1,25-dihydroxycholecalciferol, is essential for the active absorption of calcium from the gut as well as the proper synthesis of bone matrix.

During pregnancy, there is an obligatory transfer of approximately 30 g calcium to the fetus for mineralization of the skeleton. A number of factors permit this loss by combining to increase intestinal absorption.

Human placental lactogen and high levels of estrogen combine to effect an acceleration of bone metabolism and bone formation. The lower level of ionized calcium produced induces elevation of serum parathormone, which results in a balance of bone formation and resorption, and augments intestinal calcium absorption. This enhancement of bone metabolism and increase in calcium absorption provide an excellent source of calcium that becomes available to the fetus.

The placenta actively transports calcium to the fetus. At full term levels of parathormone in the fetus are low and calcitonin levels high, favoring bone formation.

The calcium reserve in the mother's skeleton is quite high in comparison to needs of the fetus. Although adequate fetal mineralization can occur without calcium supplementation, most authorities believe that the 30 g loss to the fetus should be replaced. This can be accomplished by adding 300–400 mg calcium to the 800 mg normal daily requirement. This total of 1,200 mg can be obtained by drinking 1 quart of milk daily. This amount also provides adequate levels of vitamin D and is sufficient for nursing mothers.

For patients intolerant of milk, similar intake may be provided by means of calcium supplements. In view of the controversial association of leg cramps with high serum phosphorus levels, supplements should probably be in the form of nonphosphorus salts; 500 mg calcium gluconate bid should suffice.

Zinc

Zinc is essential as a cofactor for many enzyme systems in plants and animals. Although the body contains relatively large amounts of zinc stored in bone, these supplies are not metabolically active. Dietary deficiency leads to loss of appetite and failure to grow. Gross zinc deficiency seen in the Middle East results in hypogonadism and dwarfism. Intrauterine deficiency, even when temporary, has resulted in permanent anomalies in experimental animals.

Marginal zinc deficiency seems to exist in the United States, usually in areas with low soil levels of zinc. Giving supplements to children with marginal deficiency has resulted in increased taste acuity, improved appetite, and greater growth.

Congenital lesions of the central nervous system appear to be greater in geographic areas in which zinc deficiency exists. Some studies have revealed that zinc is an essential component of the bacterial inhibitory system of the amniotic fluid. There is some suggestion that dietary availability of zinc may alter the effectiveness of this system. A case report of four pregnant women given megadose (300 mg) zinc daily during the third trimester described three preterm live births and one stillbirth.

Total body zinc increases throughout pregnancy. Levels at full term are approximately 50% above those of nonpregnant women. Plasma and hair concentrations, however, fall during this period.

The zinc content of the diet of an average American adult is 10–25 mg. Metabolic studies have revealed that balance can be maintained with an intake of 8–10 mg daily in the nonpregnant state. Subnormal maternal serum zinc levels have been reported in the first trimester among women destined to develop preeclampsia and during labor in alcoholic women.

Despite the important implications of the above-mentioned observations, little data are available on the maintenance of homeostasis in the pregnant woman. The recommended daily allowance (RDA) includes an additional 15 mg/day during pregnancy, above basal recommendations of 15 mg/day. This may indicate a need for supplementation. Of the commonly prescribed vitamin preparations, 15 mg/zinc/capsule is contained in Natalins Rx® and One-A-Day Plus Minerals®.

Chromium

Interest in chromium metabolism in pregnancy has centered around its role in glucose utilization. Chromium deficiency can be associated with decreased glucose tolerance, and its supplementation has ameliorated glucose intolerance in some clinical states. Studies have revealed lower serum concentrations during pregnancy than in the nonpregnant state. Gravid patients have failed to respond to a glucose load with the decrease in chromium level noted in nonpregnant subjects. The relationship of these findings to the impaired glucose utilization characteristic of pregnancy is unknown at this time.

Iodine

Iodine is required in the formation of the thyroid hormones, thyroxine and triiodothyronine. Iodine deficiency leads to goiter formation. For nonpregnant adult women, the minimal requirement necessary to prevent goiter formation is approximately 1 μg/kg body weight. The RDA for iodine is between 100 and 300 μg/day. The most efficient method of obtaining this amount is through iodized salt, which contains 76 μg iodine/g. Since iodized salt is rarely used in commercially prepared foods, it is recommended that this preparation be used as added table salt.

It should be noted that pharmacologic dosages of iodides may cause goiter formation in the fetus. Rapid and sustained elevation of maternal serum iodine levels has been demonstrated after vaginal application of povidone-iodine solutions used to treat vaginitis.

Copper

Copper is essential for all mammals. In rare instances, copper dietary deficiency has occurred in humans, leading to anemia, neutropenia, and bone disease. In experimental animals with copper deficiencies, major anomalies have been produced as a result of defective cross-linking in elastin and collagen. The fetus requires copper, which accumulates in certain fetal organs in much greater concentrations than are seen in adult tissue. The copper concentration in the fetal liver, for example, is 5 to 10 times that of an adult.

Copper intake of 2 mg/day seems to maintain a homeostatic balance in adults. Serum levels in the fetus rise throughout pregnancy. This may be related to elevated levels of estrogen since the increase of the two is coincident. Furthermore, exogenous estrogens raise serum levels of copper in nonpregnant women.

Multivitamin Preparations

Table 14 is a list of some commonly available prenatal multivitamin preparations. As mentioned in the text, supplementation of zinc and pantothenic acid may be required during pregnancy. Of the commonly used prenatal preparations containing 30 mg iron or more, only Natalins Rx® contains zinc.

Table 14. Content of selected vitamins and minerals of some prenatal multivitamin preparations

Multivitamin preparation	Iron[a]	Folate[a]	B$_6$[a]	D[b]	Calcium[a]	B$_{12}$[a]	Zinc[a]	Iodine[a]
Materna 1.60®	60	1	4	400	250	12	25	0.3
Natabec Kapseals®	30	0	3	400	600	5	0	0
Natabec Rx Kapseals®	30	1	3	400	600	5	0	0
Natalins®	45	0.8	4	400	200	8	0	0
Natalins Rx®	60	1	10	400	200	8	15	0.15
Stuart Prenatal®	60	0.8	4	400	200	8	0	0.15
Stuartnatal 1 + 1®	65	1	10	400	200	12	0	0.15

[a] In mg.
[b] In IU.

Recommended Reading

Bernhardt, I. B., and Dorsey, D. J. Hypervitaminosis A and congenital renal anomalies in a human fetus. *Obstet. Gynecol.* 43:750, 1974.

Brzezinski, A., Bromberg, Y. M., and Braun, K. Riboflavin excretion during pregnancy and early lactation. *J. Lab. Clin. Med.* 39:84, 1952.

Cleary, R. E., Lumeng, L., and Li, T. Maternal and fetal plasma levels of pyridoxal phosphate at term: Adequacy of vitamin B_6 supplementation during pregnancy. *Am. J. Obstet. Gynecol.* 121:25, 1975.

Cochrane, W. A. Overnutrition in prenatal and neonatal life: A problem? *Can. Med. Assoc. J.* 93:893, 1965.

Cohlan, S. Q. Congenital anomalies in the rat produced by excessive intake of vitamin A during pregnancy. *Pediatrics* 13:556, 1954.

Coursin, D. B., and Brown, V. C. Changes in vitamin B_6 during pregnancy. *Am. J. Obstet. Gynecol.* 82:1307, 1961.

Davidson, I. W., and Burt, R. L. Physiologic changes in plasma chromium of normal and pregnant women: Effect of a glucose load. *Am. J. Obstet. Gynecol.* 116:601, 1973.

Davies, N. T., and Williams, R. B. Zinc balance during pregnancy and lactation. *Am. J. Clin. Nutr.* 30:300, 1977.

Dokumov, S. I. Serum copper and pregnancy. *Am. J. Obstet. Gynecol.* 101:217, 1968.

Farris, W. A., and Erdman, J. W., Jr. Protracted hypervitaminosis A following long-term, low-level intake. *J.A.M.A.* 247:1317, 1982.

Flynn, A., et al. Zinc status of pregnant alcoholic women: A determinant of fetal outcome. *Lancet* 1:572, 1981.

Foukas, M. D. An antilactogenic effect of pyridoxine. *J. Obstet. Gynaecol. Br. Commw.* 80:718, 1973.

Friedman, W. F. Vitamin D and the supravalvular aortic stenosis syndrome. *Adv. Teratol.* 3:85, 1968.

Friedman, W. F., and Mills, L. F. The relationship between vitamin D and the craniofacial and dental anomalies of the supravalvular aortic stenosis syndrome. *Pediatrics* 43:12, 1969.

Gal, I., Sharman, I. M., and Pryse-Davies, J. Vitamin A in relation to human congenital malformations. *Adv. Teratol.* 5:143, 1972.

Geelen, J. A. G. Hypervitaminosis A induced teratogenesis. *C.R.C. Crit. Rev. Toxicol.* 6:351, 1979.

Greenberg, G. Sarcoma after intramuscular iron injection. *Br. Med. J.* 1:1508, 1976.

Heller, S., Salkeld, R. M., and Korner, W. F. Riboflavin status in pregnancy. *Am. J. Clin. Nutr.* 27:1225, 1974.

Heller, S., Salkeld, R. M., and Korner, W. F. Vitamin B_1 status in pregnancy. *Am. J. Clin. Nutr.* 27:1221, 1974.

Higginbottom, M. C., Sweetman, L., and Nyhan, W. L. A syndrome of methylmalonic aciduria, homocystinuria, megaloblastic anemia and neurologic abnormalities in a vitamin B_{12}–deficient breast-fed infant of a strict vegetarian. *N. Engl. J. Med.* 299:317, 1978.

Kitay, D. Z., and Harbort, M. S. Iron and folic acid deficiency in pregnancy. *Clin. Perinatol.* 2:255, 1975.

Lavin, P. J. M., et al. Wernicke's encephalopathy: A predictable complication of hyperemesis gravidarum. *Obstet. Gynecol.* 62(Suppl.):13S, 1983.

Lundin, P. M. The carcinogenic action of complex iron preparations. *Br. J. Cancer* 15:838, 1961.

Malone, J. M. Vitamin passage across the placenta. *Clin. Perinatol.* 2:295, 1975.

McIntosh, E. N. Treatment of women with the galactorrhea-amenorrhea syndrome with pyridoxine (vitamin B$_6$). *J. Clin. Endocrinol. Metab.* 42:1192, 1976.

Owen, G. M., et al. Use of vitamin K$_1$ in pregnancy. *Am. J. Obstet. Gynecol.* 99:368, 1967.

Pitkin, R. M. Calcium metabolism in pregnancy: A review. *Am. J. Obstet. Gynecol.* 121:724, 1975.

Pitkin, R. M. Vitamins and minerals in pregnancy. *Clin. Perinatol.* 2:221, 1975.

Recommended Daily Allowances (8th ed.). Washington, D.C.: National Academy of Science, 1974.

Rhead, W. J., and Schrauzer, G. N. Risks of long-term ascorbic acid overdosage. *Nutr. Rev.* 29:262, 1971.

Schaumburg, H., et al. Sensory neuropathy from pyridoxine abuse. *N. Engl. J. Med.* 309:445, 1983.

Schlievert, P., Johnson, W., and Galask, R. P. Bacterial growth inhibition by the amnionic fluid: VII. The effect of zinc supplementation on bacterial inhibitory activity of amniotic fluids from gestation of 20 weeks. *Am. J. Obstet. Gynecol.* 127:603, 1977.

Scott, D. E., and Pritchard, J. A. Anemia in pregnancy. *Clin. Perinatol.* 1:491, 1974.

Seligman, P. A., et al. Measurements of iron absorption from prenatal multivitamin-mineral supplements. *Obstet. Gynecol.* 61:356, 1983.

Vitamin supplements. *Med. Lett. Drugs Ther.* 27:66, 1985.

Vorherr, H., et al. Vaginal absorption of povidone-iodine. *J.A.M.A.* 244:2628, 1980.

Wald, N. J. Neural-tube defects and vitamins: The need for a randomized clinical trial. *Br. J. Obstet. Gynaecol.* 91:516, 1984.

Zimmerman, A. W., et al. Zinc transport in pregnancy. *Am. J. Obstet. Gynecol.* 149:523, 1984.

Appendix B
Effects of Industrial Chemicals
on Pregnancy

The increasing participation of pregnant women in the labor force and growing knowledge of environmental health insults have prompted considerable concern about possible hazards of workplace exposures to pregnant women. This appendix provides clinicians with available information regarding the effects of selected industrial chemicals on pregnant women and their fetuses. Since there are tens of thousands of chemicals in industrial use today, this review covers only a small fraction of potentially hazardous chemicals. The specific compounds included here are either those that have been shown to pose a hazard to reproduction or those that are commonly present in the workplace and for which some human reproductive data are available.

The format used for presenting the information on chemicals is by necessity different from that used for the drug entries. Each chemical entry begins with a list of common synonyms, the major uses of the particular compound, a listing of selected occupational groups who may potentially be exposed to the chemical in question, and current exposure standards. The OSHA/PEL refers to the current federal standard set by the Occupational Safety and Health Agency (OSHA) for the permissible exposure limit (PEL) of the particular compound in the workplace. The NIOSH recommendation is the exposure limit that the National Institute for Occupational Safety and Health has recommended to OSHA as of July 1985. Following the exposure standards is a brief description of the major routes of entry of the chemical into the worker's body. The section on biologic effects summarizes the information on general health toxicity (other than that related to the reproductive system) and thus serves as a guide for identifying symptoms that may have resulted from a particular occupational exposure.

The evidence for possible reproductive toxicity is considered under Special Considerations in Pregnancy. Although the focus is on harmful effects to the mother and fetus, notable data on possible impairments to both male and female reproductive function are also included. In addition, this section briefly describes existing evidence for human mutagenicity as well as pertinent animal evidence of adverse reproductive effects. Finally, there is an abbreviated list of recommended readings for each chemical reviewed.

It should be emphasized that the available data on chemical exposures and reproductive outcome are very sparse. As the reader may observe, a disproportionate number of reports come from the Soviet Union and eastern Europe. Since these reports often provide insufficient information regarding study design and population characteristics, it is difficult to assess the validity of their results. There are also more general methodologic problems inherent in assessing the effects of occupational exposures on reproduction, including the presence of multiple exposures, the lack of data on exposure levels, the difficulty in finding appropriate control groups, and the potential for unreliable or biased reporting of both exposures and certain pregnancy outcomes, such as spontaneous abortions. Despite these limitations, it is important for clinicians to recognize the potential effects that industrial chemicals can have on their pregnant patients.

Abbreviations

EPA   The *Environmental Protection Agency,* an independent agency within the federal government, was created in 1970 to protect the environment.

mg/m^3 Milligrams per cubic meter.

NIOSH   The *National Institute for Occupational Safety and Health* is an organization created by the OSHAct of 1970 within the U.S. Department of Health and Human Services. One of the functions of NIOSH is to develop recommendations for limits of exposure to potentially hazardous substances in the workplace.

OSHA   The *Occupational Safety and Health Agency,* created by the OSHAct of 1970 and part of the U.S. Department of Labor, is responsible for establishing and enforcing safety and health standards in the workplace.

PEL   The *permissible exposure limit* is the legal exposure standard set by OSHA. It generally represents the workshift time-weighted average (TWA) levels that should not be exceeded in the workplace.

ppb   Parts per billion.

ppm   Parts per million.

TWA   *Time-weighted average* is the permissible exposure limit (PEL) set by OSHA based on an 8-hour workday or 40-hour workweek exposure. The NIOSH TWA recommendations are generally based on up to a 10-hour workday exposure.

Aniline

SYNONYMS

Aminobenzene, aminophen, aniline oil, phenylamine, arylamine

USES

In manufacture of dyestuffs, marking inks, shoe polishes, tetryl, rubber accelerators, antioxidants, pharmaceuticals, resins, varnishes, perfumes, optical whitening agents, photographic developers; in synthesis of many organic chemicals

SELECTED OCCUPATIONAL GROUPS POTENTIALLY EXPOSED

Makers of bromide, disinfectants, inks, perfume, photographic chemicals, rocket fuel, tetryl; acetanilid workers, coal tar workers, dye workers, leather workers, lithographers, nitraniline workers, plastic workers, printers, rubber workers, varnish workers

EXPOSURE STANDARD

OSHA/PEL: 5 ppm ($19 mg/m^3$) as a TWA for an 8-hour workshift

ROUTES OF ENTRY

Inhalation of vapor; percutaneous absorption of liquid and vapor

Biologic Effects

Eye irritation, and possibly corneal damage, may result from exposure to liquid aniline. Inhalation of vapors or percutaneous absorption of the liquid can cause cyanosis and anoxia as a result of the formation of methemoglobin. Methemoglobin is a normal constituent of human blood, with a reported range of 0–0.5 g/dl and a mean of 0.09 g/dl in adults. Cyanosis is thought to occur when methemoglobin reaches levels of 1.5 g/dl or greater. The cyanosis can be accompanied by headache, weakness, nausea, drowsiness, dyspnea, and unconsciousness as oxygen deprivation increases. Death can occur if prompt treatment is not given. Intravascular hemolysis and anemia are thought to be rare sequelae of aniline–induced methemoglobinemia.

Special Considerations in Pregnancy

Concern about possible adverse reproductive effects from aniline exposure stems from aniline's ability to convert hemoglobin to methemoglobin. Fetal hemoglobin has been found in vitro to be more susceptible to methemoglobin formation than adult hemoglobin. Evidence of placental transfer of aniline in humans is not available, but enzymes necessary for aniline metabolism have been identified in human fetal liver by 6–7 weeks' gestation and in adrenal kidney and placental tissue by 8–22 weeks'. Several reports have appeared during the past century of aniline poisoning in neonates from diapers marked with indelible ink that had not been laundered before use.

Epidemiologic data are inadequate for evaluating the effect of either aniline exposure or maternal methemoglobin levels on the fetus. A single Russian study has reported an increased spontaneous abortion rate as well as more frequent menstrual and ovarian dysfunction among women employed in the aniline industry. Since the abortion rate in this study was highest (23%) among women in a low-exposure area where considerable physical activity was required, it is not clear whether the aniline exposure was responsible for the adverse effects. In a small preliminary study, methemoglobin levels were slightly higher in women who threatened to abort or subsequently aborted compared to patients whose pregnancies were maintained.

Aniline has not been found to be a mutagen in several in vitro tests, although it has been associated with an increased frequency of sister chromatid exchanges.

Recommended Reading

Barlow, S. M., and Sullivan, F. M. *Reproductive Hazards of Industrial Chemicals.* New York: Academic, 1982, Pp. 55–61.

Council on Scientific Affairs' Advisory Panel on Reproductive Hazards in the Workplace. *Effects of Toxic Chemicals on the Reproductive System.* d50:anil(1–2) (revd. 6-26-85). Chicago: American Medical Association, 1985.

Occupational Diseases: A Guide to Their Recognition. U.S. Dept. of Health, Education and Welfare, NIOSH, publication No. 77-181. Government Printing Office, 1977. Pp. 264–266.

Schmitz, J. T. Methemoglobinemia—a cause of abortions? *Obstet. Gynecol.* 17:413, 1961.

Arsenic and Its Compounds

SYNONYMS

Arsen, arsenic black, gray arsenic, metallic arsenic

SELECTED ARSENIC COMPOUNDS

Arsenic trioxide, arsenic pentoxide, calcium arsenate, calcium arsenite, potassium arsenate, potassium arsenite, sodium arsenate, disodium hydrogen arsenate, sodium arsenite

USES

In metallurgy as an alloying agent with lead and copper; in manufacture of pharmaceuticals, certain types of glass; in pigment production, textile printing, tanning, taxidermy; insecticides, herbicides, pesticides. Arsenic and its compounds are by-products of the smelting of various ores, particularly copper.

SELECTED OCCUPATIONAL GROUPS POTENTIALLY EXPOSED

Makers of alloys, brass and bronze, ceramics and enamel, drugs, dyes, fireworks, herbicides, insecticides, rodenticides, lead shot, semiconductor compounds; aniline workers; arsenic workers; Babbitt metal workers, copper and lead smelters, gold and silver refiners, printing ink workers, taxidermists, textile printers, tree and weed sprayers, type metal workers

EXPOSURE STANDARDS

OSHA/PEL: 0.01 mg/m^3 (of air as arsenic) as a TWA for an 8-hour workshift

NIOSH recommendation: ceiling of 0.002 mg/m^3 (of air as arsenic) during 15-minute sampling period

ROUTES OF ENTRY

Inhalation and ingestion of dust and fumes

Biologic Effects

Arsenic has been recognized since ancient times as a poison and, more recently, as a carcinogen in humans. Acute arsenic poisoning, which is rarely seen in industry, is generally characterized by acute gastroenteritis that is preceded by respiratory tract symptoms when inhalation is the route of entry. Shock, peripheral vascular collapse, and death can occur. Common progressive symptoms of chronic poisoning from inhalation of arsenic compounds are weakness; weight loss; mild gastrointestinal disturbances; conjunctivitis; severe inflammation of mucous membranes of the nose, larynx, and respiratory passage; perforation of nasal septum; skin lesions; peripheral neuritis; and in severe cases, motor paralysis. It is not clear whether chronic arsenic poisoning causes liver damage, but arsenic does have a depressant effect on the bone marrow.

Special Considerations in Pregnancy

Arsenic has been shown to traverse the human placenta easily with possible accumulation in the placenta, but only limited data are available suggesting adverse effects in human pregnancies. A neonatal death has been linked with maternal ingestion of a large quantity of rat poison containing arsenic trioxide. The mother survived after treatment with dimercaprol (BAL) and hemodialysis. An additional case of maternal arsenic poisoning reported in the literature resulted in both maternal and fetal death.

A series of epidemiologic investigations of exposures in and around a smelter in northern Sweden found higher rates of adverse pregnancy outcomes among female employees and populations living close to the smelter compared to more distantly located populations. Although these data are suggestive, the adverse effects cannot solely be attributed to arsenic since the smelter emits several other toxic substances including lead, mercury, cadmium, and sulfur dioxide. Furthermore, the lack of control for other variables such as age and socioeconomic status considerably weakens these studies. Nevertheless, these data as well as findings of increased frequencies of chromosomal aberrations in employees at the smelter and other groups therapeutically or occupationally exposed to arsenic underscore the need for continued evaluation of possible adverse reproductive effects of occupational exposure to this element.

Arsenic has been reported to be present in breast milk after arsenic medication, but supporting data are not available. Studies of accidental arsenic poisoning among children indicate that young infants may be particularly susceptible to arsenic toxicity with possible long-term brain damage.

Arsenic salts have been found to be both embryolethal and teratogenic in rodents, but data on maternal toxicity were not included. The malformations observed among surviving fetuses comprise a spectrum of defects, including exencephaly, encephalocele, skeletal defects, and genitourinary anomalies.

Recommended Reading

Barlow, S. M., and Sullivan, F. M. *Reproductive Hazards of Industrial Chemicals.* New York: Academic, 1982. Pp. 62–82.

Council on Scientific Affairs' Advisory Panel on Reproductive Hazards in the Workplace. *Effects of Toxic Chemicals on the Reproductive System.* d24:as(1–3) (revd. 6-19-85). Chicago: American Medical Association, 1985.

Lugo, G., Cassady, G., and Palmisano, P. Acute maternal arsenic intoxication with fetal death. *Am. J. Dis. Child.* 117:328, 1969.

Nordstrom, S., Beckman, L., and Nordenson, I. Occupational and environmental risks in and around a smelter in northern Sweden. I. Variations in birth weight. *Hereditas* 88:43, 1978.

Nordstrom, S., Beckman, L., and Nordenson, I. Occupational and environmental risks in and around a smelter in northern Sweden. III. Frequencies of spontaneous abortions. *Hereditas* 88:51, 1978.

Nordstrom, S., Beckman, I., and Nordenson, I. Occupational and environmental risks in and around a smelter in northern Sweden. V. Spontaneous abortion among female employees and decreased birth weight in their offspring. *Hereditas* 90:291, 1979.

Nordstrom, S., Beckman, L., and Nordenson, I. Occupational and environmental risks in and around a smelter in northern Sweden. VI. Congenital malformations. *Hereditas* 90:297, 1979.

Occupational Diseases: A Guide to Their Recognition. U.S. Dept. of Health, Education and Welfare, NIOSH, publication No. 77-181. Government Printing Office, 1977. Pp. 325–328.

Benzene

Benzol, benxole, phenyl hydride, coal naphtha, phene, cyclohexatriene

USES

Constituent of motor fuels; solvent for fats, oils, inks, paints, plastics, rubber; in photogravure printing; in extraction of oil from seeds and nuts; in manufacture of detergents, explosives, pharmaceuticals, dyestuffs, and other organic compounds

SELECTED OCCUPATIONAL GROUPS POTENTIALLY EXPOSED

Makers of adhesives, dry batteries, benzene hexachloride, carbolic acid, detergents, dyes, glue, linoleum, maleic acid, nitrobenzene, putty, rubber, styrene; asbestos product impregnators, burnishers, chlorinated benzene workers, furniture finishers, petrochemical workers, welders

EXPOSURE STANDARDS

OSHA/PEL: 10 ppm as a TWA for an 8-hour workshift with a ceiling concentration of 25 ppm and a maximum peak above the ceiling limit of 50 ppm for a maximum duration of 10 minutes
NIOSH recommendation: ceiling of 1 ppm over any 60-minute sampling period

ROUTES OF ENTRY

Inhalation of vapor. Percutaneous absorption is less likely as benzene is poorly absorbed through intact skin.

Biologic Effects

Vapor and liquid are irritating to skin, eyes, and respiratory tract. Acute benzene poisoning results in central nervous system depression characterized by headaches, dizziness, nausea, and convulsions that may result in coma and death. Chronic exposure is associated with myelotoxic effects including anemia, leukopenia, thrombocytopenia, and aplastic anemia. It has recently been concluded that benzene is leukemogenic.

Special Considerations in Pregnancy

Women are more susceptible to benzene poisoning than men, and pregnancy may exacerbate the hematologic changes associated with chronic benzene exposure. Accounts of benzene poisoning among female workers during the early 1900s described bleeding from the nose and gingiva, frequent and excessive menstruation, and hemorrhagic complications of pregnancy that were often fatal. Menstrual disorders and anemia as well as increased rates of spontaneous abortions, premature birth, and other pregnancy complications have been noted in more recent reports of eastern European women who were occupationally exposed to benzene. Chromosomal changes have also been recorded for both male and female workers exposed to high levels of benzene.

In addition, isolated cases of benzene-induced aplastic anemia during pregnancy have been reported. Only one of the mothers survived in a review of five such cases from 1934–1957. Fetal survival appeared to be better than maternal survival although benzene is known to cross the placenta, with concentrations in cord blood equal to or exceeding levels in maternal blood.

Embryolethal or teratogenic effects have not been observed in animal studies although reduced fetal weights have been recorded for several species.

Recommended Reading

Barlow, S. M., and Sullivan F. M. *Reproductive Hazards of Industrial Chemicals.* New York: Academic, 1982. Pp. 83–103.

Council on Scientific Affairs' Advisory Panel on Reproductive Hazards in the Workplace. *Effects of Toxic Chemicals on the Reproductive System.* d49:benz(1–2) (revd. 6-14-85). Chicago: American Medical Association, 1985.

Hunt, V. R. *Work and the Health of Women.* Boca Raton, Fla.: CRC, 1979. Pp. 204–207.

Occupational Diseases: A Guide to Their Recognition. U.S. Dept. of Health, Education and Welfare, NIOSH, publication No. 77-181. Government Printing Office, 1977. Pp. 235–238.

Beryllium and Its Compounds

SYNONYMS

None

SELECTED BERYLLIUM COMPOUNDS

Beryllium chloride, beryllium oxide, beryllium fluoride, beryllium phosphate, beryllium sulfate

USES

As a source of neutrons, moderator, and reflector in atomic energy reactions; alloying agent (e.g., in bushings, electrical contacts and switches, radio and radar components, aircraft parts, watch springs, nonspark tools); window material for x-ray tubes; in manufacture of ceramics; chemical reagent; gas mantle hardener. The use of beryllium in the manufacture of fluorescent lamps was discontinued around 1950.

SELECTED OCCUPATIONAL GROUPS POTENTIALLY EXPOSED

Beryllium alloy workers, missile technicians, nuclear reactor workers; makers of cathode ray tubes, ceramics, electrical equipment, gas mantles, refractory materials

EXPOSURE STANDARDS

OSHA/PEL: 0.002 mg/m^3 as a TWA for an 8-hour workshift with a ceiling concentration of 0.005 mg/m^3 and a maximum peak above ceiling of 0.025 mg/m^3 for no more than 30 minutes
NIOSH recommendation: not to exceed 0.0005 mg/m^3

ROUTE OF ENTRY

Inhalation of fume or dust

Biologic Effects

Beryllium and its compounds are skin, eye, and respiratory tract irritants. The major clinical manifestations of acute beryllium disease are nonproductive cough, substernal pain, and shortness of breath. Intense exposure may result in severe pneumonitis. The clinical features of chronic beryllium disease, which may not be manifested until 5–10 years after the last exposure, are initially respiratory symptoms, weakness, fatigue, and weight loss, followed by nonproductive cough, dyspnea, and bone and joint pain. Remission may occur but the disease often progresses and may involve liver and spleen dysfunction, hypercalciuria, skin lesions, spontaneous pneumothorax, severe physical wasting, oxygen desaturation, and myocardial failure. Beryllium compounds have been found to be carcinogenic in several animal species and are suspected of also being carcinogenic in humans.

Special Considerations in Pregnancy

It is believed that pregnancy may precipitate or exacerbate the symptoms of chronic beryllium disease. Among female cases in the U.S. Beryllium Registry, 40% of the women who had become pregnant after exposure experienced onset or increase of symptoms during or immediately after pregnancy. Maternal prognosis was poor, with 66% of the recorded 95 female deaths related temporally to pregnancy. Beryllium crosses the placenta, but its effect on the fetus is not known.

Animal evidence of possible teratogenic effects is lacking. Data on mutagenicity are inconclusive for animals and inadequate for humans.

Recommended Reading

Barlow, S. M., and Sullivan, F. M. *Reproductive Hazards of Industrial Chemicals.* New York: Academic, 1982. Pp. 119–125.

Hardy, H. L. Beryllium poisoning—lessons in control of man-made disease. *N. Engl. J. Med.* 273:1188, 1965.

Hardy, H. L., and Stoeckle, J. D. Beryllium disease. *J. Chron. Dis.* 9:152, 1959.

Occupational Diseases: A Guide to Their Recognition. U.S. Dept. of Health, Education and Welfare, NIOSH, publication No. 77-181. Government Printing Office, 1977. Pp. 335–338.

Cadmium and Its Compounds

SYNONYMS

None

SELECTED CADMIUM COMPOUNDS

Cadmium carbonate, cadmium chloride, cadmium oxide, cadmium sulfate, cadmium sulfide

USES

Electroplating agent; alloying agent; in electrodes of alkaline storage batteries; neutron absorber in nuclear reactors; plastics stabilizer; deoxidizer in nickel plating; amalgam in dentistry; in manufacture of fluorescent lamps, semiconductors, photocells, jewelry; process engraving; in charging Jones reductors; fungicides, insecticides, polymerization catalysts, pigments, paints, glass; contaminant of superphosphate fertilizers

SELECTED OCCUPATIONAL GROUPS POTENTIALLY EXPOSED

Makers of alloys, batteries, dental amalgam, paint; engravers, metalizers, pesticide workers, solder workers, textile printers, welders, zinc refiners

EXPOSURE STANDARDS

OSHA/PEL: 0.1 mg/m^3 for cadmium fume as a TWA for an 8-hour workshift with a ceiling concentration of 0.3 mg/m^3; 0.2 mg/m^3 for cadmium dust with a ceiling concentration of 0.6 mg/m^3
NIOSH recommendation: reduce exposure to lowest feasible level

ROUTE OF ENTRY

Inhalation or ingestion of fumes or dust

Biologic Effects

Acute poisoning has generally been associated with inhalation of cadmium fumes or dust produced from burning or heating cadmium-containing materials. Progressive symptoms are irritation of upper respiratory tract, cough, chest pain, dyspnea, weakness, and in severe cases, pulmonary edema. Chronic poisoning is usually manifested as lung damage, particularly emphysema, but cadmium absorption can also result in proteinuria and anemia. A yellow stain or ring on the teeth has also been reported after chronic exposure. Contamination of drinking water with waste cadmium has been linked to the development of a disabling bone disorder among postmenopausal Japanese women. Cadmium is also suspected of being a carcinogen.

Special Considerations in Pregnancy

There is some evidence of a partial placental barrier to cadmium transfer in humans, as blood levels in the fetus have generally been lower than those in the mother and placental concentrations have been greater than those in either maternal or fetal blood. Cigarette smoking may further increase cadmium levels in the placenta. Cadmium has also been found to be present in human breast milk. In one small-scale study, reduced birth weights along with bone and teeth abnormalities have been reported among offspring of occupationally exposed women. Levels of cadmium as well as lead were reported to be higher than expected in a series of stillbirths, but no comparison measurements were made among normal infants. Thus, existing data are inadequate for evaluating the effects of cadmium on pregnancy.

There is limited evidence from autopsies of a positive association between occupational exposure to cadmium fumes and testicular damage. Mutagenic activity has been shown in most in vitro studies, but in vivo studies of occupationally exposed men have been inconclusive.

In addition to fetotoxic, teratogenic, and embryolethal effects, parenteral administration of cadmium has produced testicular atrophy in animal experiments. Prenatal inhalation of cadmium has also been found to affect fetal and postnatal development in rats.

Recommended Reading

Barlow, S. M., and Sullivan, F. M. *Reproductive Hazards of Industrial Chemicals*. New York: Academic, 1982. Pp. 136–177.

Bryce-Smith, D., et al. Lead and cadmium levels in stillbirths. *Lancet* 1:1159, 1977.

Council on Scientific Affairs' Advisory Panel on Reproductive Hazards in the Workplace. *Effects of Toxic Chemicals on the Reproductive System*. d50:cdcl(1–3) (revd. 6-18-85). Chicago: American Medical Association, 1985.

Occupational Diseases: A Guide to Their Recognition. U.S. Dept. of Health, Education and Welfare, NIOSH, publication No. 77-181. Government Printing Office, 1977. Pp. 345–348.

Carbon Disulfide

SYNONYMS

Carbon bisulfide, dithiocarbonic anhydride

USES

In manufacture of viscose rayon, cellophane, carbon tetrachloride, ammonium salt, flotation agents, soil disinfectants, electronic vacuum tubes, optical glass, dyes, paints, varnishes, enamel, paint and varnish removers, tallow, textiles, explosives, rocket fuel, putty, preservatives, rubber cement; as a solvent; in degreasing, dry cleaning, chemical analysis, electroplating, grain fumigation, vulcanizing rubber, oil extraction

SELECTED OCCUPATIONAL GROUPS POTENTIALLY EXPOSED

Makers of ammonium salt, carbon tetrachloride, cellophane, flotation agents, preservatives, putty, rayon, resin, rocket fuel, rubber cement, tallow, textiles, vacuum tubes, varnish; degreasers, dry cleaners, electroplaters, rubber workers; processors of bromine, fat, iodine, oil, sulfur, wax

EXPOSURE STANDARDS

OSHA/PEL: 20 ppm (60 mg/m^3) as a TWA for an 8-hour workshift with a ceiling concentration of 30 ppm (90 mg/m^3) and a maximum peak of 100 ppm (300 mg/m^3) for a maximum duration of 30 minutes

NIOSH recommendation: 1 ppm as a TWA for a 10-hour workshift with a 10-ppm ceiling for any 15-minute sampling period

ROUTES OF ENTRY

Inhalation of vapor; percutaneous absorption of liquid or vapor

Biologic Effects

Carbon disulfide vapors are irritating to eyes, skin, and mucous membranes; skin contact may cause blistering and burns. Acute poisoning may lead to severe encephalopathy with psychotic manic-depressive manifestations. Chronic exposures may result in peripheral neuropathy, including sensory loss and muscle atrophy; central nervous system disorders, including personality changes; and cardiovascular disease.

Special Considerations in Pregnancy

Authors of an eastern European study have reported an excessive incidence of spontaneous abortion and premature birth among female workers in the viscose rayon industry. Since data on exposure levels in this study are not available, it cannot be determined whether adverse effects can occur at present permissible exposure limits.

Carbon disulfide is suspected of adversely affecting spermatogenesis as well as menstrual function. Significantly reduced sperm counts and abnormal sperm morphology have been reported among exposed male workers and a higher frequency of menstrual disorders among female workers in eastern European studies. However, a recent investigation undertaken by NIOSH in the United States found no evidence of impaired semen quality among carbon disulfide workers at current exposure levels.

With the possible exception of an increased frequency of sister chromatid exchanges, no evidence that carbon disulfide is a mutagen has been found in in vitro human cellular studies.

Mutagenic or teratogenic effects have not been observed with exposures up to 40 ppm in rats. However, exposure of pregnant rats to 10 mg/m^3 of carbon disulfide adversely affected postnatal viability and morphologic, sensory, and behavioral development, particularly during the early postnatal period of the offspring. Marked testicular damage has been reported in rats exposed to carbon disulfide.

Recommended Reading

Council on Scientific Affairs' Advisory Panel on Reproductive Hazards in the Workplace. *Effects of Toxic Chemicals on the Reproductive System*. d40:cs 2(1–2) (revd. 6-18-85). Chicago: American Medical Association, 1985.

Lilis, R. Carbon Disulfide. In W. N. Rom (ed.), *Environmental and Occupational Medicine*. Boston: Little, Brown, 1983. Pp. 627–631.

Meyer, C. R. Semen quality in workers exposed to carbon disulfide compared to a control group from the same plant. *J. Occup. Med.* 23:435, 1981.

Occupational Diseases: A Guide to Their Recognition. U.S. Dept. of Health, Education and Welfare, NIOSH, publication No. 77-181. Government Printing Office, 1977. Pp. 306–308.

Carbon Monoxide

SYNONYM

Monoxide

USES

Reducing agent in metallurgy (e.g., Mond process for recovery of nickel); in organic synthesis (e.g., in Fischer-Tropsch process for petroleum products and in the oxo reaction); in manufacture of metal carbonyls. Carbon monoxide is also a waste product of incomplete combustion of carbonaceous material.

SELECTED OCCUPATIONAL GROUPS POTENTIALLY EXPOSED

Acetylene workers; blast furnace, boiler room, and coke oven workers; brewery workers; carbon black makers; diesel engine operators; garage mechanics; metal oxide reducers; miners; Mond-process workers; organic chemical synthesizers; petroleum refinery workers; pulp and paper workers; steelworkers; water gas workers

EXPOSURE STANDARDS

OSHA/PEL: 50 ppm (55 mg/m^3) as a TWA for an 8-hour workshift
NIOSH recommendation: 35 ppm as a TWA for an 8-hour workshift
  with a ceiling concentration of 200 ppm

ROUTE OF ENTRY

Inhalation of gas

Biologic Effects

The toxic effects of carbon monoxide are due to its ability to combine with hemoglobin to form carboxyhemoglobin, which reduces the oxygen content of the blood and may result in tissue hypoxia. Typical progressive symptoms of acute poisoning are headache, dizziness, drowsiness, nausea, vomiting, mental confusion, collapse, coma, and death. Unconsciousness generally occurs when carboxyhemoglobin levels reach 50%. Complete recovery is possible, but severe oxygen deprivation may result in permanent brain damage. Adverse effects may be enhanced among smokers as baseline carboxyhemoglobin levels are higher in smokers than in nonsmokers.

Special Considerations in Pregnancy

Most of the reported cases of acute carbon monoxide poisoning during pregnancy have resulted in fetal or infant death or severe neurologic impairment of the offspring. Maternal prognosis appears to be better, with some cases of full recovery even after loss of consciousness. The influence of lower levels of carbon monoxide exposure on the course of pregnancy is not known, but attention has been drawn to the adverse effects of maternal smoking, which is associated with raised carboxyhemoglobin levels. Carbon monoxide crosses the placenta, with fetal carboxyhemoglobin levels similar to those in the mother. Since the fetus is more sensitive to anoxia, fetal toxicity can be expected at lower carboxyhemoglobin levels than maternal toxicity. Teratogenic effects have not been reported in humans and no data are available on the mutagenicity of carbon monoxide.

Authors of animal studies have reported fetotoxic effects at exposures beginning around 90 ppm (almost twice the OSHA/PEL standard for workers). Abnormal brain development has been observed at lower exposure levels. These effects were more apparent with exposures in later gestation and often occurred without evidence of toxicity in the dam. Experimental studies have generally found no increased risk of malformations. Adverse effects on rat spermatogenesis have only been observed at very high dosage levels, but disturbances of the estrous cycles in female rats have been reported for prolonged low-dose exposures.

Recommended Reading

Barlow, S. M., and Sullivan, F. M. *Reproductive Hazards of Industrial Chemicals*. New York: Academic, 1982. Pp. 178–199.

Council on Scientific Affairs' Advisory Panel on Reproductive Hazards in the Workplace. *Effects of Toxic Chemicals on the Reproductive System*. d40:co(1–2) (revd. 6-18-85). Chicago: American Medical Association, 1985.

Cramer, C. R. Fetal death due to accidental maternal carbon monoxide poisoning. *J. Toxicol. Clin. Toxicol.* 19:297, 1982.

Longo, L. D. The biological effects of carbon monoxide on the pregnant woman, fetus and newborn infant. *Am. J. Obstet. Gynecol.* 129:69, 1977.

Occupational Diseases: A Guide to Their Recognition. U.S. Dept. of Health, Education and Welfare, NIOSH, publication No. 77-181. Government Printing Office, 1977. Pp. 417–419.

Chloroform

SYNONYMS

Trichloromethane, methenyl chloride

USES

Solvent, especially in lacquer industry; in manufacture of fluorocarbons, plastics, artificial silk, floor polishes; in extraction and purification of penicillin and other pharmaceuticals; grain fumigant. Because of its cardiac and hepatic toxicity, chloroform is no longer used as a general anesthetic. Its use as an additive in drug and cosmetic products was banned in 1976.

SELECTED OCCUPATIONAL GROUPS POTENTIALLY EXPOSED

Chemists; makers of fluorocarbons, pharmaceuticals, polishes; lacquer and solvent workers; silk synthesizers; grain fumigators

EXPOSURE STANDARDS

OSHA/PEL: 50 ppm (240 mg/m^3) as a ceiling value
NIOSH recommendation: ceiling concentration of 2 ppm based on a 1-hour sampling

ROUTE OF ENTRY

Inhalation of vapor

Biologic Effects

Dermal contact with liquid chloroform may produce burns. Liver damage and death have been reported from administration of chloroform as an anesthetic. Vapor inhalation may result in central nervous system depression and gastrointestinal disturbances. Prolonged, intense exposures may cause hepatic and renal damage. Chloroform has been found to be carcinogenic in some animal experiments. There is limited epidemiologic evidence that chloroform may be a human carcinogen.

Special Considerations in Pregnancy

Chloroform has been shown to cross the placenta readily, but its effect on human reproduction is not known. There is a report of toxemia in two women who were working in the same laboratory and were exposed to a variety of chemicals including high concentrations of chloroform. Authors of an investigation of laboratory workers who were exposed most commonly to chloroform, benzene, and toluene found an increased frequency of chromosomal aberrations (chromatid and isochromatid breaks, sister chromatid exchange) in the workers and in children of technicians who had worked during pregnancy. The biologic importance of such aberrations, however, has not been established.

Chloroform exposure in experimental studies has resulted in increased fetal resorption and decreased fetal weight but at dosages that produced some maternal toxicity as well. Teratogenic effects that were not ascribed to maternal toxicity have been observed in rodents from inhalation exposure but not from oral dosing. In vivo studies, but not in vitro tests, suggest that chloroform may be a mutagen.

Recommended Reading

Barlow, S. M., and Sullivan, F. M. *Reproductive Hazards of Industrial Chemicals.* New York: Academic, 1982. Pp. 230–238.

Council on Scientific Affairs' Advisory Panel on Reproductive Hazards in the Workplace. *Effects of Toxic Chemicals on the Reproductive System.* d49:chlor(1) (revd. 6-14-85). Chicago: American Medical Association, 1985.

Davidson, I. W., Sumner, D. D., and Parker, J. C. Chloroform: A review of its metabolism, teratogenic, mutagenic and carcinogenic potential. *Drug Chem. Toxicol.* 5:1, 1982.

Occupational Diseases: A Guide to Their Recognition. U.S. Dept. of Health, Education and Welfare, NIOSH, publication No. 77-181. Government Printing Office, 1977. Pp. 196–197.

Chloroprene

SYNONYMS

2-Chloro-1,3-butadiene, chlorobutadiene, beta-chloroprene

USES

In manufacture of synthetic rubber

SELECTED OCCUPATIONAL GROUPS POTENTIALLY EXPOSED

Duprene, neoprene, and rubber makers

EXPOSURE STANDARDS

OSHA/PEL: 25 ppm (90 mg/m^3) as a TWA for an 8-hour workshift
NIOSH recommendation: ceiling concentration of 1 ppm during 15-minute sampling

Inhalation of vapor; skin absorption

Biologic Effects

Chloroprene is a skin and eye irritant that may result in dermatitis, conjunctivitis, and circumscribed necrosis of the cornea. Temporary hair loss has also been reported. Extensive, acute exposures may cause anesthesia and respiratory paralysis. Chronic exposure may result in injury to the lungs, nervous system, kidneys, liver, spleen, and myocardium.

Special Considerations in Pregnancy

Reports from Russia of workers exposed to chloroprene claim a variety of adverse reproductive effects including decreased menstrual flow, abnormal spermatogenesis, and excess spontaneous abortions in wives of workers. Supporting data, however, are inadequate for evaluation. There are similar anecdotal reports of increases in chromosomal aberrations in both female and male chloroprene workers in Russia.

Conflicting animal results have been presented with respect to both preconceptional and prenatal exposures. Because chloroprene at ambient temperatures readily breaks down to other toxic products, it is suspected that some of the reported effects may be due to contaminated chloroprene. Authors of studies in which the exposure may have involved impure chloroprene found testicular damage as well as embryolethal and teratogenic effects at doses of 1 ppm or even less (considerably below current OSHA/PEL standards). In contrast, exposures to pure chloroprene up to 25 ppm produced no embryolethal or teratogenic effects, and no effect on male or female fertility was found with exposures up to 100 ppm. Since workers may be exposed to both pure and contaminated chloroprene, the potential reproductive hazards of each form need to be evaluated.

Recommended Reading

Barlow, S. M., and Sullivan, F. M. *Reproductive Hazards of Industrial Chemicals.* New York: Academic, 1982. Pp. 239–252.

Council on Scientific Affairs' Advisory Panel on Reproductive Hazards in the Workplace. *Effects of Toxic Chemicals on the Reproductive System.* d50:clprn(1–2) (revd. 6-18-85). Chicago: American Medical Association, 1985.

Criteria Document for a Recommended Standard: Occupational Exposure to Chloroprene. U.S. Dept. of Health, Education and Welfare, NIOSH, publication No. 77-210. Government Printing Office, 1977.

Occupational Diseases: A Guide to Their Recognition. U.S. Dept. of Health, Education and Welfare, NIOSH, publication No. 77-181. Government Printing Office, 1977. Pp. 197–198.

Dibromochloropropane

1,2-Dibromo-3-chloropropane, DBCP

Soil fumigant; nematocide. Subsequent to reports of sterility in male workers exposed to DBCP, OSHA and the Environmental Protection Agency (EPA) restricted the use and handling of DBCP in 1977. In 1979, the EPA banned virtually all agricultural uses of DBCP because of its carcinogenic and mutagenic potential, harmful testicular effects, and persistence in the environment.

SELECTED OCCUPATIONAL GROUPS POTENTIALLY EXPOSED

Production workers and applicators of DBCP

EXPOSURE STANDARDS

OSHA/PEL: 1 ppb as a TWA for an 8-hour workshift
NIOSH recommendation (1977): 10 ppb as a TWA for a 10-hour workshift

ROUTES OF ENTRY

Inhalation of vapor; absorption through skin

Biologic Effects

Dibromochloropropane is a mild skin irritant. Hepatic and renal toxicity has been reported in laboratory animals. Since DBCP is carcinogenic in rodents, it is regarded as a potential carcinogen in humans.

Special Considerations in Pregnancy

It is well established that occupational exposure to DBCP adversely affects spermatogenesis. Studies of men employed in the manufacture and application of DBCP have documented an increased risk of both azoospermia and oligospermia. The reduction in sperm count has been found to be related to the duration of exposure. Recovery of testicular function after cessation of exposure has been reported in several of the men with previous oligospermia but in only a few who were azoospermic.

Authors of a study of wives of DBCP applicators found an excess of spontaneous abortions in pregnancies that occurred after exposure compared to before exposure, but it is not clear to what extent other factors may have been responsible for this excess. A more recent investigation found no increase in spontaneous abortions, perinatal deaths, or congenital malformations among infants born subsequent to paternal exposures. However, a significant increase in female infants was noted. It has been hypothesized that the increased frequency of Y chromosome nondisjunction, which had been reported in sperm of exposed workers, may be responsible for this decreased sex ratio.

Since few women have been occupationally exposed to DBCP, the reproductive effects of maternal exposure are not known. Animal studies suggest that females are less sensitive than males to the gonadotoxic effects of DBCP.

Apart from fetal weight reductions at maternally toxic dosages, no fetotoxic or teratogenic effects have been observed among exposed female animals. Dominant lethal activity has been shown in rats but not in mice. Dibromochloropropane is mutagenic in the Ames test with metabolic activation.

Recommended Reading

Barlow, S. M., and Sullivan, F. M. *Reproductive Hazards of Industrial Chemicals.* New York: Academic, 1982. Pp. 253–268.

Council on Scientific Affairs' Advisory Panel on Reproductive Hazards in the Workplace. *Effects of Toxic Chemicals on the Reproductive System.* d40:dbcp(1–2) (revd. 6-19-85). Chicago: American Medical Association, 1985.

Goldsmith, J. R., Potashnik, G., and Israeli, R. Reproductive outcomes in families of 1,2-dibromo-3-chloropropane–exposed men. *Arch. Environ. Health* 39:85, 1984.

Whorton, M. D., and Foliart, D. E. Mutagenicity, carcinogenicity and reproductive effects of dibromochloropropane (DBCP). *Mutat. Res.* 123:13, 1983.

Whorton, M. D., et al. Infertility in male pesticide workers. *Lancet* 2:1259, 1977.

Ethylene Dibromide

SYNONYMS

Dibromoethane, ethylene bromide, sym-dibromoethane, EDB, 1-2-dibromoethane

USES

Fumigant for ground pest control; constituent in antiknock gasoline; in fire extinguishers, gauge fluids, waterproofing preparations; solvent for celluloid, fats, oils, and waxes

SELECTED OCCUPATIONAL GROUPS POTENTIALLY EXPOSED

Makers of antiknock compounds, drugs, fire extinguishers, lead scavengers, resins, tetraethyl lead; farmers; fat processors; fumigant workers; gum processors; termite controllers; wool reclaimers

EXPOSURE STANDARDS

OSHA/PEL: 20 ppm as a TWA for an 8-hour workshift with a ceiling concentration of 30 ppm; maximum peak above ceiling for 8-hour shift is 50 ppm for no more than 5 minutes (revision being considered to reduce standard to 100 ppb for an 8-hour TWA)

NIOSH recommendation: ceiling of 0.13 ppm (1.0 mg/m^3) over any 15-minute sampling period, with a TWA of 45 ppb for an 8-hour workshift

ROUTES OF ENTRY

Inhalation of vapor; absorption through skin

Biologic Effects

Prolonged skin contact may cause erythema, blisters, and ulcers. Vapors are irritating to the eyes and mucous membranes of the respiratory tract. Vapor inhalation may result in severe respiratory injury, central nervous system depression, and severe vomiting. Ethylene dibromide is carcinogenic in rodents but its carcinogenicity in humans is not known.

Special Considerations in Pregnancy

No relevant human data link adverse pregnancy outcomes with EDB exposure. Endocrine and gonadal effects in humans are not reported in the literature, and no studies have been published on its human mutagenicity.

Evidence that EDB is an antifertility agent at nontoxic dosages exists in studies of bulls. Small-scale studies, soon to be released by NIOSH, suggest an association between occupational exposures to EDB and the reduction of several parameters of semen quality. A possible effect on reduced fertility among wives of exposed workers in one of four factories has also been reported.

Recommended Reading

Barlow, S. M., and Sullivan, F. M. *Reproductive Hazards of Industrial Chemicals.* New York: Academic, 1982. Pp. 296–309.

Council on Scientific Affairs' Advisory Panel on Reproductive Hazards in the Workplace. *Effects of Toxic Chemicals on the Reproductive System.* d49:edb(1–2) (revd. 6-14-85). Chicago: American Medical Association, 1985.

Occupational Diseases: A Guide to Their Recognition. U.S. Dept. of Health, Education and Welfare, NIOSH, publication No. 77-181. Government Printing Office, 1977. Pp. 198–199.

Ethylene Oxide

SYNONYMS

1,2-Epoxyethane, oxirane, dimethylene oxide, anprolene, ETO, oxane, dihydrooxirane

USES

Sterilizing agent for surgical instruments; pesticide fumigant; chemical intermediate in organic synthesis of ethylene glycol (for automotive antifreeze) and polyester fibers, films, and bottles; in production of nonionic surfactants (e.g., for detergents) and glycol ethers (e.g., solvents for surface coatings)

SELECTED OCCUPATIONAL GROUPS POTENTIALLY EXPOSED

Makers of acrylonitrile, butyl cellosolve, detergents, disinfectants, ethanolamine, ethylene glycol, fumigants, polyglycol, polyoxirane, surfactants; exterminators; foodstuff and textile fumigators; fungicide workers; grain elevator workers; hospital equipment and supply sterilizer operators; organic chemical synthesizers; rocket-fuel handlers

EXPOSURE STANDARDS

OSHA/PEL: 1.0 ppm as a TWA for an 8-hour workshift

NIOSH recommendation: less than 0.1 ppm as an 8-hour TWA with a short-term peak exposure not to exceed 5 ppm for more than 10 minutes/workday

ROUTE OF ENTRY

Inhalation of gas

Biologic Effects

Exposure to aqueous solutions can lead to severe forms of dermatitis and can produce burns. Eye irritation can result from vapor exposure, and severe eye damage can result from liquid splashed in the eye. Vapor inhalation can cause nausea, vomiting, respiratory irritation, or pulmonary edema. Drowsiness and unconsciousness can occur. The question of carcinogenicity is not resolved although ethylene oxide exposure has been linked with leukemia and other cancers in several small-scale studies.

Special Considerations in Pregnancy

Ethylene oxide is a mutagen in experimental studies in vitro and in vivo. Chromosomal damage (sister-chromatid exchange) has been reported in several studies of occupational exposure, although the health-related effects of these chromosomal changes are not known. Only two human pregnancy studies of ethylene oxide exposure have been reported in the literature. Each has suffered from lack of detail and possible misclassification of exposure level. The results are suggestive, however, of higher than expected rates of spontaneous abortions.

Embryo and fetal toxicity has been observed at dosages that are toxic to mice. Reduced fetal body weight in rats was observed at exposures comparable to those some workers might experience.

Recommended Reading

Barlow, S. M., and Sullivan, F. M. *Reproductive Hazards of Industrial Chemicals.* New York: Academic, 1982. Pp. 315–325.

Council on Scientific Affairs' Advisory Panel on Reproductive Hazards in the Workplace. *Effects of Toxic Chemicals on the Reproductive System.* d40:etox(1–3) (revd. 6-18-85). Chicago: American Medical Association, 1985.

Landrigan, P. J., et al. Ethylene oxide: An overview of toxicologic and epidemiologic research. *Am. J. Ind. Med.* 6:103, 1984.

Occupational Diseases: A Guide to Their Recognition. U.S. Dept. of Health, Education and Welfare, NIOSH, publication No. 77-181. Government Printing Office, 1977. Pp. 171–172.

Formaldehyde

SYNONYMS

Oxomethane, oxymethylene, methylene oxide, formic aldehyde, methyl aldehyde

USES

Fungicides, germicides; in disinfectants, embalming fluids; in manufacture of resins, woods, textiles, plastics, cellulose esters, paper and rubber products, insulating materials, protective coatings, photographic films, dyes, inks, latex

SELECTED OCCUPATIONAL GROUPS POTENTIALLY EXPOSED
Anatomists; biologists; embalmers; makers of deodorants, disinfectants, embalming fluid, formaldehyde resins, inks, latex, photographic films; hide and wood preservers; textile printers

EXPOSURE STANDARDS
OSHA/PEL: 3 ppm as a TWA for an 8-hour workshift with a ceiling concentration of 5 ppm and a maximum peak of 10 ppm for 30 minutes
NIOSH recommendation: limit exposure to lowest feasible level

ROUTE OF ENTRY
Inhalation of gas

Biologic Effects

Formaldehyde gas is an intense irritant to the respiratory tract and eyes. Dermatitis may result from repeated exposure. Systemic toxicity, which is manifested as persistent cough, shortness of breath, and possibly pulmonary edema, is less likely because of the local irritant warning signs. Formaldehyde has been found to be a carcinogen in rats, and epidemiologic evidence suggests that it may pose a carcinogenic risk to humans.

Special Considerations in Pregnancy

Epidemiologic data are inadequate for assessing the reproductive effects of formaldehyde. Authors of a Russian study have reported that female workers exposed to formaldehyde when compared to a control group had an excess of menstrual disorders (especially dysmenorrhea), pelvic inflammatory disease and secondary infertility, anemia during pregnancy, threatened abortion, and low-birth-weight infants. Although the exposure levels in this study were similar to the OSHA/PEL standards for workers, the lack of study details prevents assessment of these findings. There is also an anecdotal report from Russia of increased sexual dysfunction among male workers exposed to a variety of toxic chemicals including formaldehyde.

Animal investigations of formaldehyde exposure have generally found no effect on fertility or pregnancy outcome even at maternally toxic dosages, but most of these studies are regarded as inadequate for proper evaluation. Mutagenic effects have been observed in several cell systems and organisms.

Recommended Reading

Barlow, S. M., and Sullivan, F. M. *Reproductive Hazards of Industrial Chemicals*. New York: Academic, 1982. Pp. 334–345.

Council on Scientific Affairs' Advisory Panel on Reproductive Hazards in the Workplace. *Effects of Toxic Chemicals on the Reproductive System*. d50:hcho(1–3) (revd. 6-27-85). Chicago: American Medical Association, 1985.

Occupational Diseases: A Guide to Their Recognition. U.S. Dept. of

Health, Education and Welfare, NIOSH, publication No. 77-181. Government Printing Office, 1977. Pp. 188–190.

Report of the Federal Panel on Formaldehyde. *Environ. Health Perspect.* 43:139, 1982.

Glycol Ethers

The following review pertains to ethylene glycol ethers, specifically monoalkyl glycol ethers and their acetate derivatives.

SYNONYMS

Ethylene glycol monoethyl ether: cellosolve, 2-ethoxyethanol, 2-EE
Ethylene glycol monoethyl ether acetate: cellosolve acetate, 2-ethoxyethyl acetate
Ethylene glycol monomethyl ether: methyl cellosolve, 2-methoxyethanol, 2-ME
Ethylene glycol monomethyl ether acetate: methyl cellosolve acetate, 2-methoxyethyl acetate

USES

Solvent for resins, lacquers, paints, varnishes, gum, dyes; perfume fixative; constituent of painting pastes, cleaning compounds, liquid soaps, cosmetics, nitrocellulose; jet-fuel de-icing additive. Acetate derivatives are used as solvents; in preparation of lacquers, enamels, and adhesives; to dissolve resins and plastics.

SELECTED OCCUPATIONAL GROUPS POTENTIALLY EXPOSED

Makers of cleaning solution, enamel, film, hydraulic fluid, inks, lacquer, nail polish, plastics; cellophane sealers; dry cleaners; oil and wax processors; printers; stainers; textile dyers

EXPOSURE STANDARDS

Ethylene glycol monoethyl ether
OSHA/PEL: 200 ppm (740 mg/m^3) as a TWA for an 8-hour workshift
NIOSH recommendation: reduce exposure to lowest feasible level

Ethylene glycol monoethyl ether acetate
OSHA/PEL: 100 ppm (540 mg/m^3) as a TWA for an 8-hour workshift

Ethylene glycol monomethyl ether
OSHA/PEL: 25 ppm (80 mg/m^3) as a TWA for an 8-hour workshift
NIOSH recommendation: reduce exposure to lowest feasible level

Ethylene glycol monomethyl ether acetate
OSHA/PEL: 25 ppm (120 mg/m^3) as a TWA for an 8-hour workshift

ROUTES OF ENTRY

Inhalation of vapor; percutaneous absorption of liquid

Biologic Effects

Ethylene glycol ethers are mild skin irritants and vapors may cause conjunctivitis and upper respiratory irritation. Acute poisoning is characterized by narcosis, pulmonary edema, and renal and hepatic damage. Chronic toxicity may be manifested as fatigue, lethargy, headache, nausea, anorexia, and tremor. Hematologic abnormalities (anemia, leukopenia, and thrombocytopenia) and toxic encephalopathy have also been linked with subacute and chronic overexposure to ethylene glycol monomethyl ether. Carcinogenic effects have not been evaluated in animals or humans.

Special Considerations in Pregnancy

Only limited data are available on the reproductive effects of glycol ethers in humans. A Russian study has reported an increase in hormonal disturbances and birth defects for female workers exposed to ethylene glycol monoethyl ether (2-EE) along with other solvents. Because of the small sample size, the lack of study details, and the concomitant exposure to other solvents, it is not possible to attribute the adverse effects to the glycol ether. A small-scale study of male workers exposed to ethylene glycol monomethyl ether (2-ME) at levels below 25 ppm revealed no meaningful differences relative to the control group for a variety of fertility indices.

In various animal species, 2-EE and 2-ME have been found to be teratogenic at concentrations that do not produce maternal toxicity. The most commonly observed defects involve the axial skeleton, the cardiovascular system, and the kidneys. Behavioral abnormalities have also been noted in the offspring of rats with gestational exposure to 2-EE. Testicular atrophy and abnormal spermatogenesis, which appears to be reversible, have been observed with exposure to 2-ME. Mutagenic activity has not been demonstrated for either 2-EE or 2-ME.

Recommended Reading

Cook, R. R., et al. A cross-sectional study of ethylene glycol monomethyl ether process employees. *Arch. Environ. Health* 37:346, 1982.

Council on Scientific Affairs' Advisory Panel on Reproductive Hazards in the Workplace. *Effects of Toxic Chemicals on the Reproductive System.* d50:ece(1–3) (revd. 6-27-85); d50:mce(1–2) (revd. 6-27-85). Chicago: American Medical Association, 1985.

Occupational Diseases: A Guide to Their Recognition. U.S. Dept. of Health, Education and Welfare, NIOSH, publication No. 77-181. Government Printing Office, 1977. Pp. 161–163.

Reproductive Toxicology: A Medical Letter on Environmental Hazards to Reproduction. Reproductive Toxicity of the Glycol Ethers. Washington, D.C.: Reproductive Toxicology Center, Vol. 4, No. 4, July 1985.

Kepone

SYNONYM

Chlordecone

USES

Registration of its use as an insecticide and fungicide was canceled in 1977. The manufacture of Kepone in the United States ceased in 1975, but it is reportedly manufactured and used in other parts of the world.

EXPOSURE STANDARDS

OSHA/PEL: none
NIOSH recommendation (1976): 0.001 mg/m^3 as a TWA for a 10-hour workshift

ROUTES OF ENTRY

Inhalation; percutaneous absorption

Biologic Effects

Kepone has been found to induce acute and cumulative neurotoxic effects, manifested as nervousness, tremor, and visual disturbances. Carcinogenic effects have been demonstrated in rodents, but its carcinogenicity in humans is not known. Considerable environmental contamination was demonstrated subsequent to the closing of the major plant manufacturing Kepone in the United States.

Special Considerations in Pregnancy

Oligospermia and abnormal sperm morphology as well as neurotoxicity have been documented in workers exposed to high levels of Kepone. There is some suggestion that these reproductive effects may be reversible, as sperm counts increased and blood Kepone levels decreased in subjects treated with cholestyramine. No information is available regarding adverse effects on fertility or pregnancy outcome. Kepone has reportedly been found in breast milk.

Kepone causes testicular and ovarian damage in a wide range of avian and mammalian species. Embryolethal and teratogenic effects have only been observed at maternally toxic dosages. Its mutagenicity has only been assessed in one investigation, which reported a negative finding.

Recommended Reading

Barlow, S. M., and Sullivan, F. M . *Reproductive Hazards of Industrial Chemicals*. New York: Academic, 1982. Pp. 212–229.

Cohn, W. J., et al. Treatment of chlordecone (Kepone) toxicity with cholestyramine. *N. Engl. J. Med.* 298:243, 1978.

Council on Scientific Affairs' Advisory Panel on Reproductive Hazards in the Workplace. *Effects of Toxic Chemicals on the Reproductive System*. d49:kep(1–2) (revd. 6-14-85). Chicago: American Medical Association, 1985.

Epstein, S. S. Kepone-hazard evaluation. *Sci. Total Environ.* 9:1, 1978.

Lead (Alkyl)

SYNONYMS

Tetraethyl lead: TEL
Tetramethyl lead: TML

USES

Tetraethyl and tetramethyl lead have been widely used as antiknock ingredients in gasoline, but these additives are being phased out.

SELECTED OCCUPATIONAL GROUPS POTENTIALLY EXPOSED

Gasoline additive workers, storage tank cleaners

EXPOSURE STANDARDS

Tetraethyl lead
OSHA/PEL: 0.075 mg/m^3 (as lead) for skin as a TWA for an 8-hour workshift

Tetramethyl lead
OSHA/PEL: 0.075 mg/m^3 (as lead) for skin as a TWA for an 8-hour workshift

ROUTES OF ENTRY

Inhalation of vapor and percutaneous absorption of liquid; inhalation of dust from dried metabolic products of TEL

Biologic Effects

Inhalation of the metabolic products of TEL in dust form may cause upper respiratory tract irritation. Percutaneous contact with this dust may result in itching and burning. Acute or chronic TEL poisoning may lead to central nervous system intoxication and encephalopathy. Prognosis is poor when the time interval between termination of exposure and onset of symptoms is short (a few hours). Animal experiments suggest that TML may cause similar intoxication. Animal and human data are insufficient for evaluating the carcinogenicity of organic lead compounds.

Special Considerations in Pregnancy

No data are available regarding the effects of alkyl lead exposure on pregnancy outcome. Because of its lipid solubility it is thought that alkyl lead crosses the human placenta. In rats, TML was found to bind to maternal erythrocytes, but it reached the fetus when these binding sites were saturated.

There are two reports of abnormal spermatogenesis, reduced libido, and impotence in workers who also exhibited symptoms of tetraalkyl lead poisoning. Sperm production remained abnormal up to 5 months after exposure, although there was recovery of potency and disappearance of neurologic symptoms. Both studies lacked a control group and long-term follow-up evaluation.

Embryolethal and fetotoxic effects have been observed in rodents but only at maternally toxic dosages. There is no evidence of teratogenicity in animal studies, and experimental data on mutagenicity are inadequate for evaluation.

Recommended Reading

Barlow, S. M., and Sullivan, F. M. *Reproductive Hazards of Industrial Chemicals.* New York: Academic, 1982. Pp. 360–369.

Council on Scientific Affairs' Advisory Panel on Reproductive Hazards in the Workplace. *Effects of Toxic Chemicals on the Reproductive System.* d50:tel(1–2) (revd. 6-27-85). Chicago: American Medical Association, 1985.

Cremer, J. E. Toxicology and biochemistry of alkyl lead compounds. *Occup. Health Rev.* 17:14, 1965.

Occupational Diseases: A Guide to Their Recognition. U.S. Dept. of
Health, Education and Welfare, NIOSH, publication No. 77-181. Government Printing Office, 1977. Pp. 364–366.

Lead (Inorganic)

This review pertains to inorganic lead, specifically metallic lead and
its salts.

SYNONYMS

None

USES

Liner for equipment requiring pliability and corrosive resistance; in
petroleum refining; in halogenation, sulfonation, extraction, and
condensation processes; in building industry; ingredient in solder;
filler in automobile industry; shielding material for x rays and
atomic radiation; in manufacture of inorganic and organic lead compounds, storage batteries, pigments, paints, varnishes, enamels,
glass, ceramics, rubber, plastics, electronic devices; alloying agent

SELECTED OCCUPATIONAL GROUPS POTENTIALLY EXPOSED

Makers of batteries, ceramics, enamels, glass, imitation pearls, lubricants, matches; brass founders; insecticide workers; painters,
plumbers; solderers

EXPOSURE STANDARDS

OSHA/PEL: 0.05 mg/m^3 as a TWA for an 8-hour workshift
NIOSH recommendation: less than 0.1 mg/m^3 as a TWA for a 10-
hour workshift

ROUTES OF ENTRY

Ingestion of dust; inhalation of dust or fumes

Biologic Effects

Today, serious cases of lead poisoning are rarely seen in industry.
Early symptoms of lead poisoning are fatigue, headache, aching
bones and muscles, constipation, and abdominal pain. Progressive
symptoms include pallor, anemia, a blue-black "lead line" on the
gums, decreased hand-grip strength, "wrist-drop," intense abdominal cramping with constipation, and occasionally nausea and vomiting. Renal damage may occur. Central nervous system (CNS) depression is more likely with exposures to tetraethyl lead (see p. 346)
but may result from heavy exposure to inorganic lead. Carcinogenic
effects of lead have been documented in experimental animals. Insufficient data are available for evaluating the carcinogenicity of
lead in humans.

Special Considerations in Pregnancy

Historic accounts have linked heavy maternal exposures to lead
with a variety of adverse reproductive effects including sterility,
spontaneous abortions, stillbirths, neonatal convulsions, mental retardation, and infant death. Occasional cases of congenital lead poi-

soning continue to be reported, usually from the use of lead battery casings for home heating or maternal consumption of "moonshine" whiskey, which has a high lead concentration.

The reproductive effects of low-level lead exposure have not been established. However, one report suggests that lead concentrations in placentas of stillborn babies and babies who die after birth may be increased in comparison to those of surviving babies. Umbilical cord blood levels have also been related to minor congenital anomalies and delayed mental development. In contrast to an earlier study that reported a positive association between lead levels in cord blood and the frequency of premature rupture of membranes (PROM) and preterm delivery, a recent study found no relationship between lead concentrations in cord blood and the incidence of PROM, preterm delivery, preeclampsia, or meconium staining. The mean lead concentrations in the latter study were considerably lower than those in the former study, and the possibility of an increased risk of adverse outcomes with concentrations of lead greater than 25 μg/dl could not be excluded. As was mentioned in the section on arsenic and its compounds (see p. 327), adverse reproductive outcomes have been reported in a series of investigations in and around a smelter in northern Sweden that emitted a number of toxic substances including lead.

To prevent neurologic damage, the Centers for Disease Control have recommended that blood lead levels in children not exceed 30 μg/dl. Since lead readily crosses the placenta and a fetus may be more susceptible to the adverse effects of lead than a child, it has been recommended that maternal blood lead levels be kept under 30 μg/dl. (To ensure such levels, air lead levels must be kept below 50 μg/m^3.) Iron and calcium deficiencies may increase the susceptibility to lead toxicity. Breast milk may represent an important additional source of lead exposure to the neonate, especially in light of animal studies that suggest that lactation increases lead absorption from the gut and lead excretion via the milk.

Cytogenetic studies in male lead workers have yielded conflicting data. Studies, however, have found more positive associations between lead exposure and chromosomal aberrations than negative associations. Sperm abnormalities have been reported in one investigation of men working in a lead storage battery plant.

Lead exposure in laboratory animals has been associated with gonadal damage, impaired fertility, reduced birth weight, retarded brain growth, behavioral disorders, and decreased postnatal survival. Although an excess of animal morphologic malformations has been noted in a few investigations, the major teratogenic effect of lead is believed to be CNS injury.

Recommended Reading

Angell, N. F., and Lavery, J. P. The relationship of blood lead levels to obstetric outcome. *Am. J. Obstet. Gynecol.* 142:40, 1982.

Council on Scientific Affairs' Advisory Panel on Reproductive Hazards in the Workplace. *Effects of Toxic Chemicals on the Reproductive System.* d50:lead(1–2) (revd. 6-27-85). Chicago: American Medical Association, 1985.

Damstra, T. Toxicological properties of lead. *Environ. Health Perspect.* 19:297, 1977.

Kurzel, R. B., and Cetrulo, C. L. Chemical teratogenesis and reproductive failure. *Obstet. Gynecol. Surv.* 40:397, 1985.

Needleman, H. L., et al. The relationship between prenatal exposure to lead and congenital anomalies. *J.A.M.A.* 251:2956, 1984.

Occupational Diseases: A Guide to Their Recognition. U.S. Dept. of Health, Education and Welfare, NIOSH, publication No. 77-181. Government Printing Office, 1977. Pp. 361–363.

Rom, W. N. Effects of lead on the female and reproduction: A review. *Mt. Sinai J. Med.* 43:542, 1976.

Mercury (Alkyl)

SYNONYM

Organic mercury

SELECTED ALKYL MERCURY COMPOUNDS

Methyl mercury dicyandiamide, cyano (methyl mercury) guanidine, ethylmercuric chloride, ethylmercuric phosphate

USES

Fungicides for grain, timber preservatives, and disinfectants. The use of alkyl mercury as a fungicide has recently declined substantially.

SELECTED OCCUPATIONAL GROUPS POTENTIALLY EXPOSED

Makers of disinfectants and fungicides; seed handlers; wood preservers

EXPOSURE STANDARD

OSHA/PEL: 0.01 mg/m^3 as a TWA for an 8-hour workshift with a ceiling of 0.04 mg/m^3

ROUTES OF ENTRY

Inhalation of dust; percutaneous absorption

Biologic Effects

Skin contact, when prolonged, may cause severe burns. Systemic toxicity involves the central nervous system, including the brain. Severe poisoning may produce irreversible damage. Early signs of central nervous system damage may include tremors, slurred speech, unsteady gait, sensory disturbances of tunnel vision, blindness, and deafness. A later symptom is constriction of the visual fields, which is rarely reversible and can be associated with permanent, severe brain damage.

Special Considerations in Pregnancy

It is important to note that waterways contaminated with mercury from natural and industrial sources can constitute one of the most serious forms of toxic exposure to this compound. Microorganisms in river and lake sediments convert inorganic and organic mercurials into methyl mercury, the most toxic form of mercury. The primary sources of methyl mercury exposure in humans are consumption of contaminated fish, direct ingestion of agriculturally treated grain, or consumption of animals fed with treated grain. The major reports of toxicity in pregnancy from such contaminated sources (Japan, Iraq, and the Soviet Union) include such effects as mental retardation, ataxia, cerebral palsy, tremors, seizures, chorea, decreased birth weight, and brain damage.

Alkyl mercury compounds readily cross the placenta. Since human breast milk can also be contaminated with mercury, a neonate's body burden of mercury could theoretically be significant if neonatal blood and breast milk concentrations are considered simultaneously.

Maternal toxicity and embryotoxic and teratogenic effects have also been demonstrated in rodents.

Recommended Reading

Council on Scientific Affairs' Advisory Panel on Reproductive Hazards in the Workplace. *Effects of Toxic Chemicals on the Reproductive System.* d50:merc(1–6) (revd. 6-27-85). Chicago: American Medical Association, 1985.

Koos, B. J., and Longo, L. D. Mercury toxicity in the pregnant woman, fetus and newborn infant. *Am. J. Obstet. Gynecol.* 126:309, 1976.

Occupational Diseases: A Guide to Their Recognition. U.S. Dept. of Health, Education and Welfare, NIOSH, publication No. 77-181. Government Printing Office, 1977. Pp. 372–373.

Wolff, M. S. Occupationally derived chemicals in breast milk. *Am. J. Ind. Med.* 4:259, 1983.

Mercury (Inorganic)

SYNONYMS

Metallic mercury: quicksilver, hydrargyrum

USES

In manufacture of scientific instruments (e.g., thermometers, barometers), electrical equipment (e.g., meters, switches, batteries), mercury vapor lamps, fluorescent lamps; chemical reagent; in gold and silver extraction from ores; in manufacture of amalgams and solders; in metal plating, tanning and dyeing, textile industry, photography, paints and pigments, pharmaceuticals, and agricultural chemicals

SELECTED OCCUPATIONAL GROUPS POTENTIALLY EXPOSED

Makers of amalgams, bactericides, batteries, caustic soda, dental amalgams, fungicides, paper; gold extractors; jewelers; photographers; taxidermists

EXPOSURE STANDARDS

OSHA/PEL: 0.1 mg/m^3 as a ceiling value
NIOSH recommendation: 0.05 mg/m^3 as a TWA for an 8-hour workshift

ROUTES OF ENTRY

Inhalation of dust or vapor; absorption of elemental mercury through skin

Biologic Effects

Inorganic mercury is a skin and mucous membrane irritant. Systemic poisoning, due to vapors, affects the lungs in the form of acute interstitial pneumonitis, bronchitis, and bronchiolitis. Chronic exposure generally produces one or more classic signs: gingivitis, sialorrhea, increased irritability, and muscular tremors (often of the fingers, eyelids, lips, or tongue).

Special Considerations in Pregnancy

Inorganic forms of mercury cross the placenta but less readily than organic (alkyl) mercury. Only limited human evidence suggests a possible link between occupational exposure to inorganic mercury and reduced ovulation rate and menstrual disturbances (e.g., hypomenorrhea, hypermenorrhea, dysmenorrhea). Reduced libido and potency have also been reported in a follow-up study of a small group of men with acute mercury poisoning.

Exposure to mercury vapor has been associated with an increase in the length of the estrous cycle and a reduction in fertility in rodents. Data on the teratogenicity or mutagenicity of inorganic mercury are inadequate for evaluation.

Recommended Reading

Barlow, S. M., and Sullivan, F. M. *Reproductive Hazards of Industrial Chemicals*. New York: Academic, 1982. Pp. 386–406.

Council on Scientific Affairs' Advisory Panel on Reproductive Hazards in the Workplace. *Effects of Toxic Chemicals on the Reproductive System*. d50:merc(1–6) (revd. 6-27-85). Chicago: American Medical Association, 1985.

Occupational Diseases: A Guide to Their Recognition. U.S. Dept. of Health, Education and Welfare, NIOSH, publication No. 77-181. Government Printing Office, 1977. Pp. 370–372.

Ozone

SYNONYMS

None

USES

Oxidizing agent; disinfectant for food and water; bleaching agent for foods, textiles, minerals, paper; for aging liquor and wood; in industrial waste treatment, rapid drying of varnishes and printing inks. It should be noted that industrial exposure often occurs around ozone-generating sources, such as inert gas–shielded arc welding, x-ray or ultraviolet generators, mercury vapor lamps, and linear accelerators.

SELECTED OCCUPATIONAL GROUPS POTENTIALLY EXPOSED

Arc welders; industrial waste and sewage treaters; organic chemical synthesizers; textile, wax, and oil bleachers; liquor and wood agers

EXPOSURE STANDARD

OSHA/PEL: 0.1 ppm (0.2 mg/m^3) as a TWA for an 8-hour workshift

ROUTE OF ENTRY

Inhalation of gas

Biologic Effects

Ozone is irritating to the eyes and mucous membranes. Respiratory symptoms include dryness and irritation of upper respiratory passages, coughing, choking, bronchial irritation, substernal soreness, and possibly pulmonary edema. Subacute exposures result in headache, malaise, shortness of breath, drowsiness, reduced concentration, slowing of heart and respiration rates, visual changes, and decreased desaturation of oxyhemoglobin in capillaries. Ozone is believed to have radiomimetic characteristics in that it can alter the morphology of red blood cells.

Special Considerations in Pregnancy

Menstrual disturbances have been reported among flight attendants. However, it is not clear whether this effect is related to stress, irregular work schedules, disruption of the circadian rhythm, or exposures to increased ozone concentrations or fumes from aviation fuel. There are also undocumented claims of higher rates of spontaneous abortion and birth defects among flight attendants. Cytogenetic studies of human lymphocytes have yielded inconclusive results regarding the mutagenicity of ozone.

Ozone exposure to pregnant rodents has produced embryolethality and some fetal growth retardation at concentrations of 1.5 ppm and above. No teratogenic effects have been reported.

Recommended Reading

Barlow, S. M., and Sullivan F. M. *Reproductive Hazards of Industrial Chemicals.* New York: Academic, 1982. Pp. 422–430.

Council on Scientific Affairs' Advisory Panel on Reproductive Hazards in the Workplace. *Effects of Toxic Chemicals on the Reproductive System.* d43:ozon(1–2) (revd. 6-19-85). Chicago: American Medical Association, 1985.

Longo, L. D. Environmental pollution and pregnancy: Risks and uncertainties for the fetus and infant. *Am. J. Obstet. Gynecol.* 137:162, 1980.

Menzel, D. B. Ozone: An overview of its toxicity in man and animals. *J. Toxicol. Environ. Health* 13:183, 1984.

Occupational Diseases: A Guide to Their Recognition. U.S. Dept of Health, Education and Welfare, NIOSH, publication No. 77-181. Government Printing Office, 1977. Pp. 428–430.

Phenoxy Herbicides and Associated Dioxins

Agent Orange is composed of a 50:50 mixture of 2,4-dichlorophen-oxyacetic acid (2,4-D) and 2,4,5-trichlorophenoxyacetic acid (2,4,5-T) as well as dioxin contaminants, most notably 2,3,7,8-tetrachloro-dibenzo-*p*-dioxin (2,3,7,8-TCDD). Levels of TCDD in Agent Orange varied from 0.02–15.00 ppm with a mean of approximately 2.0 ppm. Since this contaminant is a by-product of the chemical synthesis of 2,4,5-T, other herbicides containing 2,4,5-T, silvex (2-2[2,4,5-tri-chlorophenoxy]propionic acid), and certain derivatives of chloro-phenol may be contaminated with TCDD. Current manufacturing methods are able to reduce levels of TCDD to below 0.01 ppm. The TCDD contaminant has not thus far been found to be present in 2,4-D.

SYNONYMS

Agent Orange: Herbicide Orange
2,4-Dichlorophenoxyacetic acid: 2,4-D
2,4,5-Trichlorophenoxyacetic acid: 2,4,5-T
2,3,7,8-Tetrachlorodibenzo-*p*-dioxin: TCDD, dioxin

USES

Agent Orange was used by the United States military forces in Vietnam for defoliation and crop destruction. Other phenoxy her-bicides containing 2,4,5-T have been widely used in the past in large-scale farming, forest management, landscaping, and weed control in the United States and elsewhere. The Environmental Protection Agency halted most uses of 2,4,5-T and silvex in 1979 and canceled all registrations for these herbicides in 1983–1984.

SELECTED OCCUPATIONAL GROUPS POTENTIALLY EXPOSED

Herbicide makers and applicators; chlorophenol workers; Vietnam veterans

EXPOSURE STANDARDS

Agent Orange: none

2,4,5-T
   OSHA/PEL: 10 mg/m^3

Dioxin
   OSHA/PEL: none
   NIOSH recommendation: reduce exposure to lowest feasible level

ROUTES OF ENTRY

Inhalation of vapor; percutaneous absorption

Biologic Effects

Adverse health effects of 2,4,5-T exposure are believed to be due to its contaminant, TCDD. Although TCDD is extremely toxic, it is suspected that ingestion may be necessary for development of its full toxic potential. Acute, immediate symptoms include skin, eye, and respiratory tract irritation; headache; dizziness; and nausea. Chloracne, which is the classic sign of TCDD toxicity, generally does not appear until 2–3 weeks after exposure. Other toxic effects include impaired liver function, hypertrichosis and hyperpigmentation, porphyria cutanea tarda, hirsutism, peripheral neuropathy, nervousness and irritability, and personality changes. While the chloracne has been found to persist in a large proportion of exposed workers, the other symptoms appear to subside with time. Carcinogenic effects have been observed in rodents, and there is some evidence that TCDD exposure in humans may be linked with soft tissue sarcoma.

Special Considerations in Pregnancy

There is currently no convincing epidemiologic evidence that exposure to Agent Orange or other herbicides containing 2,4,5-T adversely affects pregnancy outcome.

Investigators in Oregon report a positive correlation between spraying patterns of 2,4,5-T and spontaneous abortion rates, but the methods that were used for ascertaining exposure as well as pregnancy outcome have been criticized. Studies relating environmental or seasonal trends in birth defect rates have produced negative or conflicting findings. No consistent changes in fetal loss or birth defects have been observed since the chemical explosion in 1976 in Seveso, Italy, which resulted in considerable TCDD exposure to the surrounding population. Cytogenetic evaluations of maternal peripheral blood cells and fetal tissue from abortuses of exposed women have not revealed any abnormalities. However, it should be noted that only a small number of conceptions were available for study from the zone with the highest exposure. A follow-up study of male workers involved in the production of 2,4,5-T in a West Virginia plant revealed no evidence of adverse reproductive effects. Similarly, a survey of wives of chemical workers produced no statistically significant associations between potential paternal exposure to chlorinated dioxins and pregnancy outcome.

To date, investigations aimed at the possible association between Vietnam service and the fathering of babies with birth defects have documented no overall increased risks of major congenital anomalies, although some variation in risk was evident for specific types of defects. Preliminary results from a follow-up study of U.S. Air Force members involved in herbicide spraying missions indicate an increase in minor skin anomalies and a higher frequency of neonatal deaths and physical handicaps in the offspring of the exposed personnel when compared to nonexposed personnel. No differences, however, were reported in fertility, pregnancy loss, or major anomalies between the two groups. It should be emphasized that these studies, as well as most investigations of occupational exposures, are subject to a number of limitations, including the difficulty of quantifying exposure and identifying and controlling for concomitant exposures to other agents. As a result, a potential teratogenic effect of paternal TCDD exposure cannot be ruled out, but available data provide little if any documentation of such an effect.

Data on cytogenetic changes in humans from TCDD exposure are inadequate and equivocal. Experimental studies have yielded inconclusive results regarding mutagenic effects. Gestational exposure has been associated with embryotoxic effects in several species, but teratogenic effects (specifically, cleft palate) have only been clearly documented in mice. While reduced fertility has been reported in rats exposed to TCDD before mating, no teratogenic effects have been observed from premating exposure of male animals.

Recommended Reading

Council on Scientific Affairs' Advisory Panel on Reproductive Hazards in the Workplace. *Effects of Toxic Chemicals on the Reproductive System.* d43:ao(1–4) (revd. 6-12-85). Chicago: American Medical Association, 1985.

Erickson, J. D., et al. Vietnam veterans' risks for fathering babies with birth defects. *J.A.M.A.* 252:903, 1984.

Friedman, J. M. Does Agent Orange cause birth defects? *Teratology* 29:193, 1984.

Hatch, M. C. Reproductive Effects of the Dioxins. In W. W. Lowrance (ed.), *Public Health Risks of the Dioxins.* Los Altos, Calif.: William Kaufman, 1984.

Suskind, R. R., and Hertzberg, V. S. Human health effects of 2,4,5-T and its toxic contaminants. *J.A.M.A.* 251:2372, 1984.

Polychlorinated Biphenyls

SYNONYMS

Chlorinated biphenyl, polychlorinated diphenyl, PCB, chlordipheny

USES

Insulation for electrical cables and wires; dielectric fluids in electrical capacitors and high-voltage transformers; heat exchange fluid; hydraulic fluid; coatings in foundry uses. In the past, PCBs have been used in plasticizers, inks, adhesives, pesticide additives, and microencapsulation of dyes in carbonless copy paper.

SELECTED OCCUPATIONAL GROUPS POTENTIALLY EXPOSED

Cable coaters; makers of dyes, electrical equipment, herbicides, lacquers, plasticizers, resins, transformers; paper treaters; wood preservers; textile flameproofers

EXPOSURE STANDARDS

OSHA/PEL
  42% chlorine: 1.0 mg/m^3 as a TWA for an 8-hour workshift.
  54% chlorine: 0.5 mg/m^3 as a TWA for an 8-hour workshift.

NIOSH recommendation: 0.001 mg/m^3 as a TWA for a 10-hour workshift.

ROUTES OF ENTRY

Inhalation of fumes or vapor; dermal absorption of liquid; ingestion; skin or eye contact

Biologic Effects

Prolonged skin contact with fumes or cold wax can cause chloracne and irritation to eyes, nose, and throat. Systemic effects tend to increase in severity with an increasing degree of chlorination. Acute and chronic exposure can cause liver damage. Signs and symptoms include edema, jaundice, vomiting, anorexia, nausea, abdominal pains, and fatigue.

Special Considerations in Pregnancy

Polychlorinated biphenyls appear to have limited placental transfer particularly in the early phases of pregnancy. As fat accumulation in the fetus increases, the lipophilic nature of PCBs permits them to be stored more readily in body tissues. This may also explain the dramatic increases of blood levels of PCBs in women whose fat stores may be mobilized during reducing diets or starvation. Since milk becomes a primary excretory route for the fat-soluble PCBs, these are commonly found in breast milk. Women with occupational PCB exposure can have milk levels that are 10–100 times greater than those in the rest of the population. This is an important source of PCB exposure for offspring when the combined effects of milk and transplacental blood exposure are considered in terms of an infant's body burden.

The effects of human PCB exposure during pregnancy have been based on studies of Japanese and Taiwanese women who consumed rice oil that was accidentally contaminated with a mixture of toxic chemicals including PCBs at levels of 2,000–3,000 ppm. Infants with in utero exposures were below mean birth weight for gestational age; had a grayish-brown staining of the skin, gingiva, and nails; and had parchment-like desquamation of the skin that faded within several months. Several were stillborn. Authors of follow-up studies report temporary growth and developmental deficits lasting from 2–6 years.

Two recent studies, one in an occupational setting and the other related to dietary consumption of PCB-contaminated fish, report lower-birth-weight infants among the women with greater exposure in comparison with a low or nonexposed group. Head circumference was also reduced among the exposed group in the dietary study. Although estimated differently in each study, gradual long-term bioaccumulation of low-level PCB exposure was considered to be a more important way of defining exposure than exposure during pregnancy alone.

Recommended Reading

Barlow, S. M., and Sullivan, F. M. *Reproductive Hazards of Industrial Chemicals*. New York: Academic, 1982. Pp. 455–482.

Council on Scientific Affairs' Advisory Panel on Reproductive Hazards in the Workplace. *Effects of Toxic Chemicals on the Reproductive System*. d43:pcb(1–3) (revd. 6-9-85). Chicago: American Medical Association, 1985.

Fein, G. G., et al. Prenatal exposure to polychlorinated biphenyls: Effects on birth size and gestational age. *J. Pediatr.* 105:315, 1984.

Jacobson, S. W., et al. Intrauterine Exposure of Human Newborns to PCBs. Measures of Exposure. In F. M. D'Itri and M. Kamrin (eds.), *PCBs: Human and Environmental Hazards*. Boston: Butterworth, 1983. Pp. 311–343.

Occupational Diseases: A Guide to Their Recognition. U.S. Dept. of Health, Education and Welfare, NIOSH, publication No. 77-181. Government Printing Office, 1977. Pp. 255–256.

Taylor, P. R., et al. Polychlorinated biphenyls. Influence on birthweight and gestation. *Am. J. Public Health* 74:1153, 1984.

Selenium and Its Compounds

SYNONYMS

None

SELECTED SELENIUM COMPOUNDS

Selenium chloride, selenium hexafluoride, selenium oxychloride, selenium tetrachloride, hydrogen selenide

USES

In manufacture of selenium rectifiers; pigment for ruby-pink- and orange-colored glass; vulcanizing agent for rubber; metallic base for arc light electrodes; in manufacture of selenium photo cells, semiconductor fusion mixtures; in photographic toning baths; in dehydrogenation of organic compounds; alloy material with stainless steel, copper, and cast steel

SELECTED OCCUPATIONAL GROUPS POTENTIALLY EXPOSED

Makers of arc light electrodes, electric rectifiers, glass, pesticides, photographic chemicals, pigments, plastics, rubber, semiconductors, sulfuric acid; textile workers; pyrite workers; copper smelters

EXPOSURE STANDARD

OSHA/PEL: 0.2 mg/m^3 (as selenium) as a TWA for an 8-hour workshift

ROUTES OF ENTRY

Inhalation of dust or vapor; absorption of liquids through skin; ingestion

Biologic Effects

Elemental selenium is considered to be relatively nonirritating and poorly absorbed. However, many selenium compounds are strong skin and mucous membrane irritants. The most characteristic sign of selenium absorption is a garlic odor of the breath, probably due to the excretion of small amounts of dimethyl selenide. Other possible symptoms include pallor, lassitude, irritability, indigestion, and giddiness. Liver and kidney damage can also occur. The effects of selenium on development and its inhibitory influence on cancer are still being investigated.

Special Considerations in Pregnancy

Selenium readily passes across the placenta. It has also been measured in breast milk, but milk concentrations show geographic variation. This presumably correlates with the degree of selenium occurring naturally and entering the food chain in different areas. The outcomes of human pregnancy have not revealed systematic adverse effects of occupational selenium exposure. Suggestive data hint at an association with spontaneous abortion.

Adverse effects of selenium on fertility have only been shown in animal studies. Although some selenium compounds are normally antimutagenic and anticlastogenic, mutagenic effects have been observed under certain experimental conditions.

Recommended Reading

Barlow, S. M., and Sullivan, F. M. *Reproductive Hazards of Industrial Chemicals.* New York: Academic, 1982. Pp. 483–500.

Council on Scientific Affairs' Advisory Panel on Reproductive Hazards in the Workplace. *Effects of Toxic Chemicals on the Reproductive System.* d43:se(1–4) (revd. 6-19-85). Chicago: American Medical Association, 1985.

Occupational Diseases: A Guide to Their Recognition. U.S. Dept. of Health, Education and Welfare, NIOSH, publication No. 77-181. Government Printing Office, 1977. Pp. 387–390.

Styrene

SYNONYMS

Cinnamene, phenethylene, phenylethylene, styrene monomer, styrol, styrolene, vinyl benzene, vinyl benzol

USES

In manufacture of plastics, synthetic rubber, resins, insulators

SELECTED OCCUPATIONAL GROUPS POTENTIALLY EXPOSED

Makers of synthetic rubber, resins, polystyrene, polyesters, insulators

EXPOSURE STANDARDS

OSHA/PEL: 100 ppm (420 mg/m^3) as a TWA for an 8-hour workshift with an acceptable ceiling concentration of 200 ppm and an acceptable maximum peak of 600 ppm for 5 minutes (maximum) in any 3 hours

NIOSH recommendation: 50 ppm as a TWA for a 10-hour workshift, 40-hour workweek, with a ceiling concentration of 100 ppm as determined during any 15-minute sampling period

ROUTES OF ENTRY

Inhalation of vapor; absorption through skin

Biologic Effects

Liquid and vapors irritate eyes, nose, throat, and skin. More severe irritation of the upper respiratory tract, nose, and mouth can occur after acute exposure to high concentrations. The most severe systemic effects include symptoms of narcosis, cramps, and death due to respiratory center paralysis. Prolonged reaction time and decreased manual dexterity have been observed following short-term exposure under laboratory conditions.

Special Considerations in Pregnancy

Several investigators have reported styrene and styrene oxide to be mutagenic to human lymphocytes in vitro and to cause chromosomal damage in workers exposed to high levels for only a few months. The remaining evidence relating to reproductive effects is conflicting and relatively weak. The most recent study on menstrual dysfunction among styrene workers did not reveal a positive association, in contrast with a frequently cited study done 10 years earlier. One study suggests an increased risk of spontaneous abortion, but only six cases were investigated. A more recent study found no differences. Two other studies report increases in congenital anomalies, but these did not reach levels of statistical significance.

Apart from positive mutagenic tests, there is no convincing evidence that styrene is embryolethal or teratogenic in laboratory animals.

Recommended Reading

Barlow, S. M., and Sullivan, F. M. *Reproductive Hazards of Industrial Chemicals.* New York: Academic, 1982. Pp. 501–514.

Council on Scientific Affairs' Advisory Panel on Reproductive Hazards in the Workplace. *Effects of Toxic Chemicals on the Reproductive System.* d40:styr(1–2) (revd. 6-18-85). Chicago: American Medical Association, 1985.

Harkonen, H., and Holmberg, P. C. Obstetric histories of women occupationally exposed to styrene. *Scand. J. Work Environ. Health* 8:74, 1982.

Lemasters, G. K., Hagen, A., and Samuels, S. J. Reproductive outcomes in women exposed to solvents in 36 reinforced plastics companies: I. Menstrual dysfunction. *J. Occup. Med.* 27:490, 1985.

Occupational Diseases: A Guide to Their Recognition. U.S. Dept. of Health, Education and Welfare, NIOSH, publication No. 77-181. Government Printing Office, 1977. Pp. 241–242.

Zielhuis, R. L., et al. *Health Risks to Female Workers in Occupational Exposure to Chemical Agents.* Berlin: Springer-Verlag, 1984. Pp. 43–45.

Thallium

SYNONYMS

None

USES

Rodenticides, fungicides, insecticides; in optical lenses and instruments, photoelectric cells, mineralogic analysis; alloy with mercury in low-temperature thermometers, switches, and closures; in high-density liquids, dyes, and pigments; in manufacture of fireworks and imitation precious jewelry; alloy with silver and lead

SELECTED OCCUPATIONAL GROUPS POTENTIALLY EXPOSED

Makers of alloys, artificial diamonds, chlorinated compounds, dyes, fireworks, gems, glass, optical glass, photoelectric cells, pesticides, and insecticides

EXPOSURE STANDARD

OSHA/PEL: 0.1 mg/m^3 for skin (soluble thallium compounds) as a TWA for an 8-hour workshift

Inhalation of dust and fumes; ingestion and skin absorption of dust

Biologic Effects

Dermal contact may lead to skin irritation and sensitization. Systemic poisoning can occur with moderate or long-term exposure. Early symptoms include fatigue, limb pain, a metallic taste in the mouth, and hair loss. Late symptoms include peripheral neuritis, proteinuria, and joint pain. Acute poisoning through ingestion includes many of these symptoms, along with alopecia, gastrointestinal symptoms, and convulsions. Death can occur secondary to central nervous system damage.

Special Considerations in Pregnancy

Reports of thallium poisoning during pregnancy are rare. The reported cases are associated with attempted suicide, illegal abortion, or accidental poisoning. These case reports suggest that there may be fetal growth retardation or patches of alopecia on the baby's scalp (a typical skin condition associated with thallium toxicity in adults). These findings are not from systemic epidemiologic studies and therefore can only be taken as suggestive evidence that thallium may have had a causative role.

Recommended Reading

Barlow, S. M., and Sullivan, F. M. *Reproductive Hazards of Industrial Chemicals.* New York: Academic, 1982. Pp. 530–537.

Occupational Diseases: A Guide to Their Recognition. U.S. Dept. of Health, Education and Welfare, NIOSH, publication No. 77-181. Government Printing Office, 1977. Pp. 395–397.

Toluene

SYNONYMS

Toluol, methylbenzene, phenylmethane, methylbenzol

USES

In manufacture of benzene, benzaldehyde, explosives, dyes, and many other organic compounds; solvent for paints and coatings; component of automobile and aviation fuels; chemical feed for toluene diisocyanate (TDI)

SELECTED OCCUPATIONAL GROUPS POTENTIALLY EXPOSED

Makers of benzene, paint thinner, perfume, rubber cement, saccharin, TDI, vinyl toluene; coke oven, lacquer, petrochemical, and solvent workers; aviation fuel and gasoline blenders

EXPOSURE STANDARDS

OSHA/PEL: 200 ppm as a TWA for an 8-hour workshift with a ceiling concentration of 300 ppm; acceptable maximum peaks of 500 ppm for 10 minutes

NIOSH recommendation: 100 ppm as a TWA for an 8-hour work-shift with a ceiling of 200 ppm for a 10-minute sampling period

ROUTES OF ENTRY

Inhalation of vapor; percutaneous absorption of liquid

Biologic Effects

Toluene can result in irritation to the eyes, respiratory tract, and skin. Prolonged contact with the liquid may result in dry, fissured dermatitis. Acute exposure results primarily in central nervous system depression with symptoms that can include headache, dizziness, fatigue, drowsiness, muscular weakness, reduced coordination, skin paresthesias, and coma.

Special Considerations in Pregnancy

Toluene's conjoint use with other solvents in occupational settings has made it difficult to assess its independent effect on reproduction. Attempts have been made to determine the effect of this compound on menstrual dysfunction, fetal growth, teratogenicity, and mutagenicity. Evaluation of the findings of these studies, however, is hampered by shortcomings of their design and exposure to multiple solvents. Nevertheless, toluene remains suspect because of the similarity of reduction in fetal weight in both animal and human studies. Furthermore, this compound's lipid solubility makes it a likely candidate for placental transfer.

Recommended Reading

Barlow, S. M., and Sullivan, F. M. *Reproductive Hazards of Industrial Chemicals.* New York: Academic, 1982. Pp. 538–549.

Council on Scientific Affairs' Advisory Panel on Reproductive Hazards in the Workplace. *Effects of Toxic Chemicals on the Reproductive System.* d43:tol(1–2) (revd. 6-18-85). Chicago: American Medical Association, 1985.

Occupational Diseases: A Guide to Their Recognition. U.S. Dept. of Health, Education and Welfare, NIOSH, publication No. 77-181. Government Printing Office, 1977. Pp. 242–244.

Trichloroethylene

SYNONYMS

Ethylene trichloride, ethinyl trichloride, trichloroethene, TCE

USES

Solvent in metal and textile degreasing operations; in extraction processes for coffee and spices; dry-cleaning agent; chemical intermediate in the production of pesticides, waxes, gums, resins, tars, paints, varnishes, and organic chemicals such as chloroacetic acid. Trichloroethylene was used in the past as an anesthetic and analgesic in obstetrics and dentistry.

SELECTED OCCUPATIONAL GROUPS POTENTIALLY EXPOSED

Makers of disinfectants, drugs, dyes, perfume, shoes, soaps; caffeine processors; degreasers; dry-cleaners; electronic equipment, glass, metal, and textile cleaners; fat and oil processors; mechanics; printers; resin, solvent, and varnish workers; rubber cementers; tobacco denicotinizers

EXPOSURE STANDARDS

OSHA/PEL: 100 ppm (535 mg/m^3) as a TWA for an 8-hour work-shift with a ceiling concentration of 200 ppm and a maximum peak of 300 ppm for 5 minutes in a 2-hour period
NIOSH recommendation: 25 ppm (134 mg/m^3) as a TWA for a 10-hour workshift

ROUTES OF ENTRY

Inhalation of vapor; percutaneous absorption

Biologic Effects

Trichloroethylene vapor can be irritating to the eyes, nose, and throat. Skin contact with the liquid can cause dermatitis. Systemic toxicity is characterized by central nervous system depression with such symptoms as headache, dizziness, nausea and vomiting, incoordination, arrhythmias, and anesthesia that can lead to respiratory and cardiac failure. Alcohol consumption can exacerbate the symptoms of TCE exposure and cause "degreaser's flush." Hepatotoxicity can occur after massive exposure. An increase in hepatocellular carcinoma has been observed with TCE exposure in mice but not rats. This liquid is not believed to be carcinogenic in humans, although the available data are inconclusive.

Special Considerations in Pregnancy

A study of maternal and fetal blood levels at delivery in patients who were given TCE and nitrous oxide anesthesia demonstrated a rapid transfer of TCE across the placenta. The use of TCE as an anesthetic or analgesic during delivery has not been linked with any adverse pregnancy outcome apart from a possible increase in acidosis and hypoxia during the second stage of labor. However, no studies are available on maternal occupational exposure in pregnancy. Isolated case reports suggest that occupational exposure to toxic levels of TCE may affect endocrine and gonadal function. Cytogenetic analysis of workers also indicates that high concentrations of TCE can be mutagenic.

With the possible exception of delays in maturation and postnatal growth in rats, animal studies have not yielded convincing evidence of embryotoxic or teratogenic effects from TCE. In vitro tests for mutagenicity are conflicting.

Recommended Reading

Barlow, S. M., and Sullivan, F. M. *Reproductive Hazards of Industrial Chemicals.* New York: Academic, 1982. Pp. 556–565.
Council on Scientific Affairs' Advisory Panel on Reproductive Hazards

in the Workplace. *Effects of Toxic Chemicals on the Reproductive System*. d43:tce(1–3) (revd. 6-19-85). Chicago: American Medical Association, 1985.

Occupational Diseases: A Guide to Their Recognition. U.S. Dept. of Health, Education and Welfare, NIOSH, publication No. 77-181. Government Printing Office, 1977. Pp. 217–219.

Vinyl Chloride

SYNONYMS

Chlorethylene, chlorethene, monochloroethene, monochloroethylene, ethylene monochloride

USES

In manufacture of plastics, polyvinyl chloride, and other resins; chemical intermediate; in production of methyl chloroform; refrigerants; component of propellant mixtures

SELECTED OCCUPATIONAL GROUPS POTENTIALLY EXPOSED

Makers of polyvinyl resins and rubber; organic chemical synthesizers

EXPOSURE STANDARDS

OSHA/PEL: 1 ppm as a TWA for an 8-hour workshift with a ceiling of 5 ppm averaged over any period not exceeding 15 minutes
NIOSH recommendation: lowest reliably detectable level

ROUTE OF ENTRY

Inhalation of vapor

Biologic Effects

Vinyl chloride is a skin and eye irritant. Contact with the cooled liquid may cause frostbite on evaporation. Inhalation of vinyl chloride vapor can depress the central nervous system (CNS), resulting in symptoms that mimic mild alcohol intoxication. Death has been reported from severe, acute exposures. Chronic exposure among workers has been reported to result in the simultaneous occurrence of acroosteolysis, Raynaud's phenomenon, and sclerodermatous skin changes. Hepatic damage can also occur. Vinyl chloride is a human carcinogen and causally linked with angiosarcoma of the liver. Excess risks of cancers of the lung and lymphatic and nervous systems have also been reported. Experimental studies have demonstrated multisystemic oncogenic and toxicologic effects, including transplacental carcinogenesis in rats.

Special Considerations in Pregnancy

Communities with or near polyvinyl chloride (PVC) plants have been studied in the United States and Canada. The results of these studies suggest that there may be an association between living in such communities and an overall increased risk of congenital malformations, especially CNS defects. However, none of these studies was able to pinpoint a specific link between vinyl chloride and any particular birth defect because of flaws in study design and lack of control for the potential influence of other industrial pollutants.

Mutagenicity studies among exposed workers have produced conflicting results. However, some of the well-executed earlier studies, when exposures were higher, have provided evidence of increases in chromosomal anomalies related to duration and extent of exposure.

Recommended Reading

Barlow, S. M., and Sullivan, F. M. *Reproductive Hazards of Industrial Chemicals*. New York: Academic, 1982. Pp. 566–582.

Council on Scientific Affairs' Advisory Panel on Reproductive Hazards in the Workplace. *Effects of Toxic Chemicals on the Reproductive System*. d50:vc(1–2) (revd. 6-27-85). Chicago: American Medical Association, 1985.

Edmonds, L. D., et al. Congenital CNS malformations and vinyl chloride monomer exposure: A community study. *Teratology* 17:137, 1978.

Occupational Diseases: A Guide to Their Recognition. U.S. Dept. of Health, Education and Welfare, NIOSH, publication No. 77-181. Government Printing Office, 1977. Pp. 219–221.

Theriault, G., Iturra, H., and Gingras, S. Evaluation of the association between birth defects and exposure to ambient vinyl chloride. *Teratology* 27:359, 1983.

Waste Anesthetics

The following review relates to waste anesthetic gases and vapors in the workplace resulting from the administration of inhalation anesthetic agents. The four most commonly used agents are nitrous oxide, halothane, enflurane, and isoflurane.

SYNONYMS

Nitrous oxide: dinitrogen monoxide
Halothane: Fluothane®
Enflurane: Ethrane®
Isoflurane: Forane®

USES

Inhalation anesthetics, analgesics. Nitrous oxide is commonly used as an analgesic for dental procedures and during the first stage of labor, and in combination with other drugs for general anesthesia. Halothane has been widely used as a general anesthetic for more than 20 years; enflurane was introduced in 1973 and is increasing in popularity as a general anesthetic; isoflurane has recently become available as a general anesthetic.

SELECTED OCCUPATIONAL GROUPS POTENTIALLY EXPOSED

Anesthesiologists, nurse-anesthetists, operating room nurses and technicians, surgeons, dentists, dental assistants, veterinarians, veterinary assistants, recovery room nurses

EXPOSURE STANDARDS

Nitrous oxide
    OSHA/PEL: none

NIOSH recommendation: 25 ppm as a TWA for a 10-hour work-shift during anesthetic administration

Halogenated agents (halothane, enflurane, isoflurane)
OSHA/PEL: none
NIOSH recommendation: ceiling of 2 ppm based on a 1-hour sample

ROUTE OF ENTRY

Inhalation of gas or vapor

Biologic Effects

Complications associated with the use of these agents as inhalational anesthetics include postanesthetic hypoxia (diffusion hypoxia) in the case of nitrous oxide, and dose-related respiratory depression, uterine relaxation, and circulatory depression in the case of the halogenated agents. Investigations of occupational exposure have yielded conflicting results regarding the effects of waste anesthetics on hepatic and renal disease and carcinogenesis. There is some evidence that excess nitrous oxide exposure may increase the risk of neurologic disorders, including myeloneuropathy, possibly through inactivation of vitamin B_{12}.

Special Considerations in Pregnancy

Of all the occupational exposures, the association between waste anesthetic gases and reproductive outcome has probably received the most extensive epidemiologic assessment. Concern regarding the reproductive effects was prompted by a report in 1967 that 18 in 31 pregnancies among 110 female anesthetists in the Soviet Union had resulted in spontaneous abortion. Subsequent studies have linked exposure to waste anesthetics with a variety of adverse reproductive outcomes including infertility, spontaneous abortion, stillbirths, low birth weight, and congenital malformations. The most consistent finding is an association between maternal exposure and an increased risk of spontaneous abortion. However, since most of the studies were based on retrospective surveys that used postal questionnaires, response bias or the influence of such other factors as physical and emotional stress might be responsible for this finding.

Although no specific inhalational agent has been implicated, excess fetal loss among dental assistants has led to the suggestion that nitrous oxide may be a causative factor. Recently, nitrous oxide has been shown to interfere with methionine synthetase (which is important in myelinization of nerves) and thymidine synthetase (which is important in DNA production), both of which could have effects on a growing fetus.

Data with respect to the effects of maternal exposure on infertility, low birth weight, stillbirths, and congenital malformations in the offspring are either inconclusive or conflicting. The evidence for a paternal effect on reproductive outcome is generally weak and inconsistent.

With some exceptions, embryotoxic and teratogenic effects have generally not been observed in animal investigations except at anesthetic or near-anesthetic concentrations. Results of experimental investigations of mutagenicity have largely been negative, although authors of one study of rats with long-term exposure to a combination of halothane and nitrous oxide found an increase in cytogenetic aberrations in both bone marrow and spermatogonial cells.

According to a NIOSH report in 1977, the usual occupational exposure to halogenated anesthetics ranged from 1–10 ppm and that for nitrous oxide from 400–3,000 ppm. Current levels are presumably lower as a result of the installation of scavenging systems in operating rooms. Because of the potential for adverse health effects, it is generally agreed that levels of waste anesthetic gases be reduced to as low a level as is reasonably achievable.

Recommended Reading

Axelson, G., and Rylander, R. Exposure to anesthetic gases and spontaneous abortion: Response bias in a postal questionnaire study. *Int. J. Epidemiol.* 11:250, 1982.

Baden, J. M., et al. Thymidine and methionine syntheses in pregnant rats exposed to nitrous oxide. *Anesth. Analg.* 62:738, 1983.

Cohen, E., et al. Occupational disease in dentistry and chronic exposure to trace anesthetic gases. *J. Am. Dental Assoc.* 101:21, 1980.

Cohen, E. N., et al. Occupational disease among operating room personnel: A national study. *Anesthesiology* 41:321, 1974.

Council on Scientific Affairs' Advisory Panel on Reproductive Hazards in the Workplace. *Effects of Toxic Chemicals on the Reproductive System.* d49 halo(1–2) (revd. 6-14-85). Chicago: American Medical Association, 1985.

Criteria for a Recommended Standard—Occupational Exposure to Waste Anesthetic Gases and Vapors. U.S. Dept. of Health, Education and Welfare, NIOSH, publication No. 77-140. Government Printing Office, 1977.

Marshall, B., and Wollman, H. General Anesthetics. In A. G. Gilman, L. S. Goodman, and A. Gilman (eds.), *The Pharmacological Basis of Therapeutics* (6th ed.). New York: Macmillan, 1980. Pp. 277–283.

Vessey, M. P. Epidemiological studies of the occupational hazards of anesthesia: A review. *Anaesthesia* 33:430, 1978.

Xylene

Commercial xylene is a mixture of its three isomers, orthoxylene, metaxylene, and paraxylene, as well as small amounts of toluene, trimethylbenzene, phenol, thiophene, pyridine, and other nonaromatic hydrocarbons.

SYNONYMS

Xylol, dimethylbenzene

USES

Solvent; constituent of paint, lacquers, varnishes, inks, dyes, adhesives, cements, cleaning fluids, aviation fuels; in production of xylidines, benzoic acid, phthalic anhydride, isophthalic and terephthalic acids and their esters (for use in the manufacture of plastics and synthetic fibers); in manufacture of quartz crystal oscillators, hydrogen peroxide, perfumes, insect repellents, epoxy resins, pharmaceuticals; in the leather industry

SELECTED OCCUPATIONAL GROUPS POTENTIALLY EXPOSED

Workers in the manufacture of adhesives, aviation fuels, benzoic acid, cleaning fluids, lacquers, paints, phthalic anhydride, quartz crystal oscillators, solvents, synthetic textiles, varnishes; histology technicians

EXPOSURE STANDARDS

OSHA/PEL: 100 ppm (435 mg/m^3) as a TWA for an 8-hour work-shift

NIOSH recommendation: 100 ppm as a TWA for a 10-hour work-shift with a ceiling of 200 ppm during a 10-minute sampling period

ROUTES OF ENTRY

Inhalation of vapor; some absorption through skin

Biologic Effects

Vapor exposure can cause irritation of the eyes, nose, and throat. Prolonged skin contact can defat the skin and lead to dermatitis. Aspiration of the liquid can cause chemical pneumonitis, pulmonary edema, and hemorrhage. Acute exposures can produce central nervous system depression and reversible liver and kidney effects. At high concentrations, vapor inhalation can cause a variety of effects including dizziness, staggering, drowsiness, unconsciousness, pulmonary edema, anorexia, nausea, vomiting, and abdominal pain.

Special Considerations in Pregnancy

Since xylene so rarely occurs alone in the occupational setting, it is difficult to find groups who have not been simultaneously exposed to other solvents. Therefore, the few published studies that have implicated multiple solvent exposures as potential human teratogens and mutagens cannot be used to prove or disprove the role that xylene may play in the process.

Xylene is not teratogenic in rodents, but several animal studies have demonstrated embryolethal and fetotoxic effects at dosages that are not toxic to the mother.

Recommended Reading

Barlow, S. M., and Sullivan, F. M. *Reproductive Hazards of Industrial Chemicals*. New York: Academic, 1982. Pp. 592–599.

Council on Scientific Affairs' Advisory Panel on Reproductive Hazards in the Workplace. *Effects of Toxic Chemicals on the Reproductive System*. d43:xyl(1–2) (revd. 6-18-85). Chicago: American Medical Association, 1985.

Holmberg, P. C. Central nervous system defects in children born to mothers exposed to organic solvents. *Lancet* 2:177, 1979.

Occupational Diseases: A Guide to Their Recognition. U.S. Dept. of Health, Education and Welfare, NIOSH, publication No. 77-181. Government Printing Office, 1977. Pp. 244–246.

Appendix C
Antineoplastic Drugs

Antineoplastic drugs are covered separately in this appendix because their use during pregnancy is associated with a unique problem. All such agents are designed to attack rapidly dividing cells, and fetal organs, like neoplasms, are composed of this type of tissue. Thus, it would seem obvious that antineoplastic agents are contraindicated during pregnancy. However, the illnesses against which these drugs are directed represent urgent threats to the mother's life. Therefore, when chemotherapy offers the best chance for maternal survival, the interests of mother and fetus are at odds. In such situations, it is best to provide as much information as possible to the patient and her partner, and allow them to participate in the decision-making process. Three options are usually considered: (1) postpone the chemotherapy until after delivery, (2) use chemotherapy and allow the pregnancy to continue, and (3) use chemotherapy and terminate the pregnancy. This appendix is designed to provide information that may be helpful in choosing among the options, but it must be remembered that there rarely are absolutely right or wrong decisions in such a situation; ambivalence will inevitably accompany any choice.

Details of dosage and administration of antineoplastic drugs are not included, since such treatment is best left to experts in the field. The emphasis is on special considerations in pregnancy. Unfortunately, much of the data concerning these agents are less than optimal. For obvious reasons randomized trials do not exist, and even case series are usually small because of the limited number of pregnant women who require such treatment. Gestational timing of drug administration, critical to any discussion of teratogenicity, is frequently poorly documented. Finally, multiple agents are used more often than not, making it difficult to ascribe adverse outcomes to specific drugs. For these reasons, animal data are often cited, and as always, care must be taken in extrapolating such data to the human clinical situation.

A body of literature addresses the issue of pregnancy conceived at varying intervals *after* chemotherapy has been used, particularly for the treatment of lymphomas. Although this issue is beyond the scope of the present discussion, it is reassuring that the preponderance of evidence does not suggest increased birth defects among such offspring. However, maternal ovarian function can be adversely affected, particularly when radiation has been combined with chemotherapy.

Aminopterin

Aminopterin, a folic acid antagonist, is of historic interest only, since its use has been completely supplanted by methotrexate and other folic acid analogs. Because aminopterin was used as an abortifacient in the past, there are numerous case reports of malformed infants resulting when abortion was unsuccessful. First-trimester exposure has been associated with cranial, skeletal, facial, cardiac, and renal anomalies. Growth retardation has also been reported. In one literature survey, approximately 20% of appropriately exposed fetuses were anomalous.

Recommended Reading

Char, F. Aminopterin embryopathy syndrome. *Am. J. Dis. Child.* 133: 1189, 1979.

Gilman, A. G., Goodman, L. S., and Gilman, A. *The Pharmacological Basis of Therapeutics.* (6th ed.). New York: Macmillan, 1980. Pp. 1272–1273.

Meltzer, H. J. Congenital anomalies due to attempted abortion with 4-aminopteroglutamic acid. *J.A.M.A.* 161:1253, 1956.

Netzloff, M. L., Frias, J. L., and Rennert, O. M. Maternal aminopterin ingestion. *Am. J. Dis. Child.* 125:459, 1973.

Shaw, E. B. Fetal damage due to maternal aminopterin ingestion. *Am. J. Dis. Child.* 124:93, 1972.

Sokal, J. E., and Lessmann, E. M. Effects of cancer chemotherapeutic agents on the human fetus. *J.A.M.A.* 172:1765, 1960.

Sweet, D. L., and Kinzie, J. Consequences of radiotherapy and antineoplastic therapy for the fetus. *J. Reprod. Med.* 17:241, 1976.

Warkany, J., Beaudry, P. H., and Hornstein, S. Attempted abortion with aminopterin (4-amino-pteroylglutamic acid). *Am. J. Dis. Child.* 97:274, 1959.

Busulfan (Myleran®)

Busulfan, an alkyl sulfate alkylating agent used in the treatment of chronic granulocytic leukemia, polycythemia vera, and primary thrombocytosis, acts by myelosuppression. At low dosages, selective depression of granulocyte and platelet production occurs. At higher dosages, erythrocyte production is affected, and ultimately, pancytopenia may occur. Major toxic effects are related to both granulocytopenia and thrombocytopenia. Elevated urate levels can also occur and patients are usually treated concomitantly with allopurinol. Nausea, vomiting, diarrhea, impotence, sterility, and amenorrhea have all been reported as occasional side effects. Rarely, generalized skin pigmentation, gynecomastia, cheilosis, glossitis, anhidrosis, and pulmonary fibrosis have occurred. The drug is extremely effective, inducing remission in 85–90% of patients with chronic granulocytic leukemia.

In animal studies, cleft palate, digital defects, eye defects, growth retardation, ovarian dysgenesis, and destruction of seminiferous tubules in male fetuses exposed to busulfan have been reported. Reports on nonpregnant laboratory animals and humans receiving busulfan have shown chromosomal changes in lymphocytes and bone marrow cells.

Human case reports are, as with most antineoplastic drugs, problematic because many patients were treated with multiple drug regimens. Literature reviews have turned up reports of 24 women treated with busulfan during the first trimester. Four of the offspring manifested congenital abnormalities, including multiple malformations, cleft palate, ocular defects, and liver anomalies, and one child had mosaic trisomy 21. Among patients treated after the first trimester of pregnancy, intrauterine growth retardation was common.

Recommended Reading

Bhisey, A. N., Advani, S. H., and Khare, G. Cytogenetic anomalies in a child born to a mother receiving busulfan for chronic myeloid leukemia. *Indian J. Cancer* 19:272, 1982.

Diamond, I., Anderson, M. M., and McCreadie, S. R. Transplacental passage of busulfan (Myleran®) in a mother with leukemia. *Pediatrics* 25:85, 1960.

Gebhart, E. Comparative studies on the distribution of aberrations on human chromosomes treated with busulphan in vivo and in vitro. *Humangenetik* 21:263, 1974.

Gilman, A. G., Goodman, L. S., and Gilman, A. *The Pharmacological Basis of Therapeutics* (6th ed.). New York: Macmillan, 1980. Pp. 1268–1269.

Heller, R. H., and Jones, J. W. Production of ovarian dysgenesis in the rat and human by busulphan. *Am. J. Obstet. Gynecol.* 89:414, 1964.

Honeycombe, J. R. The effects of busulfan on the chromosomes of normal human lymphocytes. *Mutat. Res.* 57:35, 1978.

Johnson, F. D. Pregnancy and concurrent chronic myelogenous leukemia. *Am. J. Obstet. Gynecol.* 112:640, 1972.

Murphy, M. L., Delmoro, A., and Lacon, C. R. The comparative effects of polyfunctional alkylating agents in the rat fetus with additional notes on the chick embryo. *Ann. N.Y. Acad. Sci.* 68:762, 1958.

Nicholson, H. O. Cytotoxic drugs in pregnancy: Review of reported cases. *J. Obstet. Gynaecol. Br. Commonw.* 75:307, 1968.

Sweet, D. L., and Kinzie, J. Consequences of radiotherapy and antineoplastic therapy for the fetus. *J. Reprod. Med.* 17:241, 1976.

Vanhems, E., and Bousquet, J. Influence du misulban sur le développement du testicule du rat. *Ann. Endocrinol.* 33:119, 1972.

Chlorambucil (Leukeran®)

Chlorambucil, a nitrogen mustard derivative, is an alkylating agent and functions as an antineoplastic drug by disrupting nucleic acid function. It is the treatment of choice for chronic lymphocytic leukemia and primary macroglobulinemia. It has also been used to induce remissions in polycythemia vera, Hodgkin's disease, lymphomas, myelomas, and solid tumors. There have been reports of its use in vasculitis associated with rheumatoid arthritis and in autoimmune hemolytic anemia. Toxic effects include bone marrow suppression, gastrointestinal discomfort, dermatitis, and hepatic damage. It is believed to be carcinogenic, with an increased incidence of leukemias and other tumors reported at long-term follow-up study.

The exposure of pregnant rats to intraperitoneal injections of chlorambucil was associated with a variety of fetal malformations, including urinary tract abnormalities, encephalocele, facial clefts, and limb defects. There are two human case reports of unilateral renal agenesis after chlorambucil exposure throughout pregnancy. Other reported cases have been associated with apparently normal outcomes. Because chlorambucil is probably carcinogenic, concern exists about possible development of malignancies later in life after in utero exposure, but no data are currently available.

Recommended Reading

Gilman, A. G., Goodman, L. S., and Gilman, A. *The Pharmacological Basis of Therapeutics* (6th ed.). New York: Macmillan, 1980. Pp. 1267–1268.

Jacobs, C., et al. Management of the pregnant patient with Hodgkin's disease. *Ann. Intern. Med.* 95:669, 1981.

Monie, I. W. Chlorambucil-induced abnormalities of urogenital system of rat fetuses. *Anat. Rec.* 139:145, 1961.

Murphy, M. L. A comparison of the teratogenic effects of five polyfunctional alkylating agents on the rat fetus. *Pediatrics* 23:231, 1959.

Shotton, D., and Monie, I. W. Possible teratogenic effect of chlorambucil on a human fetus. *J.A.M.A.* 186:74, 1963.

Steege, J. F., and Caldwell, D. S. Renal agenesis after first trimester exposure to chlorambucil. *South. Med. J.* 73:1414, 1980.

Sweet, D. L., and Kinzie, J. Consequences of radiotherapy and antineoplastic therapy for the fetus. *J. Reprod. Med.* 17:241, 1976.

Cisplatin (Platinol®)

Cisplatin (cis-diamminedichloroplatinum, cis-DDP) is an inorganic platinum-coordination complex composed of a central platinum atom surrounded by chlorine atoms and ammonia molecules. It has some properties of an alkylating agent but primarily functions as an antineoplastic agent by interfering with DNA synthesis nonspecifically throughout the cell cycle. Cisplatin is effective against a wide array of head and neck cancers as well as carcinomas of the testes, ovary, and bladder.

Common side effects include nausea and vomiting. High-tone hearing loss can be documented by audiometric study but is rarely a clinically significant side effect. Myelosuppression is usually mild. The most significant dose-limiting toxic effect is reversible renal insufficiency.

In an autopsy study involving tissue samples from 12 patients who received varying dosages for different durations of treatment, highest platinum concentrations were found in the liver, prostate, and kidney. Lower concentrations were found in the bladder, testicle, pancreas, spleen, and muscle. Platinum was found in all tissues tested as long as 180 days after the last cisplatin administration.

Experience with cisplatin in pregnancy is extremely limited. In one patient undergoing therapeutic abortion 3 days after her third weekly intravenous treatment with 40 mg/m^2 cis-DDP, the platinum concentration in the placenta was 0.52 mg/g and 0.31 μg/g in combined parts of the 8-week-old fetus. In a second case, a woman at 10 weeks' gestation received a single intravenous dose of 50 mg/kg for cervical carcinoma. A radical hysterectomy was performed 2 weeks later, and the male fetus examined was morphologically normal for its gestational age.

The disposition of cisplatin in breast milk is not known.

Recommended Reading

Cancer chemotherapy. *Med. Lett. Drugs Ther.* 27:13, 1985.

Jacobs, A. J., et al. Oat cell carcinoma of the uterine cervix in a pregnant woman treated with cis-diamminedichloroplatinum. *Gynecol. Oncol.* 9:405, 1980.

Kiely, J. M. Clinical pharmacology (series on pharmacology in practice). 12. Antineoplastic agents. *Mayo Clin. Proc.* 56:384, 1981.

Stewart, D. J., et al. Human tissue distribution after cis-diamminedichloroplatinum. *Cancer Chemother. Pharmacol.* 10:51, 1982.

Cyclophosphamide (Cytoxan®, Neosar®)

Cyclophosphamide, a nitrogen mustard derivative, is an alkylating agent and functions as an antineoplastic drug by disrupting nucleic acid function. It is one of the most commonly used antineoplastic preparations and is often a component of multidrug protocols. It is effective orally as well as parenterally. It has been successfully employed in cases of Hodgkin's disease and lymphosarcoma. In combination with other drugs, it has been used to treat Burkitt's lymphoma and acute lymphocytic leukemia in childhood, and as adjuvant therapy in metastatic carcinoma of the breast. It has also been used in multiple myeloma, chronic lymphocytic leukemia, bronchogenic carcinoma, cervical and ovarian malignancies, neuroblastoma, and retinoblastoma. This drug is an immunosuppressant and has been used to prevent rejection in organ transplant recipients and to treat disorders such as rheumatoid arthritis, Wegener's granulomatosis, nephrotic syndrome in children, and autoallergic ocular disease.

Toxic effects of cyclophosphamide include frequent nausea and vomiting, mucosal ulcerations, dizziness, transverse ridging of the nails, and increased skin pigmentation. Alopecia is extremely common with this drug. Interstitial pulmonary fibrosis and hepatic toxicity can occur. Sterile hemorrhagic cystitis is reported in 5–10% of individuals, and is presumably due to bladder irritation from toxic products of cyclophosphamide. Inappropriate antidiuretic hormone (ADH) secretion has been reported in patients who receive high-dose therapy. Prolonged high-dose therapy is associated with bone marrow depression. Immunosuppression may be associated with opportunistic infections. The drug may be carcinogenic, similar to other nitrogren mustard derivatives. Depression of spermatogenesis and amenorrhea have been reported.

Animal experiments in various species have demonstrated skeletal defects, oral clefts, encephalocele, and limb-reduction defects after cyclophosphamide exposure in utero. Rodent studies have shown cyclophosphamide administered throughout pregnancy to be associated with delayed fetal growth.

Cyclophosphamide has been demonstrated to cross the placenta and appear in amniotic fluid at term. In one literature survey, 3 in 6 fetuses exposed during the first trimester had congenital anomalies. Case reports have included digital and toe malformations, cardiac abnormalities, imperforate anus with rectovaginal fistula, and hemangiomas. Most reported exposures have been to multiple drugs or to cyclophosphamide plus irradiation. Exposure in later pregnancy has evidently been relatively benign, except for what appears to be an increased incidence of intrauterine growth retardation. Unfortunately, no untreated disease-matched control pregnancies were available for comparison. There is a single case report of a nursing infant whose platelet and leukocyte counts were reversibly depressed during maternal cyclophosphamide therapy for Burkitt's lymphoma.

Recommended Reading

Chaube, S., Kury, G., and Murphy, M. L. Teratogenic effects of cyclophosphamide (NCA-26271) in the rat. *Cancer Chemother. Rep.* 51:363, 1967.

Coates, A. Cyclophosphamide in pregnancy. *Aust. N.Z. J. Obstet. Gynaecol.* 10:33, 1970.

D'Incalci, M., et al. Transplacental passage of cyclophosphamide. *Cancer Treat. Rep.* 66:1681, 1982.

Dubin, H. V., Courter, M. H., and Harrell, E. R. Toxoplasmosis: A complication of corticosteroid-and-cyclophosphamide–treated lupus erythematosus. *Arch. Dermatol.* 104:547, 1971.

Durodola, J. I. Administration of cyclophosphamide during late pregnancy and early lactation: A case report. *J. Natl. Med. Assoc.* 71:165, 1979.

Gibson, J. E., and Becker, B. A. The teratogenicity of cyclophosphamide in mice. *Cancer Res.* 28:475, 1968.

Gilman, A. G., Goodman, L. S., and Gilman, A. *The Pharamacological Basis of Therapeutics* (6th ed.). New York: Macmillan, 1980. Pp. 1264–1267.

Greenaway, J. C., et al. The in vitro teratogenicity of cyclophosphamide in rat embryos. *Teratology* 25:335, 1982.

Greenberg, L. H., and Tanaka, K. R. Congenital anomalies probably induced by cyclophosphamide. *J.A.M.A.* 188:123, 1964.

Hardin, J. A. Cyclophosphamide treatment of lymphoma during third trimester of pregnancy. *Obstet. Gynecol.* 39:850, 1972.

Lergier, J. E., Mimenez, E., and Maldonado, N. Normal pregnancy in multiple myeloma treated with cyclophosphamide. *Cancer* 23:1018, 1974.

Murray, C. L., et al. Multimodal cancer therapy for breast cancer in the first trimester of pregnancy. *J.A.M.A.* 252:2607, 1984.

Scott, J. R. Fetal growth retardation associated with maternal administration of immunosuppressive drugs. *Am. J. Obstet. Gynecol.* 128:668, 1977.

Toledo, T. M., Harper, R. C., and Moser, R. H. Fetal effects during cyclophosphamide and irradiation therapy. *Ann. Intern. Med.* 74:87, 1971.

Wilk, A. L., McClure, H. M., and Horigan, E. A. Induction of craniofacial malformations in the rhesus monkey with cyclophosphamide. *Teratology* 17:24A, 1978.

Cytarabine (Ara-C, Cytosar-U®, Cytosine Arabinoside)

Cytarabine, an antimetabolite, is a pyrimidine analog that is believed to act by blocking nucleic acid polymerases, and possibly by incorporation into DNA and RNA. It is commonly used, either alone or in combination with other agents, to induce remission in acute leukemias. It also may be beneficial in Hodgkin's disease and other lymphomas. Toxic effects include myelosuppression, with leukopenia, thrombocytopenia, and anemia. Gastrointestinal disturbances, stomatitis, hepatic dysfunction, thrombophlebitis at injection sites, fever, and dermatitis have also been reported.

Animal studies have demonstrated the induction of facial clefts, skeletal defects, central nervous system anomalies, ear atresia, limb-reduction defects, and renal changes with the administration of cytarabine during pregnancy.

Information about the effects of cytarabine on the developing human fetus is limited to case reports. At least 12 cases with first-trimester exposure have been described, with 3 anomalous fetuses (one with a trisomy, one with ear and limb anomalies, one with limb-reduction defects) and 9 apparently normal conceptuses resulting. An additional 17 fetuses exposed in only the second and/or third trimesters have been reported. Two of these pregnancies ended with intrauterine fetal demise, another resulted in a trisomic abortus, and at least four delivered prematurely. The remaining 10 resulted in reportedly normal offspring. Most of these exposures during pregnancy were not to cytarabine alone, but to combinations of chemotherapeutic agents. In some cases four or more different drugs were used.

Interestingly, two males taking this drug sired anomalous offspring, one with anencephaly and another with tetralogy of Fallot and syndactyly.

Recommended Reading

Blatt, J., et al. Pregnancy outcome following cancer chemotherapy. *Am. J. Med.* 69:828, 1980.

Cantanzarite, V. A., and Ferguson, J. E., II. Acute leukemia and pregnancy: A review of management and outcome, 1972–1982. *Obstet. Gynecol. Surv.* 39:663, 1984.

Chaube, S., and Murphy, M. L. The Teratogenic Effects of the Recent Drugs Active in Cancer Chemotherapy. In D. H. M. Woolam (ed.), *Advances in Teratology*. New York: Academic, 1968. Vol. 3. Pp. 204–205.

Colbert, N., et al. Leucemie aigue au cours de la grossesse: Evolution favorable de la gestation chez deux malades traitées par chimiotherapie. *Nouv. Presse Med.* 9:175, 1980.

Dara, P., Slater, L. M., and Armentrout, S. A. Successful pregnancy during chemotherapy for acute leukemia. *Cancer* 47:845, 1981.

Gililland, J., and Weinstein, L. The effects of cancer chemotherapeutic agents on the developing fetus. *Obstet. Gynecol. Surv.* 38:6, 1983.

Gilman, A. G., Goodman, L. S., and Gilman, A. *The Pharmacological Basis of Therapeutics* (6th ed.). New York: Macmillan, 1980. Pp. 1280–1281.

Gstottner, M., Frisch, H., and Dienstl, F. Normales Neugeborenes nach zytostatischer Therapie bei akuter Promyelozytenleukamie in der Schwangerschaft. (Delivery of a normal child after chemotherapy of acute promyelocytic leukemia during pregnancy.) *Blut* 36:171, 1978.

Krueger, J. A., Davis, R. B., and Field, C. Multiple-drug chemotherapy in the management of acute lymphocytic leukemia during pregnancy. *Obstet. Gynecol.* 48:324, 1976.

Manoharan, A., and Leyden, M. J. Acute non-lymphocytic leukaemia in the third trimester of pregnancy. *Aust. N.Z. J. Med.* 9:71, 1979.

Maurer, L. H., et al. Fetal group C trisomy after cytosine arabinoside and thioguanine. *Ann. Intern. Med.* 75:809, 1971.

Morgenstern, G. Cytarabine in pregnancy. *Lancet* 2:259, 1980.

Newcomb, M., et al. Acute leukemia in pregnancy: Successful delivery after cytarabine and doxorubicin. *J.A.M.A.* 239:2691, 1978.

O'Donnell, R. O., Costigan, C., and O'Connell, L. G. Two cases of acute leukaemia in pregnancy. *Acta Haematol.* 61:298, 1979.

Percy, D. H. Teratogenic effects of pyrimidine analogs 5-iododeoxyuridine and cytosine arabinoside in late fetal mice and rats. *Teratology* 11:103, 1975.

Pizzuto, J., et al. Treatment of acute leukemia during pregnancy: Presentation of nine cases. *Cancer Treat. Rep.* 64:679, 1980.

Plows, C. W. Acute myelomonocytic leukemia in pregnancy: Report of a case. *Am. J. Obstet. Gynecol.* 143:41, 1982.

Russel, J. A., Powles, R. L., and Oliver, R. T. D. Conception and congenital abnormalities after chemotherapy of acute myelogenous leukemia in two men. *Br. Med. J.* 1:1508, 1976.

Schafer, A. I. Teratogenic effects of antileukemic chemotherapy. *Arch. Intern. Med.* 141:514, 1981.

Wagner, V. M., et al. Congenital abnormalities in baby born to cytarabine treated mother. *Lancet* 2:98, 1980.

Dactinomycin (Actinomycin D, Cosmegen®)

Dactinomycin, an antibiotic that binds to DNA and interferes with transcription via RNA polymerase, inhibits rapidly proliferating cells. It is used in the treatment of rhabdomyosarcoma, Wilms' tumor, soft tissue sarcomas, and solid tumors in children. It is occasionally used to treat lymphomas, sometimes used to treat testicular carcinomas, and is commonly used for choriocarcinoma. It can cause bone marrow suppression with resultant pancytopenia (often first manifested as thrombocytopenia). Other side effects include proctitis, diarrhea, glossitis, cheilitis, oral mucosal ulcerations, alopecia, and (in areas exposed to radiation) erythema, desquamation, and increased pigmentation. Local infiltration can cause severe injury.

Because dactinomycin is extremely successful in treating trophoblastic neoplasms, it would be expected to be quite dangerous when administered during pregnancy. The two case reports that could be found described apparently normal offspring when dactinomycin was initiated in the second or third trimester. First-trimester exposure has not been reported. There are numerous descriptions of successful pregnancy subsequent to dactinomycin treatment.

Recommended Reading

Gilman, A. G., Goodman, L. S., and Gilman, A. *The Pharmacological Basis of Therapeutics* (6th ed.). New York: Macmillan, 1980. Pp. 1291–1292.

Rustin, G. J. S., et al. Pregnancy after cytotoxic chemotherapy for gestational trophoblastic tumours. *Br. Med. J.* 288:103, 1984.

Sweet, D. L., and Kinzie, J. Consequences of radiotherapy and antineoplastic therapy for the fetus. *J. Reprod. Med.* 17:241, 1976.

Weed, J. C., Roh, R. A., and Mendenhall, H. W. Recurrent endodermal sinus tumor during pregnancy. *Obstet. Gynecol.* 54:653, 1979.

Doxorubicin (Adriamycin®) and Daunorubicin (Cerubidine®)

Doxorubicin and daunorubicin are anthracycline antibiotics produced by a fungus. The mechanism of their antineoplastic action is not entirely clear, but it has been suggested that the drugs may intercalate between base pairs of DNA, inhibiting the template activity of the nucleic acid. Other hypotheses include a disruptive effect on cellular membranes and activity as an electron acceptor with the formation of free radicals.

Doxorubicin has been used successfully to treat acute leukemias and lymphomas, and it is active against a number of solid tumors. It is commonly employed in combination with other agents to treat non-Hodgkin's lymphoma, ovarian carcinoma, breast cancer, oat cell carcinoma of the lung, and various sarcomas. It is often used for metastatic carcinoma of the breast and bladder and for bronchogenic carcinoma and neuroblastoma. It is considered the best available agent against metastatic thyroid carcinoma, and it has demonstrated activity against many other carcinomas.

Daunorubicin is used in the treatment of acute lymphocytic, granulocytic, and nonlymphoblastic leukemias.

Cardiotoxicity is the major adverse effect of doxorubicin and daunorubicin. Arrhythmias and ST–T wave changes are acute and usually reversible. A more serious, chronic, cumulative dose–related cardiomyopathy resulting in congestive heart failure unresponsive to cardiac glycoside therapy has a mortality of approximately 50%. This complication is rare at total doxorubicin doses below 500 mg/m^2. It is more common in patients previously exposed to cardiac irradiation or previously treated with cyclophosphamide, and in patients with impaired hepatic function.

Myelosuppression can occur, with white cell counts reaching a nadir at approximately 2 weeks of therapy but recovering by the fourth week. Alopecia, gastrointestinal symptoms, and stomatitis often occur but are reversible.

Animal studies of doxorubicin and daunorubicin have demonstrated teratogenicity including esophageal atresia, gastrointestinal tract malformations, and cardiovascular and urinary tract anomalies.

Data on transplacental passage of doxorubicin in humans are not consistent. The amniotic fluid has been shown not to contain measurable amounts of this compound as early as 4 hours and as late as 16 hours after the administration of doxorubicin to the mother. However, in one report doxorubicin was detected in fetal liver, kidney, and lung in high concentrations when an abortion was performed 15 hours after maternal dosing. In a second report, at 34 weeks' gestation, doxorubicin was detected in umbilical cord and placenta but not in cord blood 48 hours after a maternal dose. In a stillborn who died within 36 hours after maternal dosing, doxorubicin could not be demonstrated in any fetal tissue, although a possible metabolite, which could not be further characterized, was present. Thus, it is unclear how much doxorubicin crosses the placenta or in what form it crosses.

A literature search revealed 3 cases exposed to doxorubicin during the first trimester, and 10 during later pregnancy, with structurally normal fetuses resulting. A fetus exposed to doxorubicin, cyclophosphamide, and cobalt radiation therapy during the first trimester was born with imperforate anus and rectovaginal fistula at term. One anatomically normal fetus died in utero within 36 hours of the initiation of maternal chemotherapy with doxorubicin, vincristine, and prednisone. A mother died during pregnancy while undergoing treatment with doxorubicin for metastatic malignant granular cell myoblastoma, but no fetal autopsy was obtained. Five case reports of normal human pregnancy outcomes after second-trimester exposure to daunorubicin were located. There was also a single report of a stillborn with diffuse myocardial necrosis after maternal daunorubicin treatment.

Recommended Reading

Catanzarite, V. A., and Ferguson, J. E., II. Acute leukemia and pregnancy: A review of management and outcome, 1972–1982. *Obstet. Gynecol. Surv.* 39:663, 1984.

D'Incalci, M., et al. Transplacental passage of doxorubicin. *Lancet* 1:75, 1983.

Garcia, V., San Miguel, J., and Borrasca, A. L. Doxorubicin in the first trimester of pregnancy. *Ann. Intern. Med.* 94:547, 1981.

Gililland, J., and Weinstein, L. The effects of cancer chemotherapeutic agents on the developing fetus. *Obstet. Gynecol. Surv.* 38:6, 1983.

Gilman, A. G., Goodman, L. S., and Gilman, A. *The Pharmacological Basis of Therapeutics* (6th ed.). New York: Macmillan, 1980. Pp. 1291–1293.

Gstottner, M., Frisch, H., and Dienstl, F. Normales Neugeborenes nach zytostatischer Therapie bei akuter Promyelozytenleukamie in der Schwangerschaft. (Delivery of a normal child after chemotherapy of acute promyelocytic leukemia during pregnancy.) *Blut* 36:171, 1978.

Hassenstein, E., and Riedel, H. Zur Teratogenitat von Adriamycin. *Geburtshilfe Frauenheilkd.* 38:131, 1978.

Karp, G. I., et al. Doxorubicin in pregnancy: Possible transplacental passage. *Cancer Treat. Rep.* 67:773, 1983.

Khurshid, M., and Saleem, M. Acute leukaemia in pregnancy. *Lancet* 2:534, 1978.

Maral, R. J., and Jouanne, M. Toxicology of daunorubicin in animals and man. *Cancer Treat. Rep.* 65(Suppl. 4):9, 1981.

Murray, C. L., et al. Multimodal cancer therapy for breast cancer in the first trimester of pregnancy: A case report. *J.A.M.A.* 252:2607, 1984.

Newcomb, M., et al. Acute leukemia in pregnancy: Successful delivery after cytarabine and doxorubicin. *J.A.M.A.* 239:2691, 1978.

Roboz, J., et al. Does doxorubicin cross the placenta? *Lancet* 2:1382, 1979.

Schaison, G., et al. Les risques foeto-embryonnaires des chimiotherapies. *Bull. Cancer* 66:165, 1979.

Thompson, D. J., et al. Teratogenicity of adriamycin and daunomycin in the rat and rabbit. *Teratology* 17:151, 1978.

Tobias, J. S., and Bloom, H. J. G. Doxorubicin in pregnancy. *Lancet* 1:776, 1980.

Webb, G. A. The use of hyperalimentation and chemotherapy in pregnancy: A case report. *Am. J. Obstet. Gynecol.* 137:263, 1980.

5-Fluorouracil (Adrucil®, Efudex®, Fluoroplex®)

5-Fluorouracil (5-FU) is an antimetabolite used for the palliative management of selected carcinomas, particularly of the breast and gastrointestinal tract, in patients whose disease is considered to be inoperable. In addition, beneficial effects have been reported in the treatment of hepatoma and carcinomas of the ovary, cervix, urinary bladder, prostate, pancreas, and oropharyngeal areas. Topical 5-FU is used for the treatment of multiple actinic and solar keratosis as well as for multiple superficial basal cell carcinomas in which surgical removal is impractical.

Common side effects of systemic administration of the drug include stomatitis, esophagopharyngitis, diarrhea, anorexia, nausea, and vomiting. The major toxic sequelae, however, result from bone marrow suppression with secondary leukopenia, thrombocytopenia, and anemia. Other side effects include alopecia, dermatitis, photosensitivity, lacrimation, euphoria, and acute cerebellar syndrome. The most frequent side effects of topical 5-FU are local reactions.

5-FU is known to cause hindfoot anomalies, cleft palate, microphthalmus, and omphalocele in exposed fetal mice, and intrauterine growth and retardation and fetal death in similarly exposed rhesus monkeys.

Experience with this drug in human pregnancies is extremely limited. One case of second-trimester administration resulted in a normal fetus with reversible 5-FU toxicity in the neonatal period. A second case involved first-trimester exposure to a fetus that was also exposed to 5 rads of radiation. The pregnancy was electively terminated at 16 weeks, and the fetus was found to have a single umbilical artery, hypoplastic aorta, pulmonary hypoplasia, esophageal aplasia, imperforate anus, renal dysplasia, bilateral radial aplasia, and other abnormalities. A karyotype was not obtained in this case.

Recommended Reading

Gililland, J., and Weinstein, L. The effects of cancer chemotherapeutic agents on the developing fetus. *Obstet. Gynecol. Surv.* 38:6, 1983.

Gilman, A. G., Goodman, L. S., and Gilman, A. *The Pharmacological Basis of Therapeutics* (6th ed.). New York: Macmillan, 1980. Pp. 1278–1280.

Stadler, H. E., and Knowles, J. Fluorouracil in pregnancy: Effect on the neonate. *J.A.M.A.* 217:214, 1971.

Stephens, J. D., et al. Multiple congenital anomalies in a fetus exposed to 5-fluorouracil during the first trimester. *Am. J. Obstet. Gynecol.* 136:747, 1980.

6-Mercaptopurine (Purinethol®)

6-Mercaptopurine is a purine analog chemotherapeutic agent used primarily for the treatment of leukemia. It is administered alone, or more frequently in combination with other agents, in the treatment of acute lymphocytic, acute myeloblastic, and chronic myelogenous leukemias. It is also an immunosuppressive agent and has been used in the treatment of ulcerative colitis. In obstetric patients, it should only be given when a life-threatening condition exists.

The principal toxic effect of 6-mercaptopurine is bone marrow depression, although in general this develops more gradually than with folic acid antagonists. Other side effects include anorexia, nausea, vomiting, stomatitis, and diarrhea. Hyperuricemia is a common finding and can be treated with allopurinol. One-third of the patients develop jaundice, which resolves on discontinuation of therapy. Deaths have been reported from hepatic necrosis. Dermatologic manifestations can also occur.

This drug has severe teratogenic effects in animals. In humans, it is associated with an increased incidence of abortion and prematurity, but the risk of teratogenicity in the surviving offspring is not accurately known.

A recent report reviews 34 liveborn infants exposed in utero to 6-mercaptopurine, alone or in combination therapy. In this series, 15 fetuses were exposed in the first trimester and one of the liveborn infants was anomalous. That neonate had also been exposed to busulfan and radiation therapy and was born with bilateral microphthalmia, corneal opacities, and cleft palate. None of the 19 infants exposed after the first trimester had gross malformations. No long-term follow-up data were reported for any of these infants.

Increases in chromosomal aberrations were observed in peripheral lymphocytes of most of 14 nonpregnant patients with leukemia treated with 6-mercaptopurine in cumulative doses of between 0.2 and 1.1 g.

Recommended Reading

Gililland, J., and Weinstein, L. The effects of cancer chemotherapeutic agents on the developing fetus. *Obstet. Gynecol. Surv.* 38:1,6, 1983.

Gilman, A. G., Goodman, L. S., and Gilman, A. *The Pharmacological Basis of Therapeutics* (6th ed.). New York: Macmillan, 1980. Pp. 1282–1286.

IARC Monogr. Eval. Carcinog. Risk Chem. Hum. 26:249, 1981.

Methotrexate

Methotrexate is currently the most widely utilized antimetabolite in cancer chemotherapy. It is used extensively in the treatment of acute lymphocytic leukemia, non-Hodgkin's lymphoma, osteosarcoma, choriocarcinoma, head and neck cancer, and breast cancer. It is also used in the suppression of graft-versus-host disease after bone marrow transplantation and as a therapeutic alternative in the treatment of severe psoriasis. Because this drug has been associated with spontaneous abortion, fetal death, and congenital anomalies, it should only be used in obstetric patients who have a life-threatening condition for which this is the agent of choice.

Methotrexate is a folic acid antagonist that acts by inhibiting dehydrofolate-reductase. This interferes with cellular DNA synthesis and cell multiplication and regeneration. It has been reported that chromosome breaks in cultured lymphocytes from methotrexate-treated psoriatics are significantly more frequent than in untreated control groups. These findings have not been substantiated by other investigators, but it may be true that methotrexate impairs the normal healing of spontaneously occurring chromosome breaks.

High-dose methotrexate therapy is usually well tolerated. Myelotoxicity or clinically evident nephrotoxicity is uncommon, although transient decreases in glomerular filtration rates occur in many patients. Other side effects are nausea, vomiting, and a reversible elevation of hepatic enzymes. More unusual side effects include ocular irritation, erythema and desquamation, and pleuritis.

Use of folic acid antagonists during the first trimester results in craniofacial malformations in 20–30% of live births. Other abnormalities reported include tetralogy of Fallot, multiple hemangiomas, eczema, strabismus, and multiple congenital malformations incompatible with life and leading to stillbirth. No anomalies have been reported when methotrexate was used after the first trimester, but a significantly higher incidence of prematurity has been noted.

No increased risk of congenital abnormalities has been noted in the offspring of women exposed to methotrexate before pregnancy. However, a waiting period of 1 year is generally recommended after termination of therapy before conception.

To date, no case has been reported in which a man taking this drug at the time of conception fathered a malformed child.

Recommended Reading

Baker, H. Some hazards of methotrexate treatment of psoriasis. *Trans. St. John's Hosp. Dermatol. Soc.* 56:111, 1970.

Gililland, J., and Weinstein, L. The effects of cancer chemotherapeutic agents on the developing fetus. *Obstet. Gynecol. Surv.* 38:6, 1983.

Jolivet, J., et al. The pharmacology and clinical use of methotrexate. *N. Engl. J. Med.* 309:1094, 1983.

Pessy, W. H. Methotrexate and teratogenesis. *Arch. Dermatol.* 119:874, 1983.

Schottenfeld, D. Cancer risks of medical treatment. *CA.* 32:258, 1982.

Van Thiez, D. H., Ross, G. T., and Lipsett, M. B. Pregnancies after chemotherapy of trophoblastic neoplasms. *Science* 169:1326, 1970.

Procarbazine (Matulane®)

Procarbazine is a synthetic methyl hydrazine derivative originally conceived as a monoamide oxidase inhibitor. Although its exact mechanism of action is unknown, it may function as an antineoplastic agent by depolymerizing DNA through the liberation of hydrogen peroxide produced by autooxidation of the drug. Its major application has been in combination chemotherapy for Hodgkin's disease and other lymphomas.

Acute toxicity of procarbazine consists of nausea, vomiting, central nervous system depression, and a disulfiram (Antabuse®)–like reaction with alcohol. It is known to potentiate the action of the phenothiazine class of psychotherapeutic drugs. Delayed toxicity includes bone marrow depression, stomatitis, peripheral neuropathy, pneumonitis, and leukemia. The disposition of procarbazine in breast milk is not known.

Procarbazine is both mutagenic and carcinogenic in animals. Congenital malformations are described in case reports of four in five fetuses exposed to procarbazine in the first trimester. There was no pattern of reproducible defects in these fetuses, whose mothers were also taking other chemotherapeutic agents (mechlorethamine, vinblastine, and vincristine). In one case in which a mother mistakenly took 50 mg/day procarbazine orally for 30 days during the middle trimester of pregnancy, an apparently healthy, normal male infant was delivered at term. Even when used for short periods of time in standard dosages, procarbazine alone and in combination with other antineoplastic agents is known to produce reversible ovarian and testicular dysfunction.

Recommended Reading

Cancer chemotherapy. *Med. Lett. Drugs Ther.* 27:13, 1985.

Daw, E. G. Procarbazine in pregnancy. *Lancet* 2:984, 1970.

Garrett, M. J. Teratogenic effect of combination chemotherapy. *Ann. Intern. Med.* 80:667, 1974.

Johnson, S. A., Goldman, J. M., and Hawkins, D. F. Pregnancy after chemotherapy for Hodgkin's disease. *Lancet* 2:93, 1979.

Kiely, J. M. Clinical pharmacology (series on pharmacology in practice). 12. Antineoplastic agents. *Mayo Clin. Proc.* 56:384, 1981.

Lee, I. P., and Dixon, R. L. Mutagenicity, carcinogenicity and teratogenicity of procarbazine. *Mutat. Res.* 55:1, 1978.

Mennuti, M. T., Shepard, T. H., and Mellman, W. J. Fetal renal malformation following treatment of Hodgkin's disease during pregnancy. *Obstet. Gynecol.* 46:194, 1975.

Schilsky, S. L., et al. Long-term follow-up of ovarian function in women treated with MDPP chemotherapy for Hodgkin's disease. *Am. J. Obstet. Gynecol.* 71:552, 1981.

Thomas, P. R. M., and Peckham, M. J. The investigation and management of Hodgkin's disease in the pregnant patient. *Cancer* 38:1443, 1976.

Wells, J. H., Marshall, J. R., and Carbone, P. P. Procarbazine therapy for Hodgkin's disease in early pregnancy. *J.A.M.A.* 205:935, 1968.

Appendix D
Immunization of the
Obstetric Patient

There are four types of immunizing agents: (1) toxoids, (2) killed bacterial and viral vaccines (either whole or subunit), (3) live virus vaccines, and (4) immune globulin preparations. Toxoids are preparations of chemically altered bacterial exotoxin, killed vaccines contain heat-inactivated or chemically inactivated microorganisms or portions of microorganisms, and live virus vaccines are strains of virus selected for their reduced virulence. This lowered virulence may be a selected property of the virus, or it may be produced by serial passages of the wild virus in tissue culture (attenuation). In all cases, although no significant illness is produced, the live virus vaccine has sufficient antigenic properties in common with the infectious agent to stimulate protective immunity. The fourth type of immunizing agent, immune globulin, is a protein fraction of human plasma that can produce transient, passive antibody protection in the recipient. Hyperimmune globulin, which is produced from plasma of donors with very high antibody titers to a particular agent, is useful for protection against hepatitis B, rabies, tetanus, and varicella when clinically indicated. Pooled immune globulin is useful in providing protection against hepatitis A and measles (rubeola).

A systematic approach to vaccinating women of childbearing age is needed in order to ensure that every pregnant woman and her fetus are protected from preventable, serious diseases and from the possible risk that may accompany unnecessary or hazardous vaccines. Factors to be considered include the patient's susceptibility, risk of exposure, risk from the disease, and risk from the available immunizing agents.

Most persons born prior to 1957 were infected naturally with measles, mumps, and rubella and can be considered immune. For persons born since 1957, a history of physician-diagnosed measles, documentation of vaccination with live measles vaccine on or after the first birthday, or positive serologic test results for measles antibody is considered a reliable indicator of measles immunity. A documented history of vaccination on or after the first birthday or serologic evidence of any detectable antibody specific for rubella is considered evidence of immunity to rubella. Clinical diagnosis of rubella is not reliable since many other illnesses may mimic the signs and symptoms of rubella. A history of physician-diagnosed mumps or mumps vaccination on or after the first birthday is adequate evidence of immunity to mumps. A person is considered immune to tetanus and diphtheria after receiving at least three doses of each toxoid, with the last dose administered at least 6–12 months after the preceding dose. A booster dose is required every 10 years. Other vaccines are indicated for adults in the United States only under special circumstances.

The introductory remarks and table have been reproduced with permission from Immunization during pregnancy. *ACOG Tech. Bull.* No. 64, May 1982.

Table 15. Immunization during pregnancy

Immunizing agent	Risk from disease to pregnant female	Risk from disease to fetus or neonate	Type of immunizing agent	Risk from immunizing agent to fetus	Indications for immunization during pregnancy	Dose schedule	Comments
LIVE VIRUS VACCINES							
Poliomyelitis	No increased incidence in pregnancy, but may be more severe if it does occur	Anoxic fetal damage reported; 50% mortality in neonatal disease	Live attenuated virus (OPV) and inactivated virus (IPV) vaccine*	None confirmed	Not routinely recommended for adults in U.S. except persons at increased risk of exposure	*Primary:* Three doses of IPV at 4- to 8-week intervals and a fourth dose 6–12 months after the third dose; two doses of OPV with a 6- to 8-week interval and a third dose at least 6 weeks later, customarily 8–12 months later *Booster:* Every 5 years until 18 years of age for IPV	Vaccine indicated for susceptible pregnant women traveling in endemic areas or in other high-risk situations

*Inactivated polio vaccine recommended for unimmunized adults at increased risk.
From Immunization during pregnancy. *A.C.O.G. Tech. Bull.* No. 64, May 1982. With permission.

Table 15 (continued)

LIVE VIRUS VACCINES (cont.)

Immunizing agent	Risk from disease to pregnant female	Risk from disease to fetus or neonate	Type of immunizing agent	Risk from immunizing agent to fetus	Indications for immunization during pregnancy	Dose schedule	Comments
Measles	Significant morbidity, low mortality; not altered by pregnancy	Significant increase in abortion rate; may cause malformations	Live attenuated virus vaccine	None confirmed	Contraindicated (see immune globulins)	Single dose	Vaccination of susceptible women should be part of postpartum care
Mumps	Low morbidity and mortality; not altered by pregnancy	Probable increased rate of abortion in first trimester; questionable association of fibroelastosis in neonates	Live attenuated virus vaccine	None confirmed	Contraindicated	Single dose	
Rubella	Low morbidity and mortality; not altered by pregnancy	High rate of abortion and congenital rubella syndrome	Live attenuated virus vaccine	None confirmed	Contraindicated	Single dose	Teratogenicity of vaccine is theoretic, not confirmed to date; vaccination of susceptible women should be part of postpartum care

	Risk from disease to pregnant woman	Risk from disease to fetus or neonate	Type of immunizing agent	Risk from immunizing agent to fetus	Indications for vaccination during pregnancy	Dose schedule	Comments
Yellow fever	Significant morbidity and mortality; not altered by pregnancy	Unknown	Live attenuated virus vaccine	Unknown	Contraindicated except if exposure unavoidable	Single dose	Postponement of travel preferable to vaccination, if possible
IMMUNE GLOBULINS: POOLED							
Hepatitis A	Possible increased severity during third trimester	Probable increase in abortion rate and prematurity; possible transmission to neonate at delivery if mother is incubating the virus or is acutely ill at that time	Pooled immune globulin (IG)	None reported	Postexposure prophylaxis	0.02 ml/kg in one dose of IG	IG should be given as soon as possible and within 2 weeks of exposure; infants born to mothers who are incubating the virus or are acutely ill at delivery should receive one dose of 0.5 ml as soon as possible after birth
Measles	Significant morbidity, low mortality; not altered by pregnancy	Significant increase in abortion rate; may cause malformations	Pooled immune globulin	None reported	Postexposure prophylaxis	0.25 ml/kg in one dose of IG, up to 15 ml	Unclear if it prevents abortion; must be given within 6 days of exposure

Table 15 (continued)

IMMUNE GLOBULINS: HYPERIMMUNE

Immunizing agent	Risk from disease to pregnant female	Risk from disease to fetus or neonate	Type of immunizing agent	Risk from immunizing agent to fetus	Indications for immunization during pregnancy	Dose schedule	Comments
Hepatitis B	Possible increased severity during third trimester	Possible increase in abortion rate and prematurity; neonatal hepatitis can occur if mother is a chronic carrier or is acutely infected	Hepatitis B immune globulin (HBIG)	None reported	Postexposure prophylaxis	0.06 ml/kg of HBIG immediately and 1 month later	Infants born to hepatitis B surface antigen (HBsAg)-positive mothers should receive 0.5 ml HBIG as soon after birth as possible and the same dose repeated 3 and 6 months later
Rabies	Near 100% fatality; not altered by pregnancy	Determined by maternal disease	Rabies immune globulin (RIG)	None reported	Postexposure prophylaxis	20 IU/kg in one dose of RIG	Used in conjunction with rabies killed virus vaccine
Tetanus	Severe morbidity; mortality 60%	Neonatal tetanus mortality 60%	Tetanus immune globulin (TIG)	None reported	Postexposure prophylaxis	250 units in one dose of TIG	Used in conjunction with tetanus toxoid

Varicella	Possible increase in severe varicella pneumonia	Can cause congenital varicella with increased mortality in neonatal period; very rarely causes congenital defects	Varicella-zoster immune globulin (VZIG)	None reported	Not routinely indicated in healthy pregnant women exposed to varicella	1 vial/kg in one dose of VZIG, up to 5 vials	Only indicated for newborns of mothers who developed varicella within 4 days before delivery or 2 days after delivery. Approximately 90–95% of adults are immune to varicella

TOXOIDS

Tetanus-diphtheria	Severe morbidity; tetanus mortality 60%, diphtheria mortality 10%; unaltered by pregnancy	Neonatal tetanus mortality 60%	Combined tetanus-diphtheria toxoids preferred: adult tetanus-diphtheria formulation	None confirmed	Lack of primary series, or no booster within past 10 years	*Primary:* Two doses at 1- to 2-month interval with a third dose 6–12 months after the second. *Booster:* Single dose every 10 years, after completion of the primary series	Updating of immune status should be part of antepartum care

Data on effectiveness are available for most of the agents listed in Table 15. Cholera vaccine is notable for the poor or transient immunity that it confers; influenza vaccine provides protection for about 1 year after its administration. Most other vaccines have been shown to produce long-lasting and probably permanent immunity for over 90% of those vaccinated.

Little information is available on the deleterious effects of most vaccines on a developing fetus. As of May 1982, rubella vaccine was probably the best-studied immunizing agent in this regard. A total of 111 women who were known to be susceptible and who received rubella vaccine shortly before becoming pregnant or early in pregnancy had been followed to term by the Immunization Division of the Centers for Disease Control (CDC). No infant had defects compatible with congenital rubella syndrome, although three had laboratory evidence of rubella virus infection. At that time, all three infants were developing normally. These data indicate that the risk of rubella vaccine to the fetus is negligible (an actual risk to date of 0%, with 95% confidence limits of 0–4%). Although the final decision rests with the patient and her physician, the Immunization Practices Advisory Committee of the CDC believes that rubella vaccination during pregnancy should not be a reason to routinely recommend interruption of pregnancy. Nevertheless, pregnancy is a contraindication to rubella vaccination, as well as to measles and mumps vaccination, because of the theoretic risk of damage to the fetus. In general, killed vaccines are safe. There is no evidence that they affect the fetus or increase the risk of abortion.

Live measles vaccine should not be given to the pregnant woman. Pooled immune globulin, however, usually will prevent or modify measles in the susceptible individual if given within 6 days after exposure. Conversely, pooled immune globulin has not been shown to prevent infection in a patient exposed to rubella or mumps. Pooled immune globulin is probably of little benefit, if any, for pregnant women exposed to rubella infection because subclinical infection, with attendant risk to the fetus, still may exist.

In summary, the use of immunizing agents during pregnancy should be limited to a few well-defined situations. Preferably, women should be protected from preventable diseases by vaccination before they become pregnant. Live virus vaccines, in particular, should not be given during pregnancy except when susceptibility and exposure are highly probable and the disease to be prevented poses a greater threat to the woman or fetus than does vaccination. An example would be giving yellow fever vaccine to a pregnant woman who will be living in an area in which yellow fever occurs.

In the United States the only immunizing agents recommended for routine administration during pregnancy are tetanus and diphtheria toxoids. Measles, rubella, and mumps vaccine should be given to [nonimmune] women prior to pregnancy or in the immediate postpartum period. Pregnant women in the United States should receive primary vaccination against polio only when the risk of exposure is high. As with all adults, this should be done with inactivated polio virus vaccine (IPV) when available. Live attenuated oral polio virus vaccine (OPV) can be used if time does not allow the administration of at least two doses of IPV or if IPV is not available. Physicians should evaluate a pregnant woman's need for influenza immunization on the same basis as for other persons, i.e., taking into consideration underlying high-risk conditions.

The CDC maintains a registry of women who receive live virus vaccines 3 months prior to or following conception. Physicians are urged to report such cases immediately to the CDC (404-329-3091) so the pregnancy can be prospectively followed.

Indexes

Drug Classification Index

Generic and Trade Name Index

.